Richard S. Laskin (Ed)

Total Knee Replacement

With 228 Figures

Springer-Verlag
London Berlin Heidelberg New York
Paris Tokyo Hong Kong
Barcelona Budapest

Richard S. Laskin, MD
Professor of Orthopaedic Surgery,
Albert Einstein College of Medicine,
New York, and Chairman,
Department of Orthopaedic Surgery,
Long Island Jewish Medical Center,
New Hyde Park, New York 11042, USA

With the assistance of:
Barry C. Kleeman, MD, and Andrew Turtel, MD
Department of Orthopaedic Surgery,
Long Island Jewish Medical Center,
New Hyde Park, New York 11042, USA

ISBN-13: 978-1-4471-1827-5 e-ISBN-13: 978-1-4471-1825-1
DOI: 10.1007/978-1-4471-1825-1

British Library Cataloguing in Publication Data
Laskin, Richard S., *1940*
Total Knee replacement.
1. Humans. Knees. Surgery
I. Title
617.582059
ISBN-13: 978-1-4471-1827-5

Library of Congress Cataloging-in Publication-Data
Total Knee replacement edited by Richard S. Laskin, with the assistance of Barry C. Kleeman and Andrew Turtel
p. cm. Includes index
ISBN-13: 978-1-4471-1827-5
1. Artificial knee. 2. Knee—Surgery. I. Laskin, Richard S., 1940– II. Kleeman Barry C. III. Turtel Andrew.
[DNML: 1. Knee Prosthesis—methods. WE 870 T7162]
RD561.T669 1991
617.5'820592—dc20
DNLM/DLC 90–11336
for Library of Congress CIP

Typeset by Wilmaset, Birkenhead, Wirral

28/3830-543210 Printed on acid-free paper

This book is dedicated:

To the memory of Dr Jo Miller whose keen insight, rational thinking, and good friendship I will truly miss.

To my dear wife Judge Joyce Sparrow, my mother Trudy Klein Laskin, and my sons Jonathan and Andrew.

To Mr A. Graham Apley and Dr Mark Lazansky, my first two orthopaedic teachers. Each has remained a mentor and a friend to me over the past twenty-two years.

To Dr Richard Bryan who has encouraged me through the years to continue with my investigations in total knee replacement.

To Dr John Insall whose concepts, ideas, and thoughts I feel have been the cornerstone on which I have based so much of my own work.

To Drs Ronald Rosenthal and George Mauler, who, through their own personal example, convinced me that I should make Orthopaedic Surgery my life's work.

To all my colleagues in the Knee Society for helping enrich my knowledge of knee replacement arthroplasty.

Foreword

Knee replacement can be regarded as the inevitable sequel to hip replacements, the child so to speak, of a brilliant father. As with other children, there were growing pains and a somewhat troubled adolescence, but the mature adult can now stand, proud and unashamed, alongside its distinguished forebear. Total replacement of the knee is now a highly successful operation which has enriched the lives of countless sufferers. Clearly the time is ripe for a definitive work on the subject.

Richard Laskin, whose abiding interest and profound knowledge of knee replacement are well known, has gathered together a team of notable experts who, between them, cover every aspect of the subject. The first section of this book deals with the history of knee replacement, its indications, alternative procedures, biomechanics and materials. Then follows a most important section by Laskin himself, on the surgical technique, the details of which, as he points out in his preface, are more important than differences between the various prostheses. The third section considers the results of several different prostheses and discusses some problem areas.

This is a book which surgeons in the field of knee replacement have been waiting for; those with experience will find it of absorbing interest and those who have more recently embarked on the subject will find it an invaluable guide in their quest for perfection. Dr Laskin is to be congratulated on his choice of collaborators and for producing such a masterly compilation.

A. Graham Apley

Preface

Total knee replacement is one of the most successful operations to exist in the field of orthopaedic surgery. Over the last twenty years it has become the mainstay in the treatment of the patient with advanced arthritis of the knee. Its results have become predictable and reproducible. I believe that it is now time to evaluate critically our results and techniques and to use this knowledge to guide our thinking and investigatory patterns for this new decade. It is for this reason that this, my second total knee book was conceived. The contributors are all experts in the field on knee joint surgery and among them have over three hundred years of pooled experience in knee joint replacement.

The first three chapters of the book set the stage. Dr David Murray eloquently describes the long, arduous and sometimes frustrating road we have travelled up to the present. Beginning with prosthesis which were mere hinges he progresses through the generations of constrained and then unconstrained prosthesis to the current state of the art. Dr Richard Bochner offers a comprehensive insight into the options other than total joint replacement that we can offer to the patient with advanced knee arthritis. Finally, Dr Malcolm Pope and Mr Braden Fleming discuss the relevant biomechanics of the knee and the choice of materials used in implant design.

The next section deals with surgical technique. With no disrespect for any knee prosthesis designer, I feel that it is the technique, rather than the small nuances of any one prosthesis that in the long run accounts for the success or failure of most total knee replacements. I have written two chapters on "How I do a Knee Replacement". One relates to the soft tissue technique, the other to the bony cuts. They are generic chapters, applicable to almost any total knee prosthesis that the surgeon chooses to implant. The surgical tips and ideas are a potpourri of those that have been described by my colleagues in the Knee Society, as well as some that I probably conceived personally.

In the third section there is a description of the long term results of many of the most widely used implants. Drs John Insall, Kelly Vince, Giles Scuderi and Russ Windsor draw upon the extensive and ground breaking work done at the Hospital for Special Surgery for three chapters covering the cemented Total Condylar and Insall-Burstein Posterior Stabilized prostheses. The "fathers" of the uncemented total knee, Drs Kenneth Krackow and David Hungerford, describe the long term results with their PCA prosthesis. Professor Stock reports on the long term experience of his group in Braunsweig, using unicompartmental prostheses with localized arthritis of the knee. Finally, I have included a long term evaluation of the Tricon-M uncemented prosthesis, and a description of its successor, the Genesis uncemented total knee, the implants that I have been using when performing uncemented total knee replacement surgery.

The fourth section covers the problem areas in total knee replacement. Dr Hugh Cameron describes the Canadian experience with patellar problems in total knee replacement. Dr Edward Habermann evaluates the problem with infection and the current concepts of its treatment. Dr Thomas Sculco presents an algorithmic approach to evaluating the patient who has had a total knee replacement, but who still continues to have knee pain. Dr Leif Ryd of Sweden gives an in-depth analysis of the problem of his seminal work with the problem of subsidence and its causes. His Swedish colleague Dr Anders Wigren writes of his extensive experience in treating rheumatoid patients, and of their special problems. Bone loss from the tibia or femur occurs often in the patient with advanced arthritis. The chapter on bone loss describes how bone loss is handled by three different surgeons: Dr Thomas Sculco from the Hospital for Special Surgery, Drs Springorum, De Nicola and Lowe from the University of Heidelberg, and myself.

The material in this book should act both as a source of ideas and a springboard for further thought and investigation in the field of total knee replacement. It should enable all of us to progress and advance in the 1990s, further refining and perfecting this excellent surgical procedure.

New York, May 1990 Richard S. Laskin

Acknowledgements

I would like to thank the administrative and nursing staff of the Department of Orthopaedic Surgery at Long Island Jewish Medical Center for their unceasing help and assistance in the preparation of this book. I would also like to thank all the orthopaedic residents in my Department and my colleagues Dr Ronald Rosenthal, Dr John Handelsman, Dr Cathleen Raggio, and Dr Richard Bochner for their guidance, patient understanding, and professional advice. Finally I would like to thank Drs Barry Kleeman and Andrew Turtel. After working long hard hours as senior orthopaedic residents they somehow always found the extra hours to assist me with the reviewing, editing, and the layout of the book.

Richard S. Laskin

Contents

Section IV Problem Areas in Total Knee Replacement

Contributors

Richard Bochner, MD
Assistant Professor of Orthopaedic Surgery, Albert Einstein College of Medicine, Long Island Jewish Medical Center, New Hyde Park, NY 11042, USA

Hugh U. Cameron MB, ChB, FRCS(C)
Assistant Professor of Orthopaedic Surgery, University of Toronto, 43 Wellesley St. E., NY4 1H1 Toronto, Canada

R. Fabiasiak, MD
Orthopädische Klinik Melverode, Leipziger Strasse 24, 3300 Braunschweig-Melverode, Germany

Ugo De Nicola, MD
Caritaskrankenhaus, Ulandstrasse, Bad Mergenthim 6990, Germany

Braden C. Fleming, MS
University of Vermont, Burlington, VT 05405, USA

Edward T. Habermann, MD
Professor of Orthopaedic Surgery, Albert Einstein College of Medicine, 111 E. 210 St. Bronx, NY 10467, USA

David S. Hungerford, MD
Professor of Orthopaedic Surgery, Johns Hopkins University, 5601 Loch Raven Blvd., Baltimore, MD 21239, USA

John N. Insall, MD
Professor of Orthopaedic Surgery, Cornell University Medical College, Attending Orthopaedic Surgeon and Director of Knee Service, Hospital for Special Surgery, 535 E. 70th St., New York, NY 10021, USA

Robert V. Kenna
Johns Hopkins University, 5601 Loch Raven Blvd., Baltimore, MD 21239, USA

Kenneth A. Krackow, MD
Professor of Orthopaedic Surgery, Johns Hopkins University, 5601 Loch Raven Blvd., Baltimore, MD 21239, USA

Richard S. Laskin, MD
Professor of Orthopaedic Surgery, Albert Einstein College of Medicine, and Chairman, Department of Orthopaedic Surgery, Long Island Jewish Medical Center, New Hyde Park, NY 11042, USA

Walter J. Lowe, MD
Caritaskrankenhaus, Ulandstrasse, Bad Mergenthim, 6990 Germany

David G. Murray, MD
Professor of Orthopaedic Surgery, State University of New York, Upstate Medical Center, 115 Circle Rd., Syracuse, NY 13210, USA

A. Niezgoda, MD
Orthopädische Klinik Melverode, Leipziger Strasse 24, 3300 Braunschweig-Melverode, Germany

Malcolm H. Pope, PhD, Dr MedSc
Professor of Orthopaedics and Rehabilitation, Director of Research, University of Vermont, Burlington, VT 05405, USA

Lief Ryd, MD
Department of Orthopaedics, Lund University Hospital Ort Likn, S221 85 Lund, Sweden

Giles R. Scuderi, MD
Attending Orthopaedic Surgeon, South Nassau Community Hospital and Mercy Hospital, Rockville Centre, NY 11570, USA

Thomas P. Sculco, MD
Associate Clinical Professor of Orthopaedic Surgery, Cornell University Medical College, Assistant Director of Orthopaedic Surgery, Hospital for Special Surgery, 535 E. 70th St., New York, NY 10021, USA

Professor Hans W. Springorum, MD
Caritaskrankenhaus, Ulandstrasse, Bad Mergenthim, 6990 Germany

Professor D. Stock, MD
Chefarzt d Klinik, Orthopädische Klinik Melverode, Leipziger Strasse 24, 3300 Braunschweig-Melverode, Germany

Kelly G. Vince, MD, FRCS(C)
Orthopaedic Surgeon, Kerlan-Jobe Orthopaedic Clinic, 501 E. Hardy St., Englewood, CA 90301, USA

Anders Wigren, MD
Assistant Professor of Orthopaedic Surgery, University of Uppsala, Funbo, Enhojden S 755 97 Uppsala, Sweden

Russell E. Windsor, MD
Assistant Professor of Orthopaedic Surgery, Cornell University Medical College, and Attending Orthopaedic Surgeon, Hospital for Special Surgery, 535 E. 70 St., New York, NY 10021, USA

Section 1

The Basics

Chapter 1

History of Total Knee Replacement

David G. Murray

Introduction

"Arthroplasty of the knee has as yet, no standard technique. It is still an open chapter in joint surgery and one which offers much promise" (Albee 1928). F. H. Albee made this statement in 1928 in his description of an arthroplasty with "an improved prognosis". His conclusion reflected (and still reflects to some degree) the frustrations associated with attempting effectively to replace one of the most complex joints in the body. As the joint in the body which is furthest removed both proximally and distally from the next adjacent articulation, it is subjected to major stresses. Deficiencies in mobility cannot be easily compensated for by the hip or the ankle. The incongruity of the opposing joint surfaces with the additional complexity of the patellofemoral articulation have presented a challenge for over a century to those surgeons attempting to provide relief from major disabilities involving the knee. For the most part, until the last fifteen years, these efforts have been characterized more by ingenuity than by success. Allison and Brooks in 1923 conceded that it was impossible to restore the normal gliding of the articular surfaces of the knee, either experimentally or in surgically reconstructed joints. This attitude of course did not dissuade the pioneers in the field from individually or collectively pursuing the "impossible".

As might be expected, the approaches taken toward the restoration of function to the impaired knee varied widely. The direction adopted by a particular surgeon was as much influenced by current technology as by imagination. The availability of X-ray, the development of biocompatible materials, the discovery of antibiotics as well as the evolution of specialists primarily concerned with the musculoskeletal system, all played a role. As one reviews the history of this subject the importance of the contributions made at each step emerge. The present is built on the past. An understanding of what has gone before is essential in planning effectively for the future.

Resection and Interposition Arthroplasties

The modern record concerning arthroplasty of the knee dates back to the middle nineteenth century. Fergusson (1861) described a case in which he resected the knee with creation of a pseudoarthrosis and, according to his report, "a useful limb". The results of resection arthroplasty however were frequently compromised by ankylosis or fusion. If excessive bone was resected, the resultant instability provided a significant problem. Because of this, a variety of methods were introduced to attempt to recreate a joint surface. Among the earliest descriptions was that of Verneuil (1860) who suggested using soft tissue interposed between the raw bone ends after joint resection. His initial report discussed arthroplasty of the temporomandibular joint. In 1863 he described arthroplasty of the knee using joint capsule as the tissue for interposition (Verneuil 1863). Ollier in 1886 described a similar procedure using muscle instead of joint capsule. Helferich (1894) also reported success in treating an ankylosis of the knee with a resection arthroplasty using muscle as the interposed tissue. Luck reported the use of skin for resurfacing the raw bone ends but his results were inconsistent. J.B. Murphy (1905) introduced arthroplasty to the United States describing the treatment of five ankylosed knees which he treated by using fat and fascia to recreate a joint lining. Murphy (1905) conceded in his article that "the knee is the most difficult joint in which to secure perfect restoration of function". Sporadic reports describing interposition arthroplasty appeared during the first third of this century (Gluck 1902; Henderson 1918; Hofman 1908). Various materials were used including chromaticized pig's bladder (Baer 1918; Campbell 1921), fascial flaps or grafts (Murphy 1905; Putti 1920–21) and fat (MacAusland 1933). The major problems associated with these various techniques were summed up by Albee in 1928 commenting upon Dr. Murphy's patients (as well as his own!). "These patients either had insufficient motion to satisfy them, or more often the degree of mobility was satisfactory but lateral instability was present and proved so troublesome as to offset the advantages of mobility." Even as late as 1950, good results were being described by Kuhns and Potter (1950) using nylon membrane as the interpositional material. By 1964, however, the authors had abandoned this procedure because of a high rate of recurrent deformity. The results were severely compromised, not only by instability or stiffness, but also by a tendency for the nylon to deteriorate and disintegrate within the joint. Although interpositional arthroplasty was reported as being done in various forms into the 1950s (Brown et al. 1958; Hass 1944; Samson 1949; Skolnick et al. 1976b), the results were never uniformly satisfactory. Persistent attempts were based more on the absence of a satisfactory alternative than any indication that continued refinements were leading to improved results.

Biologic Replacement

The concept of replacing the entire knee with an allograft attracted attention early in the twentieth century. Erich Lexer (1925) claimed that "Joint transplantation is essential in repairing joint defects, and further plays a role in the treatment of ankylosis". He described in detail the transplantation of a knee including the cruciate ligaments from an amputation specimen to a patient with sarcoma of the joint (1909). His description alludes to the fact that the donor and recipient knees were opposite sides but that this did not seem to constitute a problem. The reconstructed joint was noted to be slightly loose on weight bearing initially but ultimately was well incorporated and exhibited very good motion. In spite of "the best clinical results" this particular patient subsequently had an amputation of the limb less than two years later (Professor Lexer suggested that this was for "religious purposes" and was not related to the results of the transplant). The amputation provided an opportunity for histologic analysis of the transplant. "The specimen showed complete union with the diaphysis: the spongy part of the epiphysis was well restored and nourished in the periphery, it was dry and necrotic only in the middle . . . the capsular attachments were well united, and there were no adhesions in the joint cavity. The joint cartilage was everywhere well maintained, indeed, regenerated." Apparently encouraged by early results he continued to perform knee transplants using a variety of techniques over the next two decades. Although his description of results included references to good function and freedom from pain, he also documented severe complications and a high incidence of failure. His series constituted the largest published group of cases until Parrish (1966) revived the use of massive homologous grafts for the treatment of bone tumors in the 1960s. Improved methods of preservation, effective antibiotics, and dramatic improvements in surgical techniques have led to the adoption of this form of replacement by others (Meyers, Mankin, Friedlaender, and Gross). Although reserved primarily for the treatment of malignancies about the joint, Meyers (Meyers et al. 1989) and Gross (Gross et al. 1975; Zukor et al. 1989) in particular have discussed the use of allografts for the treatment of osteoarthritis. As better techniques for preservation of cartilage and for tissue typing evolve, allografts for the treatment of benign diseases of the knee may become the procedure of choice.

Endoprostheses

Initial attempts at knee replacement with endoprostheses involved resurfacing procedures for the tibia or the femur. This represented a distinct departure from pre-existing arthroplasty techniques using biologic or artificial materials in the reconstruction of the joint. Using durable materials which were relatively non-reactive in the biologic environment, prostheses were created to *replace* a joint surface as opposed to simply *separating* the surfaces while the damaged or revised bone ends healed. The initial approach involved the implantation of a relatively anatomically configured device to replace one side of the joint, relying on the natural counter surface to complete the articulation. The opposing surface could be remodeled to some extent to achieve better conformity.

Drawing from the experience of Smith Peterson with cup arthroplasty of the hip, Willis Campbell (1940) designed a vitallium prosthesis for the distal end of the femur. Although he decribed an early satisfactory result in 1940, he abandoned the procedure after four cases because of generally poor results. The technique of distal femoral condylar prosthetic replacement was revived in 1952 by Lacheretz (1953) using an acrylic device. Kraft and Levinthal (1954) also used an acrylic prosthesis for the distal end of the femur with good results over a short term follow-up. Jones et al. (1967) (Fig. 1.1) introduced a vitallium prosthesis for the distal end of the femur molded to duplicate the contours of the femoral condyles and fixed with an intramedullary stem. Although this prosthesis did not achieve wide popularity, several reports (Jones 1969; Murray and Barranco 1974) indicated a reasonable degree of success over an intermediate term of 3–5 years. The design of the prosthesis necessitated removal of the cruciate ligaments, pre-disposing to some degree of instability. Of more concern however was the effect of the metallic femoral condylar replacements on the opposite cartilage or bone. Over varying periods of time, the prosthesis tended to erode the articulating cartilage and create a depression in the tibial plateau. This was particularly troublesome where the normal alignment of the joint had been incompletely restored. Furthermore, adequate fixation of the femoral prosthesis depended upon a close fit between the prosthesis and the reshaped ends of the distal femur. A membrane routinely formed at the interface which tended to be erosive and painful in some cases (Platt and Pepler 1968). A large proportion of these cases underwent eventual conversion to total knee replacements.

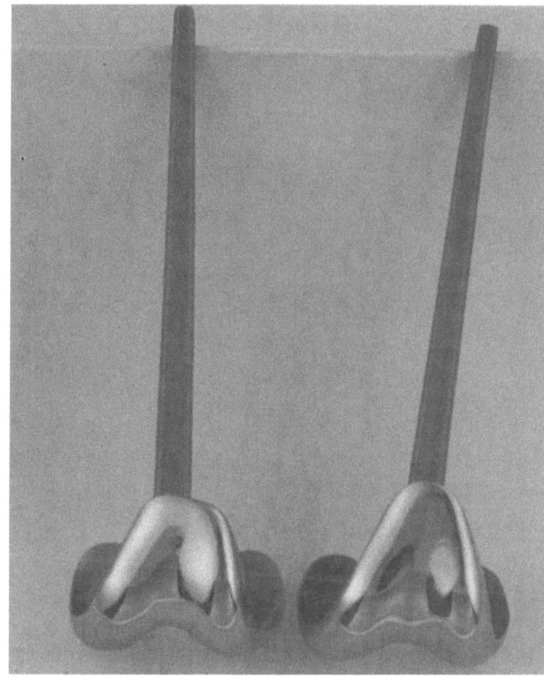

Fig. 1.1 MGH femoral condylar replacements.

It was a natural corollary that prostheses would be developed for replacing the articulating surfaces of the proximal tibia. Beginning in 1950, replacement prostheses for the tibial plateaus were described by DePalma (1954), McKeever (1955), MacIntosh (1958), and Townley (1964) in North America. The tibial plateau replacements consisted of a unicondylar or bicondylar vitallium plate fixed in place either by a flange (McKeever), screws (Townley), or surface irregularities (MacIntosh). The plateau prostheses were widely used with reports of good to excellent results in 60%–80% of the cases (Lowe et al. 1972; Potter et al. 1972). The technique involved resection of the defective tibial surface and insertion of a replacement of appropriate thickness. As opposed to the femoral condylar prosthesis, tibial replacements could be used for one compartment disease and facilitated realignment of the knee by selecting the thickness of prosthesis that would correct excessive valgus or

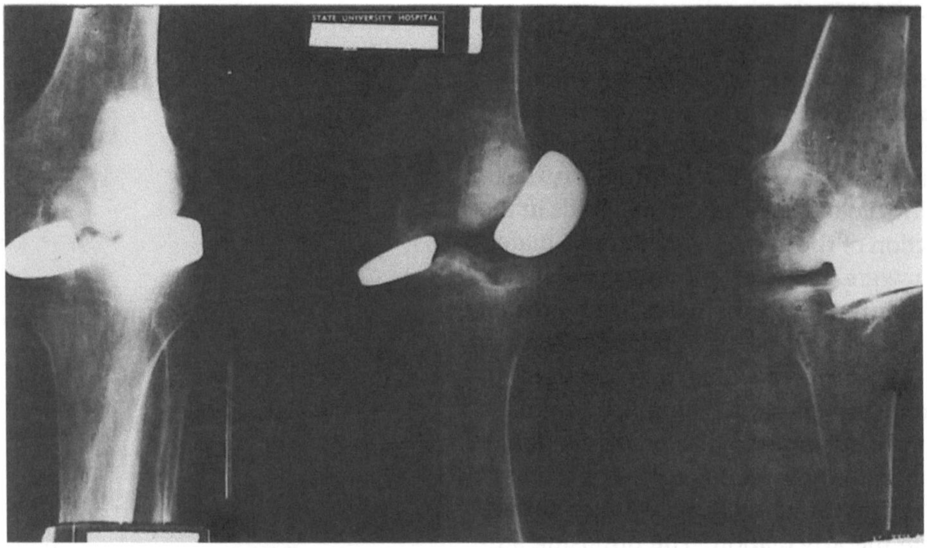

Fig.1.2. MacIntosh prostheses – sequential displacement over three years.

varus. Although the MacIntosh and McKeever prostheses were basically designed for unicompartment replacement, they were often used in pairs to replace both tibial plateaus, (Hastings and Hewitson 1973; Potter et al. 1972). In such cases the cruciate ligaments were left undisturbed and continued to provide stability to the joint. Fixation of the prosthetic devices remained a problem with migration or subsidence emerging as a significant complication with time (Fig. 1.2). As with the femoral condylar replacement, the reaction of the opposing articular cartilage was unpredictable. In some cases the opposing cartilage would wear out. In other cases a shift of stress to the opposite compartment would result in deterioration on the other side of the joint. In either case the knee tended to be uncomfortable and the result suboptimal.

In spite of numerous optimistic early reports, the frequency of complications and the emergence of semiconstrained total knee replacement arthroplasty spelled the end of the use of the resurfacing techniques by the early 1970s.

Total Knee Replacement Prostheses

The general dissatisfaction with interpositional arthroplasty and human allografts for treating arthritis of the knee led to the development of total joint endoprostheses beginning in the late 1940s. Majnoni d'Intignano (1950) reported on the insertion of a hinge joint knee prosthesis constructed of acrylic. The result was apparently unsuccessful and his series ended at one. Moeys (1954) described a metallic hinge prosthesis which he used experimentally in dogs. He was encouraged in his search for a suitable knee prosthesis by "the fact that a search of the literature failed to reveal any record of successful metal alloplasty due to the technical difficulties of the procedure". He was convinced that an appropriate design could be developed which would provide stability, adequate fixation, and at the same time be relatively simple to insert. Based on three experiments, two of which failed, he concluded that the hinge knee prosthesis showed promise but required further development.

Walldius (1957, 1960) reported on the use of a hinged acrylic prosthesis, later modified to be constructed of vitallium. This device was basically a simple hinge with a single axle and separate femoral and tibial components. The femoral component had a flange for articulation with the patella. Both sections had straight stems about 4 in in length to provide some stability in the bone. The tibial component also had a posterior flange which aided in resisting rotational displacement about the long axis of the leg. The maximum range of motion intrinsic in the artificial joint was from 5° of hyperextension to 90° of flexion. The linked characteristic of the prosthesis made loss of the cruciate ligaments of no significance. In a report of a prospective study using the Walldius prosthesis, Wilson (1972) described predominantly good results, acknowledging loosening and settling of the prosthesis as observations which apparently did not severely compromise the result.

Modifications of the hinge knee prosthesis were developed and reported by Shiers (1954, 1961), Young (1963, 1965), and a group in France which developed the prosthesis known as the Guepar (Mazas 1973) (Fig. 1.3). The Shiers and Young prostheses were introduced prior to the advent of cement fixation and relied predominantly on long intramedullary stems for stability. Neither prosthesis provided an articular surface for the patella. Both designs allowed a greater degree of flexion than the Walldius prosthesis. The axis of rotation in the Shiers device was offset posteriorly resulting in alignment of the tibia somewhat anterior to the femur. This gave a theoretic mechanical advantage to the extensor mechanism and allowed unrestricted flexion in the prosthesis. By contrast the Guepar hinge was developed for use with cement and had an attenuated articular extension for the patella. The axis of the hinge was located posteriorly and superiorly to simulate the tibial "rolling" characteristic during flexion. A silastic bumper was introduced to dampen the extension stop, and the stem on the femoral component was angled 7° to conform to the natural valgus angle of the knee. The long femoral stem was slightly bent at its proximal end to adapt to the bow of the femur. This seemingly simple design characteristic was rarely mentioned in descriptions of the prosthesis but could create enormous problems when trying to remove the prosthesis when it was tightly fixed in the femur with cement.

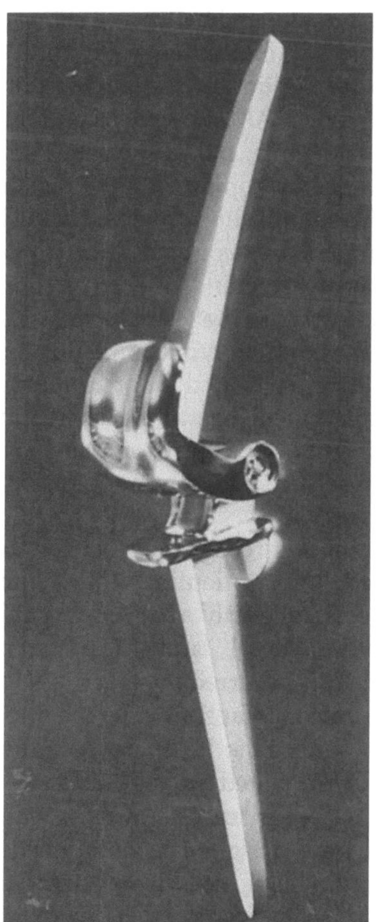

Fig. 1.3. Guepar hinge prosthesis. Note slight angle at upper end of femoral stem.

The early enthusiasm for the hinged replacements began to pall in the 1960s as the disability associated with almost universal loosening and settling became recognised (MacAusland 1957). The introduction of polymethylmethacrylate bone cement for fixation brought about a transient resurgence of interest in the hinge. It was during this period that the Guepar emerged as well as some other short lived hinge type inventions such as Taverneti Tennant, "LL" (Le Tournel and Lagrange 1973) and Stanmore (Lettin et al. 1978). Brady and Garber (1974), and Insall et al. (1976) were among those who published encouraging reports with a warning that results were still short term. Phillips (1973) was prophetic when he concluded, "While no example of prosthetic disintegration is reported here, there are already indications that the lifespan of Shiers prosthesis is limited . . . the Shiers knee hinge may be no more than of historical significance." Thereafter it became quickly accepted knowledge that the fixed hinge, regardless of the location of the axle, the intrinsic range of motion, or the method of fixation was highly subject to symptomatic loosening beginning about two years after insertion. The inability to absorb rotational stresses about the long axis of the limb except at the bone/cement interface constituted an insurmountable flaw.

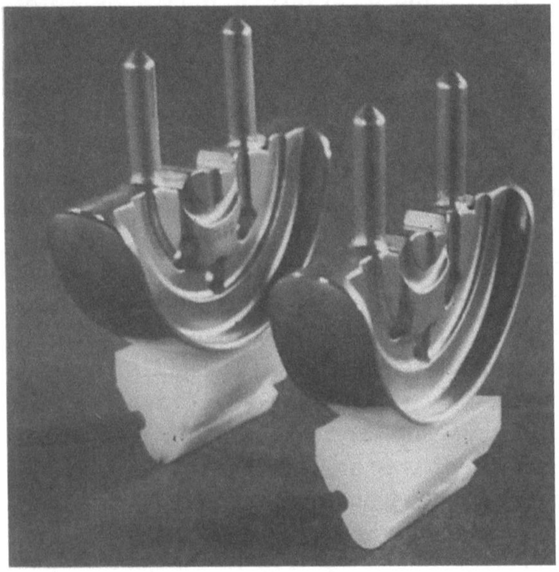

Fig. 1.4. Modified polycentric (Gunston) prosthesis.

Cemented Endoprostheses

With the introduction of cement for fixation of hip prostheses, the possibilities for similar fixation of knee prostheses seemed to be a natural sequel. Actually it was a surprisingly long time before the transfer of the technique to the knee took place. Gunston (1971, 1973) (Fig. 1.4) receives credit for the first series describing a nonconstrained knee arthroplasty with cemented prosthetic components. The polycentric knee prosthesis consisted of two metallic semicircular runners inserted into slots in the femoral condyles which articulated with two high density polyethylene tracks cemented into slots in the tibial plateaus. The patellofemoral joint was not involved with the replacement. Gunston reported one failure in his first 21 cases making his procedure far and away the most successful arthroplasty described to that point (despite multiple designs and improvements in techniques, his results have rarely been equaled since.) His use of cemented components attracted wide attention. The polycentric design was used in a number of centers but its acceptance was inhibited by the complexity of the surgical technique (Skolnick et al. 1976a). Four separate components were involved, each of which was seated independently. Aligning jigs were available to assist in placing the components in the femur and tibia respectively. Part of the difficulty in placement related to the fact that the femoral components were semicircular in shape making a precise match with the femoral condyles impossible. The shape of the prosthesis was apparently dictated by the fact that Gunston produced his prosthesis himself in the initial stage and was limited by equipment which consisted of a metal turning lathe. Gunston's pioneering work with the polycentric cemented prosthesis sent the orthopaedic world to the drawing board. The next decade brought forth the best and the worst in innovative thinking applied to the design of a knee prosthesis.

The first types to emerge were largely refinements of Gunston's modular concept. The Marmor (1973) Savastano, Liverpool (Cavendish and Wright 1973), Unicondylar, Sledge, and Manchester (Shaw and Chatterlee 1978) to name a few of the better recognized designs, all improved on the polycentric concept with more anatomic configuration of the femoral components, broader and better fixed tibial plateaus, and improved instruments for insertion. All provided the option of resurfacing one or both compartments. All allowed retention of both cruciate ligaments, but at the same time, made no allowance for coping with the patellofemoral joint. The complexities involved with inserting four components, coupled with an increased incidence of loosening of one or more of the pieces has led over the years to virtual abandonment of the modular type for treating bicompartmental arthritis. Whether or not unicompartment replacement has a role in treating single compartment osteoarthritis remains an ongoing and unresolved debate among reconstructive knee surgeons.

It was quickly recognized that the difficulties associated with orienting four components could be significantly reduced by linking the respective femoral and tibial components together. This occurred in stages in some cases, with the unicondylar spawning the duocondylar (Ranawat and Shine 1973) in which the femoral runners were joined and the tibial tracks were separate. In most cases however, single components were designed to be applied to cover medial and lateral condyles of both femur and tibia. The Geometric prosthesis (Coventry et al. 1972; Skolnick et al. 1976a) (Fig. 1.5) emerged as one of the most popular and was basically a modification of the modular types with a con-

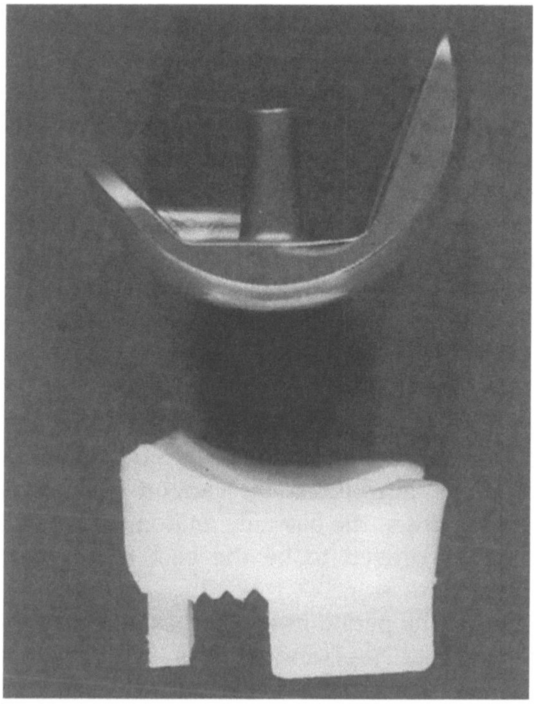

Fig. 1.5. Geometric prosthesis.

necting strut between the two metal femoral runners and a polyethylene bridge between the tibial sockets. Although the design allowed for retention of the anterior and posterior cruciate ligaments, the axis of flexion dictated by the prosthetic configuration was incompatible with the gliding/rolling motion proscribed by intact cruciates, leading to the routine sacrifice of the anterior cruciate. The UCI prosthesis (Waugh et al. 1973) (Fig. 1.6) was a modification which accommodated rotation about the long axis of the leg with a horseshoe shaped tibial articulating surface, a distinct advance over the Geometric which was quite constrained with regard to rotation. Neither prosthesis addressed the problem of patellofemoral arthritis.

Freeman and Sawnson (Freeman et al. 1973, 1978) coincidentally developed the ICLH prosthesis (Fig. 1.7), representing a departure from the modular concept. The ICLH prosthesis required sacrifice of both cruciate ligaments, somewhat simplifying insertion. A flange was added to the femoral component to accommodate the patella. Initially this extension was rudimentary with two knobs to guide the patella, but quickly was altered to provide a very broad, if nonanatomic, surface for the kneecap.

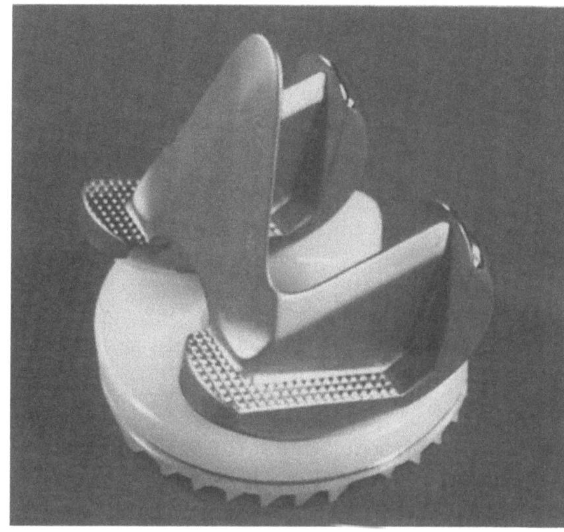

Fig. 1.6. UCI prosthesis. Designed at the University of California, Irvine by Dr T. Waugh and co-workers.

Stability was afforded by the breadth of the prosthesis and a shallow transverse V configuration to the tibial surface.

Prostheses up to this point were typically designed with metal femoral components and polyethylene tibial counter surfaces which were fixed to the bone by a layer of cement. Tibial fixation of the polyethylene was enhanced by fins, grooves, slots, or other shallow irregularities on the undersurface of the prosthesis.

The first prosthesis incorporating a metallic tibial tray with interchangeable polyethylene

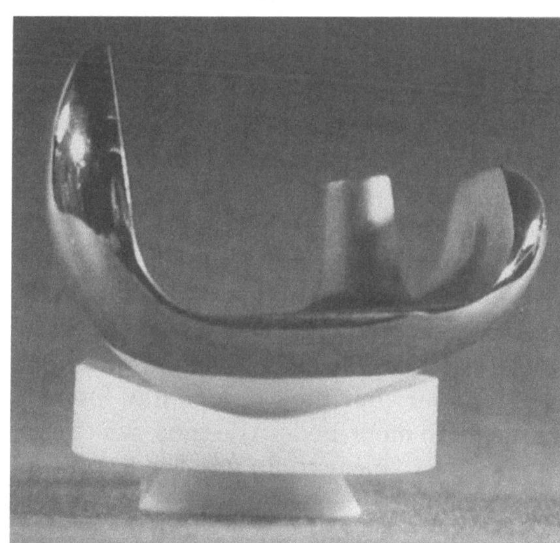

Fig. 1.7. Freeman-Swanson prosthesis. One of the earliest designs to have a patellar flange.

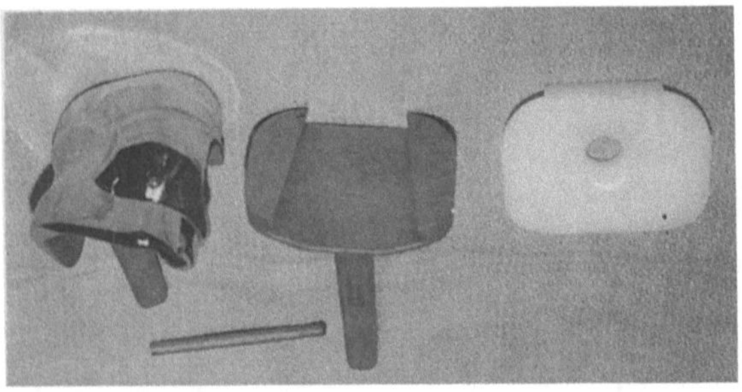

Fig. 1.8. Variable Axis prothesis. The tibial surface was replaceable and came in several thicknesses.

inserts was introduced as the Variable Axis prosthesis in 1974 (Murray 1982) (Fig. 1.8). The metal components had stems to enhance fixation. The interchangeable polyethylene tibial surfaces were designed to allow adjustments for stability and alignment after the metal parts had been fixed in place. Subsequently, an added advantage emerged as the design permitted replacement of worn polyethylene without disturbing the cement. Rotational stability was provided by a shallow central ball and socket characteristic. This minimal constraint coupled with stem fixation markedly reduced the incidence of loosening but the central spherical prominence on the femoral side tended to compromise flexion beyond 95°. This constituted a limiting flaw in the overall design.

Goodfellow (1978; Goodfellow and O'Connor 1978) introduced the concept of moveable tibial components inserted between curved femoral and flat tibial metallic surfaces. The plastic inserts were designed to move posteriorly in flexion consistent with the "roll-back" phenomenon of the normal knee. This was proposed as a method to increase the range of motion with a more normal arc, and relieve stress on the prosthesis–cement–bone interfaces. The application demanded precise technique to avoid subsequent displacement of the "floating" components. This requirement tended to limit the use of this particular device beyond the hands of the developer, but the concept has found a resurgence in more modern designs, which capture the tibial "menisci" in grooves to prevent dislodgement.

Insall and colleagues (1976, 1979) provided a breakthrough in the mid 70s with the evolution of a prosthetic design from "Unicondylar" through "Duocondylar" and "Patellocondylar" to "Total Condylar" configuration. The Total Condylar design (Fig. 1.9) with the addition of a patellar resurfacing polyethylene button became the "generic" knee replacement. The basic concepts included a relatively anatomic metallic replacement of the distal femur, articulating with shallow sockets in a polyethylene tibial component which included a tibial peg for fixation. Subsequent modifications have included the addition of metallic backing, stems of various length for fixation of the tibial and/or femoral components, modifications of the tibial surface to increase stability, and replaceable polyethylene inserts. Although many models are now available to choose from with minor individual alterations introduced by various designs or manufacturers, the basically anatomic configuration has proved to be the best for primary replacement.

During the period in which the condylar type of prosthetic replacement was evolving, the problem of instability associated with semiconstrained prostheses attracted considerable attention. The failure of the hinge prosthesis was attributed largely to the absence of rotation between the femoral and tibial components in the long axis of the prosthesis. Rotational stresses applied to the legs were therefore concentrated at the bone–cement interface, promoting early failure. Ingenious designs were developed to provide for some degree of rotation

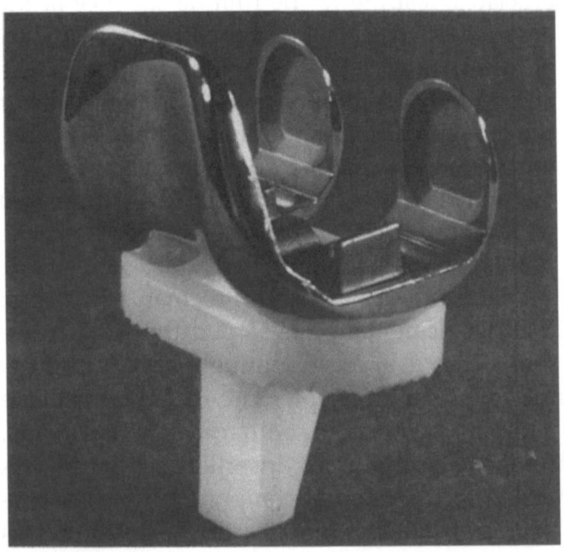

Fig. 1.9. Total Condylar prosthesis. This evolved from earlier "Uni-" and "Duo-" condylar designs.

about this axis either through a spherical articulation between the femoral and tibial components (Spherocentric [Matthews et al. 1973; Fig. 1.10], Herbert [Herbert and Herbert 1973; Fig. 1.11]), through rotation about a separate axle in a tibial receptacle (Attenborough [1978; Fig. 1.12], Noiles [Fig. 1.13], Kinematic Hinge [Walker et al. 1982]), or through some degree of "sloppiness" in the femoral tibial linkage (Sheehan [O'Rourke and Sheehan 1987; Fig. 1.14], Stabilocondylar [Fig. 1.15]). Each of these modifications increased the durability of the linked prosthetic replacement, none however, have begun to approach the semiconstrained type of prosthesis in terms of longevity of the device after implantation. Failure continues to occur primarily at the bone–cement interface in either the tibia or femur. The prosthetic designs with a longitudinal tibial axle in a polyethylene receptacle have also failed through deformation and fracture of the polyethylene around the tip of the axle. The development of a constrained pros-

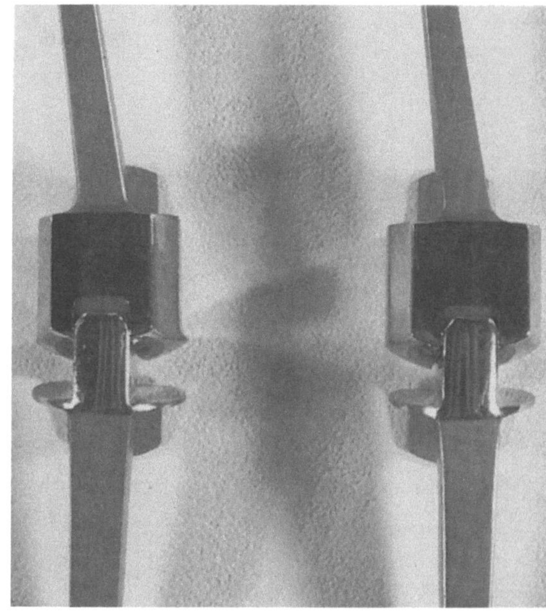

Fig. 1.11. Herbert prosthesis. The femoral housing was strengthened (prosthesis on right) because of breakage.

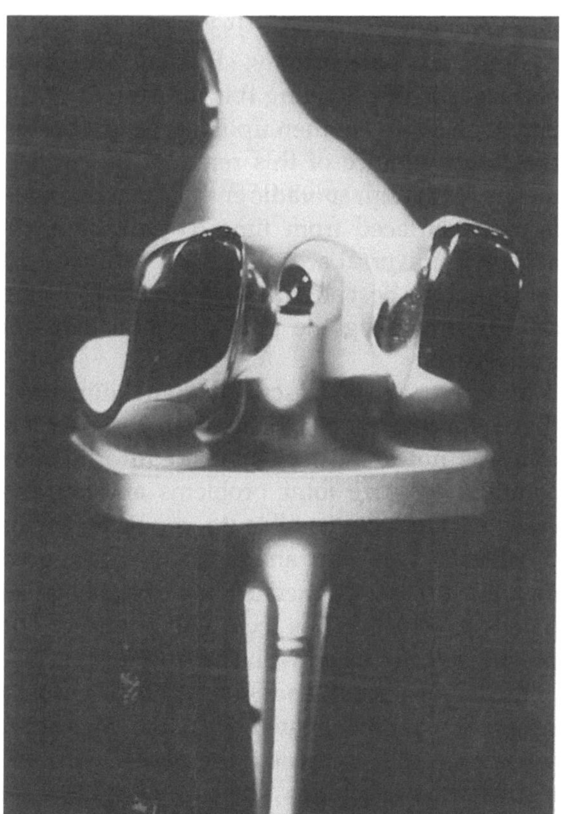

Fig. 1.10. Spherocentric prosthesis. Central ball and socket allowed internal and external rotation.

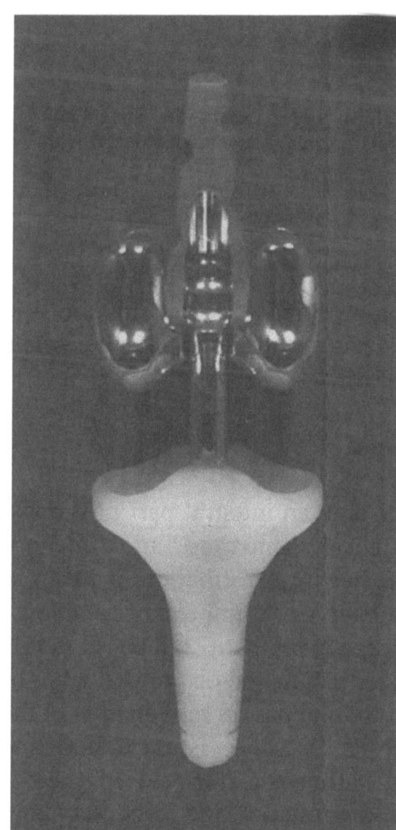

Fig. 1.12. Attenborough prosthesis. The linkage occurred with a stem which slid into a polyethylene tibial sleeve.

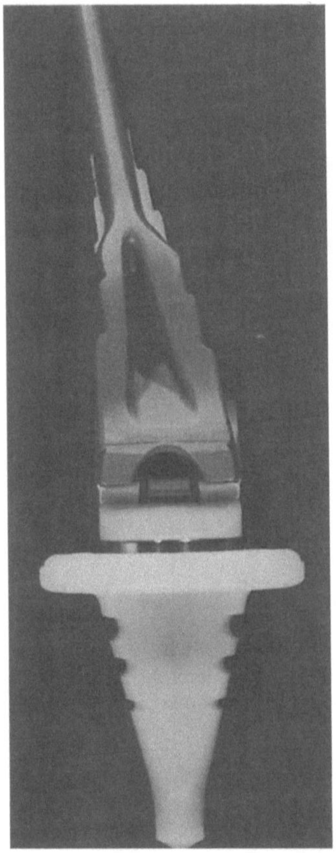

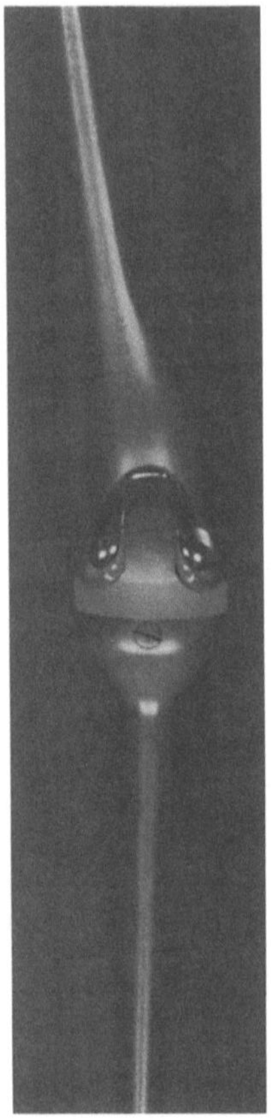

Fig. 1.13. (left) Noiles prosthesis. The tibial component allowed rotation through a stem in a polyethylene housing.

Fig.1.14. (right) Sheehan prosthesis. This design allowed some rotation by a "sloppy" fit between femoral and tibial components.

thesis, in contradistinction to the semiconstrained design, continues to be a challenge.

The Patella

"The patella is an integral part of the skeleton, phylogenetically inherited, and function plays no part either in its formation or its growth. In man it subserves no important function. It is a morphological remnant which is tending to undergo reduction and disappear. It has become modified to take part in movements of the knee joint but its presence is incidental and is a deterrent rather than an aid to these movements. Experimental and other evidence has been advanced to show that in its absence the efficiency of the knee joint is, if anything, increased, both as regards to rapidity of movement and power" (Brooke 1937). Not the first to recommend patellectomy, Brooke was most enthusiastic in providing this indictment of the patella in 1936. He thereupon set out to hasten the disappearance of this remnant by surgical means. Although sporadic enthusiasm for patellectomy surfaced from time to time, it never achieved universal acceptance. Nevertheless, it remained the best alternative for treating severe arthritis involving the patellofemoral joint for many years.

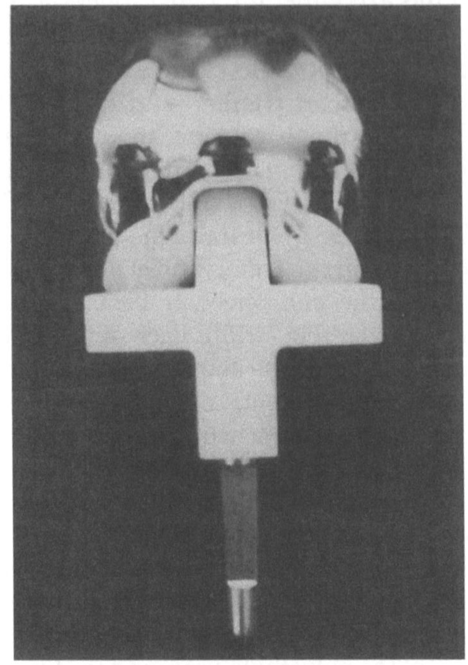

Fig. 1.15. Stabilocondylar prosthesis. Some rotation could occur between the linked components at the axle.

McKeever (1955) described a vitallium prosthesis for the patella, stating that "(patellectomy) is not a satisfactory procedure in more complicated knee joint problems and, in any case, it must be possible to do better". His prosthesis was an anatomically configured metallic surface designed to fit over the reshaped patella to which it was fixed with a screw. The prosthesis articulated with the trochlear surface of the femur. Pickett and Stoll (1979) described a series of patients treated with the McKeever prosthesis and compared the result with the results of patellectomy. Their conclusions were that preserving the patella with a prosthesis was preferable to patellectomy in terms of cosmesis and range of motion.

The availability of cement for fixation promoted several revisions in patellar prosthetic design. A metal "button" was described in a report by Insall et al. (1980) with limited success due to residual pain. Blazina and colleagues (1979) added a metallic counter surface to the trochlear groove of the femur in an attempt to prevent pain associated with the artificial patellar surface articulating with the natural surface of the femur. The follow-up was not encouraging, in part because of continued or associated deterioration of the rest of the knee. Worrell (1979) reported somewhat better results with metallic resurfacing of the patella but his length of follow-up was relatively short.

Independent patellar resurfacing procedures gave way to incorporating patellar surfaces with total knee replacement prostheses during the latter part of the 1970s. Scott et al. (1978) compared total knee prosthetic replacements with and without a plastic patellar surface. The results of their analysis showed a statistically valid improvement in results when the patella was resurfaced. Based on this and other data, patellar resurfacing became a standard part of knee replacement surgery. Although various designs have emerged, the principle remains established. The patella is, after all, an important part of the knee.

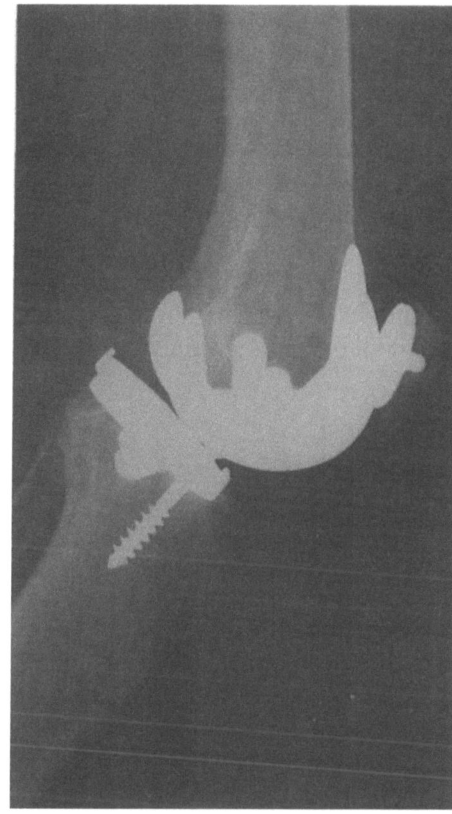

Fig. 1.16. PCA prosthesis. Fixation occurs by bone ingrowth.

Prosthetic Fixation

The availability of cement for fixation of knee prostheses opened the door for the successful treatment of arthritic conditions of this joint. Attempts at replacement without cement in the 1950s and 1960s were met with a high degree of failure due to loosening, settling, or displacement of the devices as noted earlier. With the advent of cement fixation, the primary failures in the early 1970s were markedly reduced or delayed in occurrence. Further refinements in design improved the durability of fixation with few failures reported solely due to loosening. Despite this fact, the introduction of porous coating for bone ingrowth to fix hip prostheses resulted in a second look at fixation methods for knee prostheses (Hungerford et al. 1982). Porous coating of femoral, tibial and patellar prostheses (Fig. 1.16) or the addition of specially designed polyethylene pegs (Fig. 1.17) have

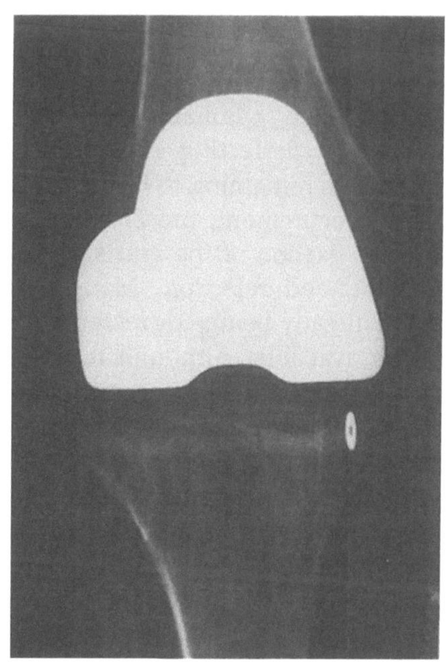

Fig. 1.17. Freeman prosthesis. The tibial component is fixed by press fit serrated polyethylene pegs in the tibial metaphysis.

been adopted with various types of devices. Experience is still accumulating but suggests that the porous coating can be relied upon for fixation of the femoral component but is less dependable for fixation of the tibial tray. The problems associated with the metal backed patellar surface prostheses have precipitated a return to the use of the pure polyethylene surface, precluding porous coated surfaces for fixation. The ultimate role of porous coating or other alternate types of fixation, avoiding cement, is still being determined.

Conclusion

The evolution of arthroplasty of the knee from the use of interpositional membranes of one sort or another to the modern prosthetic replacement represents a dramatic advancement in the treatment of arthritis of the knee. Current techniques when applied as primary procedures will provide good to excellent results in over 90% of patients treated. In the residual 5%–10% poor or indifferent results, the failure due to prosthetic design alone is uncommon. On the other hand, revision cases, those involving severe bone destruction or tumor, or cases involving young persons or individuals of excessive weight, still provide a challenge. Ultimately this will most likely be met by perfecting allografting techniques. Problems remaining to be solved in this area include procurement, preservation, anatomic matching, fixation of the grafts, incorporation, infection, and rejection. Many of these concerns are already being addressed with partial solutions available. Although it seems unlikely that allografts will replace semiconstrained prostheses for the treatment of the uncomplicated impaired knee, such transplants may provide the ultimate solution to replacing those knees which now require a linked prosthesis because of multiple failures of semiconstrained devices, or extensive resection of bone for tumor control.

References

Albee FH (1928) Original features in arthroplasty of the knee with improved prognosis. Surg Gynecol Obstet 47:312–328

Attenborough CG (1978) The Attenborough total knee replacement. J Bone Joint Surg (Br) 60:333–338

Baer WS (1918) Arthroplasty with the aid of animal membrane. Am J Orthop Surg 16:1–29

Blazina ME, Fox JM, Del Pizzo W, Broukhim B, Ivey FM (1979) Patello-femoral replacement. Clin Orthop 144:98–102

Brady TA, Garber JN (1974) Knee joint replacement using the Shiers knee hinge. J Bone Joint Surg (Am) 56:1610–1614

Brooke R (1937) The treatment of fractured patella by excision. A study of morphology and function. Br J Surg 24:733–747

Brown JE, McGaw WH, Shaw DT (1958) Use of cutis as an interposing membrane in arthroplasty of the knee. J Bone Joint Surg (Am) 40:1003–1018

Campbell WC (1940) Interposition of vitallium plates in arthroplasties of the knee. Preliminary report. Am J Surg 47:639–641

Cavendish ME, Wright JTM (1973) The Liverpool mark II knee prosthesis. J Bone Joint Surg (Br) 60:315–319

Coventry MB, Finerman GAM, Riley LH et al. (1972) A new geometric knee for total knee arthroplasty. Clin Orthop 94:171–184

DePalma AF (1954) Diseases of the knee. JB Lippincott Co, Philadelphia, London, Montreal

Fergusson W (1861) Excision of the knee-joint. Recovery with a false joint and a useful limb. Med Times and Gaz 1:601

Freeman MAR, Swanson SAV, Todd RC et al. (1973) Total replacement of the knee using the Freeman Swanson Prosthesis. Clin Orthop 94:153–170

Freeman MAR, Todd RC, Bamert P et al. (1978) ICLH arthroplasty of the knee: 1968–1977. J Bone Joint Surg (Br) 60:339–344

Gluck TT (1902) Zur Behandlung der Ankylose des Kiefergelenkes. Verh Dtsch Ges Chir 1:67

Goodfellow J (1978) The mechanics of the knee and the prosthesis design. J Bone Joint Surg (Br) 60:358–369

Goodfellow J, O'Connor J (1978) Kinematics of the knee and prosthesis design. J Bone Joint Surg (Br) 59:119

Gross AE, Silverstein EA, Falk J et al. (1975) The allotransplantation of the partial joint in the treatment of osteoarthritis of the knee. Clin Orthop 108:7–14

Gunston FH (1971) Polycentric knee arthroplasty. J Bone Joint Surg (Br) 53:272–275

Gunston FH (1973) Polycentric knee arthroplasty. Clin Orthop 94:128–135

Hass J (1944) Functional arthroplasty. J Bone Joint Surg 26:297–306

Hastings DE, Hewitson WA (1973) Double hemiarthroplasty of the knee in rheumatoid arthritis. J Bone Joint Surg (Br) 55:112–118

Helferich E (1894) Ein neues Operation verfahren zur Heilung der knöcherne Kiefergeleuksankylose. Arch Klin Chir 48:864

Henderson MS (1918) What are the real results of arthroplasty? Am J Orthop 94:202–210

Herbert JJ, Herbert A (1973) A new total knee prosthesis. Clin Orthop 94:202–210

Hofman M (1908) Weitere Untersuchungen und Erfahrungen über Periosttransplantation bei Behandlung knöcherner Ankylosen. Beitr Klin Chir 59:717

Hungerford DS, Kenna RV, Krackow KA (1982) The porous coated anatomic total knee. Orthop Clin No Am 13:103–122

Insall JN, Ranawat CS, Aglietti P et al. (1976) A comparison of four models of total knee replacement prostheses. J Bone Joint Surg (Am) 58:754–765

Insall J, Scott WN, Ranawat CS (1979) The total condylar knee prosthesis. J Bone Joint Surg (Am) 61:173–180

Insall J, Tria AJ, Aglietti P (1980) Resurfacing of the patella. J Bone Joint Surg (Am) 62:933–936

Jones WN (1969) Mold arthroplasty of the knee joint. Clin Orthop 66:82–89

Jones WN, Aufranc OE, Kermond WL (1967) Mold arthroplasty of the knee. J Bone Joint Surg (Am) 49:1022

Kraft GL, Levinthal DN (1954) Acrylic prosthesis replacing lower end of the femur for benign giant-cell tumor. J Bone Joint Surg (Am) 36:368–374

Kuhns JG, Potter TA (1950) Nylon arthroplasty of the knee joint in chronic arthritis. Surg Gynec Obstet 91:351–362

Lacheretz M (1953) Traitement des ankylose. Rev Chir Orthop 39:495

LeTournel E, Lagrange J (1973) Total knee replacement with the "LL" type prosthesis. Clin Orthop 94:249–256

Lettin AW, Deliss LJ, Blackburne JS et al. (1978) The Stanmore hinged knee arthroplasty. J Bone Joint Surg (Br) 60:327–332

Lexer E (1909) Uber Gelenktransplantation. Langenbecke Archiv für klinische Chirurgie 90:263

Lexer E (1925) Joint transplantation and arthroplasty. Surg Gynec and Obstet 40:782–809

Lowe LW, Kates A, Kay AGL (1972) MacIntosh arthroplasty in the rheumatoid knee. J Bone Joint Surg (Br) 54:170

MacAusland WR (1933) Knee joint arthroplasty. J Am Med Assoc 101:1699–1702

MacAusland WR (1957) Total replacement of the knee joint by a prosthesis. Surg Gynec Obstet 104:579–583

MacIntosh DL (1958) Hemiarthroplasty of the knee using a space-occupying prosthesis for painful varus and valgus deformities. J Bone Joint Surg (Am) 40:1431

Majnoni d'Intignano JM (1950) Articulation totales en resine acrylique. Rev d'Orthop 36:535–537

Marmor L (1973) The modular knee. Clin Orthop 94:242–248

Matthews LS, Sonstegard DA, Kaufer H (1973) The spherocentric knee. Clin Orthop 94:234–241

Mazas FB (1973) Guepar total knee prosthesis. Clin Orthop 94:211–221

McKeever DC (1955) Patellar prosthesis. J Bone Joint Surg (Am) 37:1074–1084

Meyers MH, Akeson W, Convery R (1989) Resurfacing of the knee with fresh osteochondral allograft. J Bone Joint Surg (Am) 71:704–713

Moeys EJ (1954) Metal alloplasty of the knee joint. An experimental study. J Bone Joint Surg (Am) 36:363–367

Murphy JB (1905) Ankylosis. Arthroplasty, clinical and experimental. J Am Med Arthrop 44:1573

Murray DG (1982) Total knee replacement with a variable axis prosthesis. Orthop Clin North Am 101:155–172

Murray DG, Barranco S (1974) Femoral condylar hemiarthroplasty of the knee. Clin Orthop 101:68–73

O'Rourke K, Sheehan JM (1987) The Sheehan knee arthroplasty: long term results. J Bone Joint Surg (Br) 69:488

Parrish FF (1966) Treatment of bone tumors by total excision and replacement with massive autologous and homologous grafts. J Bone Joint Surg (Am) 48:969–990

Phillips RS (1973) Shiers arthroplasty of the knee. Clin Orthop 94:122–127

Pickett JC, Stoll DA (1979) Patellaplasty or patellectomy? Clin Orthop 144:103–106

Platt G, Pepler C (1968) Mold arthroplasty of the knee. J Bone Joint Surg (Am) 54:1–23

Potter TA, Weinfeld MS, Thomas WH (1972) Arthroplasty of the knee in rheumatoid arthritis and osteoarthritis. J Bone Joint Surg (Am) 54:1–23

Ranawat CS, Shine JJ (1973) Duocondylar total knee arthroplasty. Clin Orthop 94:185–195

Samson JE (1949) Arthroplasty of the knee joint. J Bone Joint Surg (Br) 31:50–52

Scott WN, Rozbruch JD, Otis JC et al. (1978) Clinical and biomechanical evaluation of patella replacement in total knee arthroplasty. Orthop Trans 2:203

Shaw NE, Chatterlee RK (1978) Manchester knee arthroplasty. J Bone Joint Surg (Br) 60:310–314

Shiers LGP (1954) Arthroplasty of the knee. Preliminary report of a new method. J Bone Joint Surg (Br) 36:553–560

Shiers LGP (1961) Hinge arthroplasty for arthritis. Rheumat 17:54–62

Skolnick MD, Bryan RS, Peterson LFA et al. (1976a) Polycentric total knee arthroplasty. A two-year follow-up study. J Bone Joint Surg (Am) 58:743–748

Skolnick MD, Coventry MB, Ilstrup DM (1976b) Geometric total knee arthroplasty. J Bone Joint Surg (Am) 58:749–753

Townley CO (1964) Articular-plate replacement arthroplasty for the knee joint. Clin Orthop 36:77–85

Verneuil A (1860) De la creation d'une fausse articulation par section ou resection partielle de l'os maxillaire inferieur, comme moyen de remedier a l'ankylose vraie ou fausse de la machoire inferieure. Arch Gen Med 5e serie 15, 174, 284

Verneuil AS (1863) Affection articular du genou. Arch Med

Walker PS, Emerson R, Potter T et al. (1982) The kinematic rotating hinge: biomechanics and clinical application. Orthop Clin North Am 13:187–199

Walldius B (1957) Arthroplasty of the knee using an endoprosthesis. Acta Orthop Scand [Suppl] 24

Walldius B (1960) Arthroplasty of the knee using an endoprosthesis. Eight years' experience. Acta Orthop Scand 30:137–148

Waugh TR, Smith RC, Orofino CF et al. (1973) Total knee replacement. Clin Orthop 94:196–201

Wilson FC (1972) Total replacement of the knee in rheumatoid arthritis. J Bone Joint Surg (Am) 54:1429–1443

Worrell RV (1979) Prosthetic resurfacing of the patella. Clin Orthop 144:91–97

Young HH (1963) Use of a hinged vitallium prosthesis for arthroplasty of the knee. J Bone Joint Surg (Am) 45:1627–1642

Young HH (1965) Use of a hinged vitallium prosthesis for arthroplasty of the knee. A preliminary report. J Bone Joint Surg (Am) 45:1627–1642

Zukor DJ, Oakeshott RD, Gross AE (1989) Osteochondral allograft reconstruction of the knee. Am J Knee Surg Z:182–191

Chapter 2

Indications and Alternatives to Total Knee Replacement

Richard Bochner

Introduction

Over 50,000 knee replacements are performed in the United States each year. In order to obtain optimal results, the surgeon must properly choose the patient and weigh the benefits and risks of the surgery and its alternatives. This chapter will discuss these factors.

Indications for Knee Replacement

Symptoms and Signs

The primary indication for performing a total knee replacement is pain. The "ideal" candidate for surgery has moderate or severe knee pain that will be present during routine daily activities. Most patients also have pain at rest or at night, although usually of a lesser degree than activity pain. The pain is chronic, often progressive, and is refractory to all non-surgical modalities.

Frequently, the painful knee will lack a normal arc of motion. Patients will have both a block to full extension as well as a restriction of full flexion. Although loss of motion alone is rarely an indication for knee replacement, the stiffness can be problematic especially in patients with arthritis in the adjacent joints of the lower extremities. In these situations arthroplasty may be indicated even if the pain is not severe.

Patients may present initially with a significant angular deformity such as genu varum or valgum. This may be associated with instability of the joint and with pain in the ipsilateral hip or foot. Cosmesis alone should never be the indication for a knee replacement. Improvement in outward appearance is often a secondary benefit after surgery performed for other indications.

Disease Process

The triad of knee pain, stiffness and deformity can be seen in a variety of diseases. Patients with osteoarthritis will form the largest group of patients needing total knee replacement. This group includes those with progressive idiopathic degenerative joint disease as well as those with osteonecrosis or secondary degeneration after old ligamentous or meniscal injuries. In deciding whether or not to offer knee replacement to these patients, the surgeon must consider the patient's age, size, activity and goals. Since even the most skillfully performed knee arthroplasty has a finite lifetime, the younger the patient when the procedure is performed, the higher the likelihood that revision surgery (or surgeries) will be necessary. Younger patients are also more likely to engage in vigorous sports and heavy labor which put more stress across the arthroplasty and tend to shorten its lifetime. Similarly, the obese patient is at increased risk to have a failed arthroplasty regardless of the age at implantation. When faced with the younger, heavier, more active patient, the alternatives to total knee replacement should be examined carefully.

Knee replacement is often indicated in patients with rheumatoid arthritis when medical therapy or other surgical procedures such as synovectomy have failed. The patient with rheumatoid disease often has polyarthritis and may require replacement of more than one joint. Generally, the demands that the rheumatoid patient places on the joint is less than that of other patients and arthroplasties can be performed at a younger age and be expected to exhibit less mechanical failure. Unfortunately, the nature of the disease, as well as the immunosuppressive therapy frequently required makes the rheumatoid patient more susceptible to such complications as delayed wound healing and sepsis. Because the patient with rheumatoid arthritis tends to have osteopenic bone from disuse, corticosteroids and the disease process itself, there can be an increased incidence of intra-operative complications as well (Hirsh et al. 1981). Recovery is often delayed secondary to muscle weakness.

Total knee replacement is often indicated in patients with one of the sero-negative spondyloarthropathies. Patients with ankylosing spondylitis often have bilateral knee and hip deformities which are similar to those seen in advanced osteoarthritis. Patients with psoriatic arthropathy have a more inflammatory picture, much akin to that seen in rheumatoid arthritis. The knee arthritis associated with chronic bowel disease (i.e. ulcerative colitis and Crohn's disease) may present with either of the above clinical pictures.

Total knee replacement may be indicated in patients with post-traumatic arthritis secondary to intra-articular fracture. These patients usually have more diminution in range of motion than do those with non-traumatic arthritis. They are often younger and more active than the osteoarthritic or rheumatoid. The caveats that were applicable to the osteoarthritic patient apply here as well. In some cases, however, the choice of a potentially failed arthroplasty must be weighed against a severely impaired lifestyle.

Arthritis may progress after an otherwise successful high tibial osteotomy and knee replacement may then be performed. Such a conversion may pose some technical problems but studies have reported results comparable to those following knee replacement on the virgin knee (Staeheli et al. 1987).

Patellofemoral arthritis can usually be treated well by non operative means. If surgery is indicated, arthroscopic debridement (Schonholtz and Ling 1985), tibial tubercle advancement (Maquet 1976) or patellectomy (Lewis et al. 1976) may suffice. In some elderly patients who are severly disabled by patellofemoral disease, however, total knee replacement may be indicated even in the face of a lesser degree of tibiofemoral disease.

Contraindications to Total Knee Replacement

Active sepsis is an absolute contraindication to performing a knee replacement. The introduction of prosthetic material into a septic knee almost assures an increase in the severity of the inflammatory process and an eventual progression into a chronic osteomyelitic process. Prior infection in a knee joint may be only a relative contraindication to surgery. Thorough debridement of all the necrotic material and appropriate antibiotic treatment of the susceptible organisms may have eradicated the infection thus permitting implantation of a prosthesis. Infection of the knee with streptococcus, gonococcus, and some strains of staphylococcus may in many cases be treated in this manner. At the other end of the spectrum is the knee that has been involved in a severe gram negative infection. Rarely is that joint truly cleansed bacteriologically. Later total knee replacement is therefore usually not applicable. Before any arthroplasty is performed in a knee with a history of prior sepsis a proper workup must be performed to assure that no residue of the infection remains. At the minimum, this workup will include a white cell count, an erythrocyte sedimentation rate and a culture of the synovial aspirate. At surgery these procedures may have to be supplemented by a synovial frozen section biopsy.

Absent quadriceps function is a contraindication to knee replacement – arthrodesis or bracing are much better alternatives. An exception may be made after en bloc resection of tumors about the knee. In these cases an articulated prosthesis may be used as an intercalary spacer in an attempt to salvage the extremity.

A painless arthrodesis in a good functional position should not be converted to a total knee replacement. Likewise, the proper treatment for a pseudoarthrosis following an attempted knee fusion is re-arthrodesis, not knee replacement. The chances of successful conversion of an arthrodesis to a knee replacement are small because of muscle and skin contractures and profound quadriceps weakness that occur after an arthrodesis. Some patients with rheumatoid and other inflammatory arthropathies may have a fibrous ankylosis of the knee. Although it is possible to perform a total knee replacement in these patients, the functional results are never as good as those seen in the patients in whom there have been at least 90° of motion pre-operatively (Apyan et al. 1989).

A relative contraindication to a total knee replacement is the triad of youth, obesity, and a job requiring heavy use of the leg. In assessing the patients' age, it is obviously the physiological and not the chronological factor which is most important. A young patient with end stage renal disease or a juvenile rheumatoid arthritis patient may not be "too young" for a total knee once the life expectancy, limited activity level, and limited goal expectations are considered.

The obese patient is at an increased risk for peri-operative anesthesia and vascular problems, intra-operative technical problems, and postoperative prosthetic loosening. It is tempting to state that surgery in such a patient should not be done until weight reduction is accomplished. However, disability from arthritis may be so profound that even walking is too painful, and without exercise significant weight reduction is not possible. In some cases arthroplasty will be performed in the obese patient despite the risks as an adjunct to a weight reduction program. Before this decision is made, consultation with appropriate medical specialists is necessary.

It would be optimal if all the patients undergoing knee replacements were thin, over seventy years of age, in excellent health, and sedentary. Such is rarely the case, however. The unanswered question is what to offer the 55-year old laborer with severe tricompartmental arthritis in one knee which has proved to be refractory to all conservative therapy. This patient could have another ten productive years if his knee functioned better. Must he suffer for another 10 years until he is "old enough" to have total knee replacement at retirement age, or should we suggest that he accept the risk of loosening, reoperation and possible long-term failure in order to enable him to work now? The answer may become more clear as our collective experience with both cemented and non-cemented arthroplasty grows.

Alternatives to Total Knee Replacement

Nonsurgical Treatment

Nonsurgical treatment of knee arthritis should be the first step for all patients. The treatment plan is based on the individual patient, the presenting complaints, and the physical findings. If pain is the primary complaint treatment should help to alleviate the pain. If stiffness or weakness are the prime complaints, therapy should focus on these factors. Radiographs are an important part of the diagnostic regimen, but it is the patient we are treating, not the X-ray. If the patient is comfortable, it matters little how narrow the joint space is on the radiograph.

Anti-inflammatory drugs are, theoretically, most effective when treating signs and symptoms of inflammation. They are, therefore, most applicable in rheumatoid and psoriatic arthritis, and least applicable for cases of osteoarthritis. Almost all of the anti-inflammatory drugs are also analgesics and at times it is difficult to tell whether the diminution of pain is due to one or the other action of the drug. For patients with rheumatoid arthritis, oral steroids, gold, penicillamine, methotrexate and other immunosuppressive drugs may be used under the care of a rheumatologist.

Aspirin remains the most effective, least expensive and most readily available analgesic and anti-inflammatory agent. Even at dose levels of 10–12 tablets per day, the side effects are minimal. The major side effect is gastric intolerance, although tinnitus, and platelet dysfunction may occur.

When aspirin is ineffective or poorly tolerated, the various families of nonsteroidal anti-inflammatory drugs (NSAIDs) may be used. Aspirin and the NSAIDs are both prostaglandin inhibitors and may cause a similar increase in gastrointestinal acid secretion. In some cases, this may be ameliorated by switching NSAIDs, taking them after meals or with antacids or prostaglandin agonists so as to offer some protection to the gastric mucosa. The metabolites of the NSAIDs may have potential for hepatic and renal toxicity and patients on long term NSAID therapy should be monitored for the above. Phenylbutazone has fallen out of favor as an anti-inflammatory and analgesic agent because of its potential to cause aplastic anemia in some patients.

An occasional intra-articular corticosteroid injection may be useful in diminishing inflammation in the arthritic knee. Steroids themselves can cause osteonecrosis in the subchondral bone and should therefore be used sparingly. Opiate analgesics are to be avoided except in short term instances.

Physical therapy modalities often play a beneficial role in the nonsurgical treatment of arthritis. Local heat, cold and ultrasound may give temporary symptomatic relief and can be used instead of or in combination with oral medication. All of these may assist the patient in regaining or improving quadriceps and hamstring muscle strength and control. This may be helpful for mild to moderate tibiofemoral arthritis and particularly for isolated patellofemoral disease. Even in patients for whom surgery is planned, a well directed exercise program can help to maintain muscle tone and accelerate postoperative progress.

Joint Debridement

Open joint debridement was a popular procedure for the patient with advanced osteoarthritis during the pre-total knee replacement era. Both Haggart (1940, 1947) and Magnuson (1941) described "house cleaning" techniques which included synovectomy, meniscectomy, articular cartilage shaving, osteophyte resection and at times patellectomy. The goal of these procedures was to remove mechanical irritants in order to alleviate pain and slow the progress of the disease. Haggart reported success in 27 of 30 patients. The recuperation from such an extensive open procedure was often very painful and the period of rehabilitation could take up to 6 months.

As the popularity of arthroscopy increased in the 1970s and 1980s, arthroscopic debridement of the arthritic knee became possible. The hope was that an arthroscopic technique would eliminate the problems associated with open surgery while accomplishing the same goals. Sprague (1981) and Shahriaree et al. (1982) reported approximately 75% good results in two of the earliest reports. Although not all patients were improved by the procedure, and some who were had only temporary relief, the complications were few, the rehabilitation was swift, and later reconstructive surgery could still be done if required.

Pridie (1959) and Insall(1974) had initially described drilling or abrading the eburnated bone during the time of open knee debridement in an attempt to encourage reformation of cartilage in the arthritic knee. Johnson (1986), and Friedman et al. (1984) reported that 60%–70% of their patients were improved following abrasion arthroplasty performed arthroscopically. Johnson demonstrated that there was an increase in the width of the joint space roentgenographically following abrasion arthroplasty, suggesting the regrowth of some type of cartilage. Second look arthroscopies and gross specimens analyzed after knee replacement have shown, however, that following abrasion arthroplasty, articular cartilage defects are filled with smooth tissue which has the appearance, but not the consistency or resistance to compressive forces, of normal hyaline cartilage. The collagen type and histological appearance of the new material are consistent with that of fibrocartilage rather than hyaline cartilage.

Clinically it has been difficult to assess the efficacy of abrasion arthroplasty alone since it is generally performed in conjunction with arthroscopic debridement of loose bodies and degenerative menisci. Bert and Maschka (1989), however, reported on two large groups of patients who underwent arthroscopic debridement, one with and one without abrasion arthroplasty. The group with abrasion arthroplasty had fewer good to excellent results and significantly more poor results. Part of the reason for the poorer results of abrasion arthroplasty may have been the fact that many of the postabrasion arthroplasty patients could not or would not comply with instructions to remain nonweightbearing for 6–8 weeks post-surgery. Johnson (1986) claims better compliance in his series. This need for a prolonged period of protected weight bearing may make abrasion arthroplasty a less viable option in the elderly population.

Although arthroscopic debridement is offered as an alternative to high tibial osteotomy, there may be some circumstances in which the two may be done together. Salisbury et al. (1985) found that results from debridement were much better in normally aligned knees than in varus knees. It may be inferred that a combined procedure would be beneficial. MacIntosh and Welsh (1977) described their technique of combining open joint debridement with high tibial osteotomy. Realizing that the immobilization required for routing healing of the tibial osteotomy would encourage stiffness in a freshly arthrotomized knee, they held the osteotomy with an external fixator and encouraged early motion of the knee. Unfortunately, this protocol resulted in an infection rate of 9% and a non-union rate of 4%. Certainly an advantage of arthroscopic debridement is that it does not pose as great a risk of arthrofibrosis as arthrotomy does.

Coventry (1979) has noted improvement in the articular surface and growth of some type of cartilage following tibial osteotomy without any concomitant intra-articular procedure. Fujisawa et al. (1979) have confirmed this arthroscopically with second looks. Arthroscopic surgery at the time of osteotomy may be needed especially in the face of mechanical blocks in the knee, but may not be necessary for every case.

At this stage in its development, it can be said that arthroscopic debridement of the knee has a place in the treatment of osteoarthritis of the knee. It offers an alternative to the patient unwilling or unable to have a high tibial osteotomy or a total knee replacement because of their youth, weight, medical or activity status. Although its efficacy in any given patient is somewhat unpredictable, good results are more likely in patients with normal knee alignment (Salisbury et al. 1985), unicompartmental disease (Bert and Maschka 1989), and those with a localized area of underlying osteonecrosis (Miller et al. 1986). The role of arthroscopic abrasion arthroplasty is somewhat less clear. Some of the patients who might theoretically benefit the most from abrasion will be unable to remain truly nonweightbearing for 6–8 weeks.

The candidate for arthroscopic debridement needs to realize that he or she is receiving a palliative procedure which may give them only temporary relief, and that additional surgery, i.e. tibial osteotomy, knee replacement or repeat arthroscopic debridement, may be needed.

Osteotomy

Osteotomy of the proximal tibia as a treatment for arthritis of the knee was initially described by Jackson (1958) and Wardle (1962) before being popularized in the 1960s by Mark Coventry (1965). Coventry modified the previously performed procedures by performing the osteotomy proximal to the tibial tubercle. This had several advantages. The osteotomy was performed closer to the area of the deformity, the bone involved was cancellous and tended to heal rapidly, and the patient could bear weight on the leg since the pull of the quadriceps tended to compress the osteotomy.

The rationale behind the procedure was to correct the angular deformity at the knee and therefore decrease the excessive weight bearing loads across the affected compartment (usually the medial one) which was most affected by the arthritic process. Early clinical results were encouraging and radiographs demonstrated the transference of weight bearing load to the uninvolved tibial condyle and often a widening of the involved joint space. Since alternative treatments for severe arthritis of the knee in the 1960s were limited, tibial osteotomy was used for osteoarthritis, rheumatoid arthritis and post-traumatic arthritis regardless of the magnitude of the angular deformity.

After several years' experience, Coventry (1973), Insall et al. (1974) and others narrowed the criteria for tibial osteotomy. By the late 1970s high tibial osteotomy was felt to be indicated for the younger more active patient in whom total knee replacement was thought to be unwise. Osteotomy would be best done for primarily unicompartmental osteoarthritis in knees with generally well maintained motion (at least 90° of flexion, less that a 15° flexion contracture). Tibial osteotomy should probably not be done in patients with rheumatoid arthritis, patients with very unstable knees, nor in knees with greater than a 12° valgus deformity. Insall felt that osteotomy should not be performed in varus knees with greater than 15° of deformity because these knees were associated with greater ligamentous laxity and subluxation.

There is no universal agreement as to the proper position to which the leg should be corrected after a tibial osteotomy. Coventry originally recommended that the valgus osteotomy performed for medial compartment disease should be such that the resultant femoraltibial angle was several degrees greater than the normal 7° (Coventry 1973). Others have suggested that the results are comparable whether or not the leg is overcorrected or brought to a neutral 7° alignment (Insall et al. 1984). All agree, however, that undercorrection is associated with failure.

Valgus deformity of over 15° of femoral-tibial valgus associated with lateral compartment disease is best treated by a distal femoral osteotomy. For lesser degrees of valgus either a femoral or tibial osteotomy may suffice. Again there is no universal agreement as to what the position is to aim for after such an osteotomy, although most agree that the neutral 7° of valgus is probably optimal.

The complications from high tibial osteotomy include loss of fixation of the fragment, fracture into the knee joint, and non union. There are also the general complications of any knee surgery, i.e. deep venous thrombosis, pulmonary embolism, arterial occlusion, wound infection and peroneal nerve palsy.

Some of the initial enthusiasm for high tibial osteotomy has waned as long term studies have demonstrated deterioration of results with time. Cass and Bryan (1988) at the Mayo Clinic found that although 94% of their patients were doing well at 2 years, this number deteriorated to 87% at 5 years and 69% at 10 years. Others (Coventry 1979, Insall et al. 1984) have reported only 60% of patients being pain free at 10 year follow-up.

With this in mind, high tibial osteotomy remains a viable alternative to total knee replacement in the young, active, athletic patient. A successful tibial osteotomy permits unlimited activity; total knee replacement does not. The prospective candidate must be aware that good results very well may be time limited, and he may require arthroplasty within 10 years. There is some evidence that prior tibial osteotomy may lower the success rate of knee replacement (Katz et al. 1987; Windsor et al. 1988), however, this factor is probably outweighed by the advantages of osteotomy in the young patient.

Arthrodesis

In the days prior to the development of tibial osteotomy, arthrodesis was offered to patients with severe, disabling knee disease which was refractory to medical management and such lesser operative procedures as debridement or synovectomy. Arthrodesis of the knee did not attain the popularity of hip arthrodesis because patients did not attain the same functional level of activity. Using public transportation or sitting in a theater was extremely difficult with an arthrodesed knee. Putting on shoes and socks was also very difficult without special equipment.

In current practice the indications for knee arthrodesis are limited. It is performed in cases of septic arthritis when destruction is significant and arthroplasty is contraindicated, in cases of failed knee replacement when revision is not possible due to sepsis or loss of extensor function, and in the occasional young person with tricompartmental arthritis, minimal motion, and intractable pain, for whom knee replacement is not a viable alternative.

Synovectomy

Synovectomy alone is mainly of value as a treatment for rheumatoid arthritis of the knee. This has been performed classically via arthrotomy with good results in appropriately selected patients. Arthroscopic synovectomy, in the hands of the skilled arthroscopist, can offer the same benefits of open synovectomy with less morbidity. A thorough exploration of anterior and posterior compartments can be carried out and synovium and damaged menisci can be excised. The procedure can be quite tedious and at times visualization may be very difficult because of the proliferative synovitis. Early postoperative range of motion is possible and desirable, sometimes with the aid of a continuous passive motion machine in the postoperative period.

Although synovectomy is a useful treatment modality in the care of the patient with rheumatoid arthritis, it cannot be accurately described as an alternative to knee replacement. The ideal candidate for synovectomy is at an earlier stage in the course of the disease and has not yet developed the bony changes and joint space narrowing present in the total knee candidate. Most appropriately, synovectomy should be offered to patients in an attempt to forestall the progression of the disease and postpone the need for knee replacement.

Tibial Tuberculoplasty

The procedure of tibial tubercle advancement was described in 1963 by Paul Maquet as treatment for osteoarthritis of the patellofemoral joint (Maquet 1963). Through the years various authors have reported results which have ranged from excellent to poor (Maquet 1976; Rozbruch et al. 1979; Leach et al. 1981). The common thread running through these reports is the high rate of complications. These have ranged from skin necrosis secondary to the 1.5–2 cm bone graft placed beneath the tibial tubercle, to tibial fractures, compartment syndrome, and pain with kneeling. When performed well, without complication, this has been an effective procedure. Modifications to the procedure such as those described by Ferguson (1982) and Fulkerson (1983) may prove to diminish the complication rate. The combination of tibial tubercle advancement and tibial osteotomy, although intellectually appealing for the patient with bicompartmental disease, has not proven to be very clinically successful. Most patients do not have patellar complaints following tibial osteotomy, regardless of the preoperative state of their patellofemoral joint.

Summary

After all alternative options have been exhausted, total knee replacement is a logical choice for those patients with painful knees secondary to arthritis or trauma. Age, level of activity, patient weight and realistic goals all must be considered if the patient is to be properly advised to undergo a total knee replacement.

References

Apyan PM, Rorabeck CH, Bourne RB, Nott L, (1989) Factors affecting postoperative range of motion in primary cemented total knee arthroplasty. Presented at American Academy of Orthopaedic Surgeons Annual Meeting, Las Vegas

Bert JM, Maschka K (1989) The arthroscopic treatment of unicompartmental gonarthrosis. Arthroscopy 5:25–32

Cass JR, Bryan RS (1988) High tibial osteotomy. Clin Orthop 230:196–199

Coventry MB (1965) Osteotomy of the upper portion of the tibia for degenerative arthritis of the knee. J Bone Joint Surg (Am) 47:984–990

Coventry MB (1973) Osteotomy about the knee for degenerative and rheumatoid arthritis. J Bone Joint Surg (Am) 55:23–48

Coventry MB (1979) Upper tibial osteotomy for gonarthrosis. Orthop Clin N Am 10:191–210

Ferguson AB (1982) Elevation of the insertion of the patellar ligament for patellofemoral pain. J Bone Joint Surg (Am) 64:766–771

Friedman MJ, Berasi CC, Fox JM et al. (1984) Preliminary results with abrasion arthroplasty in the osteoarthritic knee. Clin Orthop 182:200–205

Fujisawa Y, Masuhra K, Shiomi S (1979) The effect of high tibial osteotomy in osteoarthritis of the knee: an arthroscopic study of 54 knee joints. Orthop Clin N Am 3:585

Fulkerson JP (1983) Anteromedialization of the tibial tuberosity for patellofemoral malalignment. Clin Orthop 177:176–181

Haggart GE (1940) The surgical treatment of degenerative arthritis of the knee joint. J Bone Joint Surg (Am) 22:717

Haggart GE (1947) Surgical treatment of degenerative arthritis of the knee joint. N Engl J Med 236:971

Hirsh DM, Bhalla S, Roffman M (1981) Supracondylar fracture of the femur following total knee replacement. J Bone Joint Surg (Am) 63:162–163

Insall JN (1974) The Pridie debridement operation for osteoarthritis of the knee joint. Clin Orthop 101:61

Insall JN, Shoji H, Mayer V (1974) High tibial osteotomy, a five year evaluation. J Bone Joint Surg (Am) 56:1397–1405

Insall JN, Joseph DM, Msika C (1984) High tibial osteotomy for varus gonarthrosis. J Bone Joint Surg (Am) 66:1040–1048

Jackson JP (1958) Osteotomy for osteoarthritis of the knee. In:Proceedings of the Sheffield Regional Orthopaedic Club. J Bone Joint Surg (Br) 40:826

Johnson LL (1986) Arthroscopic abrasion arthroplasty:

historical and pathologic perspective:present status. Arthroscopy 2:54 -69
Katz MM, Hungerford DS, Krackow KA, Lennox DW (1987) Results of total knee arthroplasty after failed proximal tibial osteotomy for osteoarthritis. J Bone Joint Surg (Am) 69:225–233
Leach RE, Paul GR, Yablon IG, Schepsis AA (1981) Anterior displacement of the tibial tubercle:the Maquet procedure. Cont Orthop 3:119–124
Lewis MM, Fitzgerald PF, Jacobs B (1976) Patellectomy: An analysis of one hundred cases. J Bone Joint Surg (Am) 58:736
MacIntosh DL, Welsh RP (1977) Joint debridement – a complement to high tibial osteotomy in the treatment of osteoarthritis of the knee. J Bone Joint Surg (Am) 59:1094–1097
Magnuson PB (1941) Joint debridement: surgical treatment of degenerative arthritis. Surg Gynecol Obstet 73:1
Maquet P (1963) Considerations biomechaniques sur l'arthrose femoropatellaire. L'avancement du tendon rotulien. Rev Rhum 30:779–783
Maquet P (1976) Advancement of the tibial tuberosity. Clin Orthop 115:225–230
Miller GK, Maylahn DJ, Drennan DB (1986) The treatment of idiopathic osteonecrosis of the medial femoral condyle with arthroscopic debridement. Arthroscopy 2:21–29
Pridie KH (1959) A method of resurfacing osteoarthritic knee joints. J Bone Joint Surg (Br) 41:618
Rozbruch JD, Campbell RD, Insall JN (1979) Tibial tubercle elevation. Orthop Trans 3:291
Salisbury RB, Nottage WM, Gardner V (1985) The effect of alignment on results in arthroscopic debridement of the degenerative knee. Clin Orthop 198:268–272
Schonholtz GJ, Ling B (1985) Arthroscopic chondroplasty of the patella. Arthroscopy 1:92–96
Shahriaree H, O'Connor RL, Nottage W (1982) Seven years' follow-up on arthroscopic debridement of the degenerative knee. Field of View 1:1
Sprague NF (1981) Arthroscopic debridement for degenerative knee joint disease. Clin Orthop 160:118–123
Staeheli JW, Cass JR, Morrey BF (1987) Condylar total knee arthroplasty after failed proximal tibial osteotomy. J Bone Joint Surg (Am) 69:28–31
Wardle EN (1962) Osteotomy of the tibia and fibula. Surg Gynecol Obstet 115:61–64
Windsor RE, Insall JN, Vince KG (1988) Technical considerations of total knee arthroplasty after proximal tibial osteotomy. J Bone Joint Surg (Am) 70:547–555

Chapter 3

Knee Biomechanics and Materials

Malcolm H. Pope and Braden C. Fleming

Introduction

"Biomechanics is the study of forces and the effects that these forces have on the human body" (LeVeau 1984). From the orthopaedist's perspective, there is a normal equilibrium between mechanical stress on the musculoskeletal system and its response to that stress. Any disturbance to this balance will eventually result in remodeling, degeneration, or failure of a structure. Within the realm of total knee replacement, it is necessary to understand fully the biomechanics of the normal joint since the objective of total knee arthroplasty is to re-establish normal joint function.

The biomechanics of the knee involves three interacting categories: geometry, kinematics, and kinetics. The geometry is defined by the anatomical structures and the orientation of these structures within the knee. The limitations of motion, or kinematics, are determined by the geometry of the knee. Kinetics is the study of force and the effects of forces on the structure, kinematics and function of the knee. Any alterations to any one of the three categories will result in pathologic changes of the whole system. For example, a torn anterior cruciate ligament leads to instability and alters the kinematics of the knee. As a result, the load distribution across the joint is altered, which in turn, accelerates the degenerative process (Liljedahl and Nordstrand 1969; Palmer 1938).

The success of total joint arthroplasty over the last 10 years is the result of the development of sophisticated biomechanical concepts, biomaterials and surgical techniques. The goals of total joint arthroplasty to eliminate pain and restore mechanical function have more or less been achieved for the older sedentary patient, however, total joint arthroplasty continues to be plagued by a high incidence of aseptic loosening and failure, especially in younger patients (Lewis and Galante 1985). Continued biomechanical research is required to improve instrumentation and implantation techniques of currently available devices, and to develop total joint arthroplasty systems which will restore normal joint function to the young athletic individual without failure.

The objective of this chapter is to provide an overview of the biomechanics of the knee as it relates to total joint arthroplasty. The specific aims are (1) to examine the biomechanics of the normal knee relevant to total knee arthroplasty, (2) to understand the biomechanics of the arthritic knee and the need to correct these alterations, (3) to present an overview of the biomechanics of the total joint arthroplasty, and (4) to discuss materials used in total joint arthroplasty.

Biomechanics of the Normal Knee

The human knee has two primary functions: to provide mobility, and to provide stability to the lower extremity. The knee joint must allow both flexion and axial rotation to occur while still maintaining stability. The knee is actually composed of two articulating joints; the patello-femoral and the tibiofemoral joint. The tibio-femoral joint defines the kinematics of flexion, extension and axial rotation while the patello-femoral joint increases the efficiency of the extensor mechanism. Some compromises must be made in the structure of the knee in order to optimize both mobility and stability. The knee is thus susceptible to sprains, tears, dislocations, and general wear which may eventually lead to degenerative joint disease.

Joint stability is provided by both intrinsic and extrinsic anatomical mechanisms. The intrinsic stability of the knee joint is provided by the four primary ligaments, the capsule, the shape of the bony structures, and the menisci. The ligaments act as tensile check reins which permit motion to occur within limits. The limits of motion are dependent on orientation of these ligaments. The two cruciates provide stability in the sagittal plane, resisting anterior and posterior shear, whereas the collaterals provide resistance to varus and valgus angulation. The intercondylar tubercles are bony structures on the tibial plateau which interlock with the intercondylar notch of the distal femur. Their interference fit provides stability to medial and lateral shear stresses and prevents hyperextension without inhibiting flexion or axial rotation. The tibial plateau in conjunction with the menisci provide channels for the femoral condyles that add stability in flexion and axial rotation without overconstraining the joint. The radius of curvature of the femoral condyles increases anteriorly. With extension, there is increased compression on the tibiofemoral joint and increased tension in the ligaments. This force couple is another check to hyperextension.

The muscles of the thigh and calf give extrinsic stability to the knee. The muscles provide both the force to articulate the knee, and the check-rein stability to resist abnormal stresses. The act of extension is achieved through the quadriceps mechanism transmitted through the patella. The patella is a sesamoid bone which acts as a pulley mechanism to increase the efficiency of the extension effort and to direct the action of these quadriceps forces.

In 1836, Weber described knee motion as a combination of rolling, sliding, and axial rotation of the tibiofemoral joint (Muller 1938). Unfortunately, as yet there have been few three-dimensional models described in the literature which incorporate this axial rotation with the rolling and sliding of the joint (Wismans et al. 1980). The kinematic principles of the knee have therefore been reduced to a two-dimensional midsagittal plane model known as the "cruciate" linkage (Goodfellow and O'Connor 1978; Huson 1974; Kapandji 1970; Menschik 1974; Muller 1938; O'Connor and Shercliff, unpublished report 1980). The four links of this linkage represent the neutral fiber of the ACL, the neutral fiber of the PCL, a tibial link between the tibial cruciate attachment sites and a femoral link between the femoral cruciate attachment sites (Fig. 3.1). If the femoral link is articulated about the fixed tibial link, a graphic representation of knee joint motion can be obtained. Kapandji (1970) has concluded that "the shape of the femoral condyles are geometrically determined by the lengths of each of the cruciate ligaments, as well as by the ratio of their individual lengths and the arrangement of their insertions".

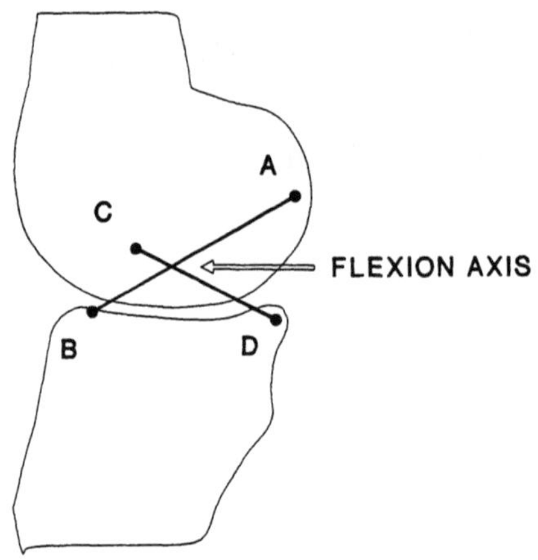

Fig.3.1. The cruciate linkage comprises four links: AB is the neutral fiber of the ACL, CD is the neutral fiber of the PCL, BD is the link between the tibial attachment sites, and CA designates the femoral insertion points. The flexion axis is the point of intersection between the links AB and CD. (From Kampandji 1970.)

As the knee is flexed from full extension, the point of intersection of the ACL and PCL links moves posterior. A two-dimensional model has been constructed for a situation in which the tibia rotated on a stationary femur and the femur rotated on a stationary tibia (Huson 1974; Menschik 1974; O'Connor and Shercliff, unpublished report 1980). These curves developed by plotting the centers of rotation in each situation are called centroids. The tibial centroid approximates a straight line whereas the femoral centroid is elliptical. As the two bones move on each other they undergo both rolling and sliding. It is obvious that the femur must slide forward on the tibia during flexion; a pure rolling motion would result in the femur falling off the back of the tibia as the knee was flexed over 100°. During the early phases of flexion, rolling is the predominant motion, while as flexion continues, sliding tends to predominate (Kapandji 1970). Activities such as walking and running occur when the knee is near full extension, where the motion is predominantly rolling. Standing from a seat and squatting down occur when the knee is flexed, during which point the femur and tibia are mainly sliding with respect to each other.

Axial rotation of the tibia relative to the femur is the result of the application of the ground reactive force (passive rotation), the rotation applied by the musculature (manual rotation), and the screwhome mechanism (automatic rotation). The ligaments and capsular structures act as restraints to this rotation. The musculature of the lower limb serves both as a passive restraint against rotation, and to provide the force to cause rotation.

The screwhome mechanism (external rotation of the tibia on the femur) occurs automatically as the knee is extended. In the sagittal plane, the radius of curvature, or evolute, of the medial plateau is different from the lateral plateau. The medial tibial plateau is concave superiorly and the lateral is convex. Therefore, the articulating surfaces of the tibiofemoral joint are not congruent. When viewed distally, the lateral femoral condyle is longer than the medial. The unequal lengths and radii of curvature of the two femoral condyles, the shape of the tibial plateaus, and the position of the four primary ligaments force the tibia to rotate externally with extension (Kapandji 1970).

The loading mechanisms of the knee joint are important in the study of the arthritic knee. The success or failure of the total joint arthroplasty is dependent on the forces exhibited at the knee joint. These are the forces which will ultimately determine the stresses aplied to the prosthesis–bone interface. Joint load can be divided into two components: a normal or compressive force (applied perpendicular to the surfaces), and a shearing force applied tangential to the joint surfaces (Nisell 1985).

Joint forces have been determined through experimental methods and modeling (Calderale and Scelfo 1987; Harrington 1976; Kettlekamp and Chao 1972; Mena et al. 1981; Mikosz 1985; Mikosz et al. 1988; Minns 1981; Morrison 1968, 1970a, b; Seireg and Arvikar 1975; Simon et al. 1981; Whittle 1985). These models use experimental data and mechanical laws to make approximations of joint forces. The major differences between the various models are the assumptions made regarding the center of rotation of the knee joint. Such joint load analyses are particularly important in the design of knee prostheses. The implants must remain well fixed while being subjected to a multitude of deleterious loading conditions. They must function under these constraints while still maximizing the kinematics of the joint.

Maquet (1984a) used the models of Braune and Fischer to illustrate the forces exerted on the knee joint during static activities. They had determined that when a person stood on both legs, each knee joint carried 43% of the body weight. When standing on one leg, the supporting knee had to support the partial body weight suspended vertically from the center of gravity of the body. To maintain equilibrium, a force had to be generated in the lateral tension band. The resultant force across the joint surface was more than twice body weight. This resultant force was located between the centers of curvature of the medial and lateral femoral condyles through the center of the weight bearing surfaces (Fig. 3.2).

In a more dynamic situation such as walking, the models increase in complexity. Seireg and Arvikar (1975) determined that compressive forces up to six times body weight and shear forces up to twice body weight were developed at the knee joint. With the patient walking on a level surface, the resultant forces across the joint were as high as seven times body weight. Considering that an average individual takes over 1 900 000 steps a year, it is easy to understand why friction in the normal (and prosthetic) knee must be kept to a minimum (Walker 1977a).

The anatomy and physiology of articular cartilage, the presence of the menisci, and the natural lubricating properties of synovial fluid are responsible for the normal knee having an extremely low coefficient of friction. Derangement of any of these structures can lead to increased friction and increased wear.

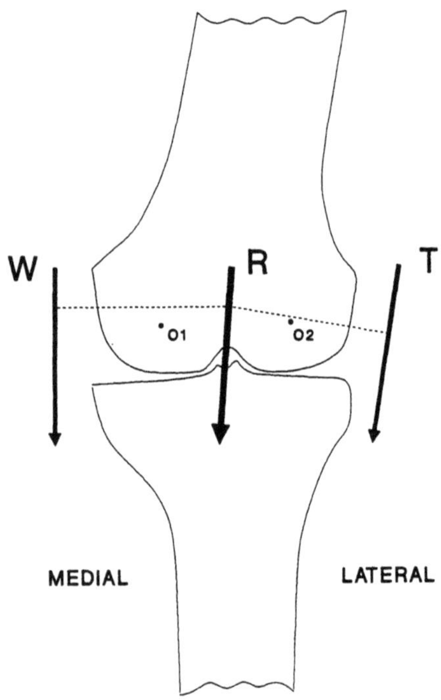

Fig. 3.2. The forces generated in the knee while standing on one leg (coronal plane). The partial body weight, W, is held in equilibrium by the lateral tension band, T. Thus, the resultant force, R, is located through the center of the medial and lateral weight bearing surfaces between the centers of curvature of the medial and lateral femoral condyles, 01 and 02. (From Maquet 1984a.)

Articular cartilage is a viscoelastic bearing surface with excellent lubrication properties. The coefficient of friction of articular cartilage is many times less than that of Teflon on Teflon (Fung 1981). The structure of the collagen fibril orientation within the cartilage may convert shear forces on the articular surface to compressive forces at the bone–cartilage interface (Bullough and Goodfellow 1968).

Synovial fluid is a lubricant which bathes the articular cartilage. It is a non-newtonian fluid which demonstrates high viscosity at low shear rates and low viscosity at high shear rates. The viscoelastic properties of synovial fluid led Balazs and Gibbs (1970) to hypothesize that the biologic function of synovial fluid is to serve as a shock absorber. Under impulse loadings (i.e. heel strike), synovial fluid has a higher viscosity, preventing the boundary layer of fluid between the tibial and femoral condyles from squeezing out from the articulating surfaces. During flexion, low viscosity is required to lubricate the sliding surfaces adequately (King 1966).

The menisci are cartilaginous load bearing "washers" that increase the load bearing surface area between the tibia and femur (Bullough et al. 1970; Kettlekamp and Jacob 1972; Mathur et al. 1949; Walker and Hajek 1972). As described earlier, the articulating surfaces of the femoral and tibial condyles are noncongruent. Stress is equal to force per unit area. The menisci function to increase the contact area between the femoral and tibial condyles, reducing the stress on the load bearing surfaces. A reduction in stress eliminates the detrimental degenerative effects of point loading.

The regenerative properties of the joint tissues enable the knee to function for many decades with little or no degenerative changes. As with any biomechanical system, the knee is prone to failure from exposure to excessive loading, trauma, ageing, and disease. Singularly or in combination, these may result in degenerative joint disease.

Biomechanics of the Arthritic Knee

A failure in any structure of the knee will alter the joint kinematics and the load bearing characteristics, resulting in arthritis. Several theories exist on the origins of arthritis (Goodfellow and Bullough 1967; Harrison et al. 1953); however, the mechanical wear theory seems most accurate (Walker 1977b). The work of Bennett et al. (1942) suggests that osteoarthritis is a degenerative process of hyaline cartilage which increases with increasing age.

The effects of degeneration of the articular surfaces can be demonstrated using the simple model of the force exerted on the knee while standing on one leg described earlier (Maquet 1984b). Despite the fact that this model is much less complex than that involving normal gait, the alterations due to arthritis that it predicts are still severe.

Osteoarthritis of the medial compartment will lead to loss of cartilage from the medial femoral condyle and tibial plateau and will result in a varus deformity. This forces the partial body weight to act on a longer moment arm than normal since the position of the knee places it far

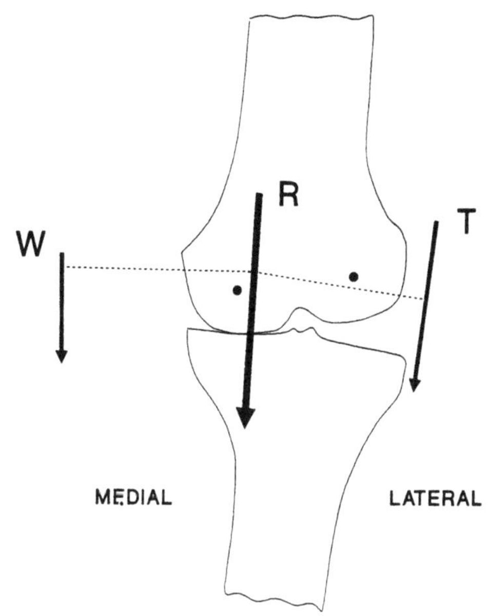

Fig. 3.3. Osteoarthritis of the medial compartment forces the limb into varus alignment shifting the resultant force to the medial compartment. Thus, the stress in the medial compartment increases. (From Maquet 1984b.)

lateral from the line of the center of gravity of the torso. Concomitantly, the balancing force in the iliotibial band is increased. The resultant of these two forces is shifted to the medial plateau. The overall stress on the medial compartment is increased since the force is greater and that force is exerted through a smaller than normal surface area (Fig. 3.3). This increase in stress causes the degenerative process to accelerate even further. An unstable varus deformity will eventually occur when the resultant vector shifts medial to the center of curvature of the medial femoral condyle (Maquet 1984b).

Arthritis of the lateral compartment leads to similar problems. The lower limb alignment becomes valgus, shifting the resulting load vector to the lateral side to maintain equilibrium. The contact stress on the lateral femoral condyle and lateral tibial plateau is increased and the arthritic process further accelerates.

Arthritic changes pose a serious clinical problem since once the damage is initiated, the pathologic changes accelerate the degeneration. There is no cure for arthritis. The alignment deformities may be corrected, however, with a high tibial osteotomy. Unfortunately, deterioration of good clinical results after a tibial osteotomy can be expected to occur within a 6–10 year period (Vainionpaa et al. 1981).

Theoretically, a total knee replacement should be the optimal answer to correct the problems in the knee since it eliminates the degenerative tissues, reduces pain and restores some function to the afflicted joint. However, a total knee replacement itself may pose many biomechanical problems which must be solved if initial short term successes are to be transformed into long term good results, particularly for the younger patient.

Materials for Total Knee Arthroplasty

Tribology is the study of friction and wear. The natural tribological principles of the normal knee have been discussed previously. Materials chosen for the prosthetic knee should demonstrate similar friction and wear characteristics approaching that of normal cartilage. This choice poses a very difficult problem since the normal knee is composed of biologic tissues which can remodel in response to applied stress. The materials used in prosthetic devices are inanimate. The material properties of the ideal material for total joint arthroplasty must endure the physiological demands without subsequent degeneration.

Materials used in total joint arthroplasty must meet three criteria: (1) a high resistance to wear, (2) a low coefficient of friction, and (3) biocompatibility. The material must be wear resistant to improve the prosthesis wear life. A low coefficient of friction enables smooth flexion–extension, reduces stresses transmitted to the prosthesis–bone interface and reduces the amount of wear of the prosthesis. The material must be biocompatible so as not to cause inflammation in the surrounding tissues.

The materials currently used in prosthetic design are either metallic or polymeric. The two metals commonly used are cobalt-chromium (CoCrMo) and titanium alloy (usually Ti-6A1-4V). The metallic crystals in both types of alloys are hexagonal in structure and may be polished so as to have a low coefficient of friction (Walker 1977a). The polymer that is used is ultra high molecular weight polyethylene (UHMWPE).

Some of the earlier prostheses consisted of metal implants articulating with other metal implants. As wear progressed, small dark wear particles developed. These caused inflammation in the soft tissues (Walker 1977a) and led to progressive loosening of the prostheses. The wear particles themselves, due to their inherent hardness, caused three body wear between the metal surfaces, causing more wear products to form. As a result of these problems, metal on metal bearing surfaces for total knee prostheses have been abandoned.

All prostheses now have a metal surface (usually the femoral component) articulating with polyethylene implants (usually the tibial and patellar components). Synovial fluid is the lubricant (Mears 1979). The modulus of elasticity of the polyethylene is similar to that of bone and cartilage. This adds a damping effect to the system during shock loading. The coefficient of friction of these metal on plastic bearings varies from 0.1 to 0.4 for both CoCrMo and titanium alloys (Mears 1979; Walker 1977a). (The coefficient of friction of normal articular cartilage on normal articular cartilage is 0.009 : Table 3.1).

Table 3.1. Coefficients of friction for various combinations of materials

Material	Lubrication	Coefficient
Metal/metal (smooth)	Dry	100
Tire/road	Dry	1
Nylon/steel	Dry	0.2
PTFE/PTFE	Dry	0.07
PTFE/PTFE	Water	0.04
CoCR/CoCr	Water	0.38
CoCr/HDPE	Water	0.04
Human hip joint (in vitro)	Water	0.009

HDPE, high density polyethylene.
CoCr, cobalt-chromium alloy.
PTFE, polytetrafluoroethylene (Teflon).

Ultra high molecular weight polyethylene (UHMWPE) has certain limitations. The results from many post-mortem retrieval studies indicate the UHMWPE tends to creep or cold flow and is subjected to many types of wear disorders. UHMWPE is prone to scratching, gouging, wear polishing, pitting, delamination, shredding, and cracking (Hood et al. 1983; Landy and Walker 1985; Mirra et al. 1982; Rose et al. 1979; Rostoker et al. 1978; Walker 1977a; Wright and Bartel 1986; Wright et al. 1988).

Polyethylene wear in the total joint arthroplasty can be caused by several different mechanisms. The most important factor is excessive stresses in the component. The wear rate increases with an increase in contact pressure. The wear of UHMWPE is inversely proportional to the contact area (Treharne et al. 1981). An increase in the molecular weight of UHMWPE will increase the wear resistance of the tibial component. The method of prosthesis fixation is also important in reducing wear. The retrieval studies indicate that polymethylmethacrylate (PMMA) fragments can gouge and abrade the UHMWPE articular surface. Bone fragments are very abrasive to UHMWPE. Wear may also be caused by irregularities and intergranular defects formed in polyethylene during the manufacturing process (Walker 1977a).

The study of wear mechanisms in total joint arthroplasty has important clinical significance. Wear can cause the prosthesis to subside improperly, which in turn will change the angulation of the lower limb. The contact stress on the medial or lateral portion of the prosthesis increases, accelerating the wear process and fatigue fracture of the component. Studies by Mirra et al. (1976, 1982) have determined that long term complications such as loosening and infection are linked to the biological response elucidated by polyethylene and PMMA debris in the surrounding tissues. Wear particles from CoCr have been shown to elicit similar biological responses (Barbos and Benvenuti 1983; Bartel et al. 1982; Walker 1977a).

Currently, only UHMWPE, CoCr, and titanium alloys are used in prosthetic knees. Many R and D groups are studying alternative materials to improve the results of total joint arthroplasty. There are some prosthetic hips available that are made of ceramic materials. Although they are not available in prosthetic knees, these materials show great potential as total joint arthroplasty possibilities. Although ceramics have the tendency to be brittle and expensive, the quality of ceramics is improving and the cost is diminishing every year (Walker 1977a).

Work is presently underway to study new alloys for use in the femoral component. For the polymeric components, a composite of carbon fiber reinforced UHMWPE is now available. The increased modulus of the material is intended to improve the wear resistance. Studies have shown, however, that there was no improvement in the resistance to surface damage over standard UHMWPE. Ultimately the carbon fibers increased the susceptibility of the components to delamination and crack propagation (Connelly et al. 1984; Wright et al. 1981, 1988). Some investigators are modifying UHMWPE, further increasing its molecular weight to see if this can increase its wear properties.

Biomechanical Considerations of Total Knee Arthroplasty

The goals of total joint arthroplasty are to eliminate pain and restore function of the knee joint. To achieve these goals, total knee components are engineered using biomechanical concepts to optimize many variables. Design criteria for total knee prostheses must be established from a data base derived from normal knee biomechanics and past clinical experience so as to re-establish the anatomical alignment, normal kinematics and normal function of the knee.

The evolution of total joint arthroplasty began with the uniaxial hinged prosthesis which permitted only flexion and extension of the knee. The normal kinematics of the knee are not uniaxial, however. Consequently forces applied to the device along another axis (for instance the rotatory axis) are transmitted to the prosthesis–bone interface. This can lead to loosening. In 1969, the first nonhinged metal on plastic device was introduced by Gunstun. It too, however, had a high rate of loosening due to its configuration and the inability to fix it properly to bone (Walker 1989). At present, almost all the total knee prostheses are either semiconstrained or nonconstrained. The semiconstrained devices provide inherent joint stability, and compensate for the loss of the anterior (and at times the posterior) cruciate ligament. The nonconstrained devices are designed to recreate normal joint kinematics with the use of anatomical surface designs and intact collateral and cruciate ligaments. Both types of prostheses have advantages and disadvantages.

Stability

Normal kinematics are required for normal joint function. In attempting to recreate the kinematics and normal function of the knee, the stability of the prosthesis must not be ignored. Most semiconstrained implants require sacrifice of the anterior cruciate ligament. This will reduce the stability of the knee in the anteroposterior plane. If there is no constraint in the implant to resist this sliding, large tibial excursions will occur and these will rock the tibial component. This process may cause subsidence and expose the anterior and posterior portions of the implant to cyclic tension and compression loading. A semiconstrained device usually has an articular configuration so as to inhibit anterior sliding of the tibia on the femur, but as a consquence shearing forces will be transmitted to the prosthesis–bone interface and this may increase the rate of loosening.

The stability of the prosthesis is dependent on many factors. The intrinsic mechanisms involve the design of the prosthesis and the way that it is inserted. As noted previously, the shape of the articulating surface can compensate for a lack of stability. Precise instrumentation is required so as to properly implant the prosthesis in the correct orientation to the bones. Accurate cuts which will restore the normal joint line, re-establish the proper tension in the remaining ligaments, and preserve the posterior tilt of the tibial component are extremely important in insuring stability in the knee. This stability is enhanced by tension in the remaining ligaments, joint capsule and musculature.

Many studies have been performed evaluating the surface topography of different total knee prostheses. The intrinsic stability of prostheses has been compared using a material testing system. Compressive loads are applied axially across the prostheses while shear and torsional forces are applied to one of the components. The results demonstrate a wide range of stability depending on the conformity of the particular total knee prosthesis system (Greenwald et al. 1981; Thatcher et al. 1987).

At the University of Vermont, nine total condylar type prostheses were compared which had been implanted in cadaveric knee specimens (Fleming et al. 1987). The stability was evaluated for both anteroposterior (A/P) and mediolateral

(M/L) shear at 20° and 30° of flexion, and of axial rotation of the tibia with respect to the femur (I/E) at 20° of flexion. A Genucom knee evaluation system was modified for use in these cadaveric knees. No axial compressive load was placed across the joint. The results indicated that only one of the semiconstrained devices was able to recreate normal joint stability in the A/P plane; all the other devices were more lax than the normal knee in this plane. During M/L and I/E testing, some devices were more constrained than the normal knee, others were equal to it, and some were more lax. The degree of constraint was dependent on the surface geometry. In a cadaveric evaluation by Shoemaker et al. (1982), similar results were obtained when they tested the knee also without a compressive load across the joint. They found, however, that with a compressive load of 920 N across the knee, the laxity of all the prostheses was significantly less than the normal knee (they all were intrinsically more stable).

At the University of Vermont, an in vivo comparison of the stability of four different knee prostheses was performed following the same protocol as the forementioned cadaveric study. The results were compared to a group of ten normal patients for statistical evaluation. The Variable Axis prosthesis was significantly more constrained that the normal knee. This prosthesis utilizes a central ball and socket configuration to compensate for the lack of both cruciate ligaments. No difference existed, however, between the Tricon-M, PCA and Anametric knees, all of which sacrificed the anterior but retained the posterior cruciate ligaments. These results were in variance from those found in the cadaveric study, indicating that in vivo other structures such as the musculature may compensate for deficiency of the anterior cruciate ligament (Stein et al. 1987).

Total knee function has been evaluated in vivo using gait analysis laboratories (Andriacchi et al. 1982; Andriacchi 1988; Collopy et al. 1977; Rittman et al. 1981; Simon et al. 1983). Functional comparisons of semi- and nonconstrained prostheses were done by Andriacchi (1988; Andriacchi et al. 1982). He determined that patients with excellent clinical results demonstrate abnormalities during gait with either type of device. Patients with the least constrained prostheses, however, demonstrated the greatest range of motion while climbing stairs. Patients with posterior cruciate resecting prostheses performed poorly during stair climbing since the femur was allowed to rock back, decreasing the lever arm of the quadriceps mechanism (Andriacchi 1988).

There obviously are many total knee prostheses available with a wide variety of kinematic properties. Devices that are nonconstrained rely on ligamentous load sharing and healthy musculature to compensate for the ACL deficiency. It should be noted that nonconstraining devices have other inherent disadvantages which will be discussed later. Biomechanical research has shown that there is wide variety in stability of semiconstrained devices. The more constrained a prosthesis, the greater the forces that are transmitted to the bone–prosthesis interface. Choice of an implant should therefore be dependent on ligament integrity and musculature, as well as the patient's life style and activity level.

Contact Stresses

As discussed earlier contact stress is a significant variable affecting the success of total joint arthroplasty. As the contact area between the femoral and tibial components is reduced, there is a significant increase in UHMWPE wear. Polyethylene wear has been shown to reduce the fatigue life of the tibial component and cause mechanical or aseptic loosening. Wear debris may initiate inflammatory responses which may enhance septic loosening.

There have been many methods described to measure the contact area of the normal tibiofemoral and patellofemoral joint at different load levels. Only a few reports exist, however, measuring the contact area of total knee implants. Seedhom et al. (1972) calculated contact stresses using an acrylic casting method and from this developed a total joint arthroplasty prototype. Walker and Seitelman (1978) and Walker and Zhou (1987) performed a comparative study of the contact area of different prostheses and found them to vary considerably. They determined that a reduction in prosthesis conformity resulted in decreased contact areas and large contact stresses in the tibial component. These stresses often exceeded the compressive

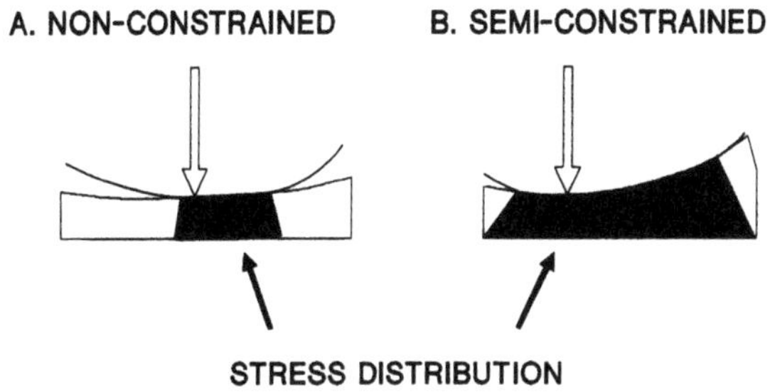

Fig. 3.4. The transfer of stress through the tibial plateau is dependent on the contact area between the tibial and femoral components. The contact area of the nonconstrained device (**a**) is much less than the semiconstrained total knee (**b**). The smaller contact area distributes the compressive load through a smaller region of the tibial component, increasing the stresses throughout this region.

strength of the plastic. Nonconstrained prostheses also demonstrated a substantial reduction in anterior shear stability when compared to more conforming implants (Walker and Hsieh 1977).

The distribution of stress through the UHMWPE component is dependent on the area of contact. The ideal prosthesis will distribute stress equally throughout the tibial component without exceeding the yield strength of UHMWPE. A device with a low contact area, however, transfers the large compressive forces through a smaller region of the UHMWPE to the tibial surface. An increase in contact area will result in the application of the forces through a large surface area (Fig. 3.4). This is important since optimal component fixation can best be obtained when there is a uniform distribution of stress at the prosthesis–cement–bone interfaces.

A thicker tibial component will provide greater stress distribution at the interface than that of a thinner component (Fig. 3.5). Furthermore, implants thinner than 6 mm are too flexible and may physically deform at the interface. As the thickness of the component increases, however, there is an increase in the effective lever arm to shearing forces at the articulating surface. This longer lever arm will increase the moment on the tibial interface, increasing the risk of component loosening.

In summary an increase in contact area will improve the fatigue life of the prosthesis. However, the more conforming and thicker the prostheses, the greater the shear stresses and bending moments applied to the prosthesis–bone interface. Consequently, we need to continue to search for a material to replace UHMWPE which will improve material wear resistance without over constraining the design.

Stress Distribution

Loosening is the primary mechanism of failure of a total knee implant. The two major mechanisms responsible for loosening are excessive stress and micromotion at the bone–prosthesis interface. The long term success of total knee

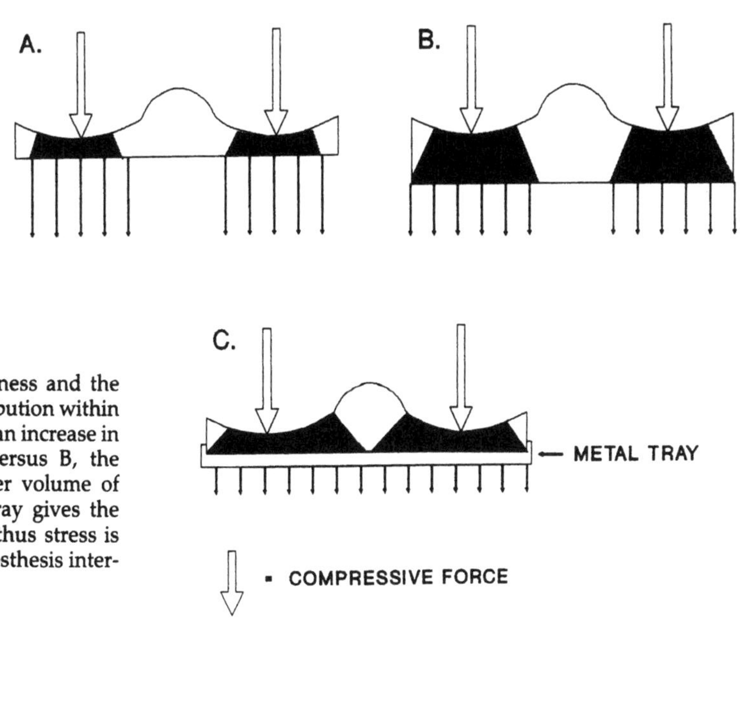

Fig. 3.5. The effects of component thickness and the addition of a metal tray on the stress distribution within the tibial component are illustrated. With an increase in thickness of the tibial component, A versus B, the stresses are distributed through a greater volume of polyethylene. The addition of a metal tray gives the polyethylene a much stiffer foundation, thus stress is distributed uniformly across the bone–prosthesis interface.

replacement is partially dependent on the optimum stress distribution at prosthesis–bone interface. Stress exceeding the failure strength of the components, surrounding structures and the prosthesis–bone interface will result in component micromotion. Because of the lack of rigidity of UHMWPE, the stress distribution in the tibial component is the primary concern when one talks about loosening of a total knee prosthesis (Mears 1979). Clinically this is obvious since failure and loosening typically occur in the tibial component.

Many models and experimental methods have been developed to determine the stresses exhibited at the bone–prosthesis interface while different variables (i.e. fixation technique, bone stiffness, and component sizing) are examined (Bartel et al. 1982; Beaupre et al. 1986; Cheal et al. 1985; Garg and Walker 1986; Johnson et al. 1983; Lewis et al. 1977; Miegel et al. 1986; Vasu et al. 1986; Walker et al. 1980). Comparisons have been made between those prostheses stablilized by biological ingrowth and those fixed with cement. Miegel et al. (1986) determined experimentally that cementing provides a more uniform distribution of the contact stress over the entire tibial resection surface than does bone ingrowth. Bone ingrowth into the tibial component is not uniform, therefore portions of the resected surface are subjected to stress shielding and others to excessive stress.

In the two-dimensional finite element model (FEM) of Vasu et al. (1986) and Garg and Walker (1986), no differences were found in the stress distributions in the proximal tibia when cemented and uncemented implants were compared. To the contrary, the three-dimensional FEM of Cheal et al. (1985) examined the stress distribution on the tibial interface and found that the injection of PMMA into the proximal tibia increased the rigidity of the cancellous bone resulting in an increase in stress. Cheal's model did not demonstrate a difference in stress distribution in those tibia with a stiff cortical rim. The criticism of these finite element models is that they assume a perfectly level tibial cut. Clinically, perfectly smooth bone resection is difficult to achieve. If the cut is not smooth, high stresses will be concentrated at the high points and stress shielding will occur at the low points.

The need for a metal tray to distribute stress

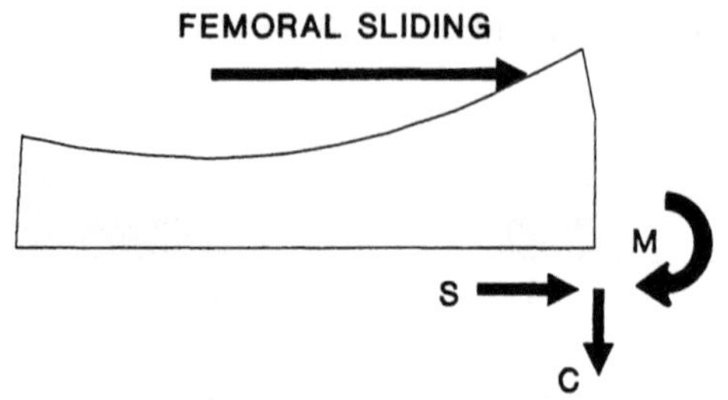

Fig. 3.6. As the femoral component slides anterior relative to the femur, a shearing force, S, a compressive force, C, and a moment, M, are generated at the bone–prosthesis interface. The more constrained the device, the greater the forces at the bone–prosthesis interface.

uniformly across the tibial surface was noted by Bartel et al. (1982). Unlike UHMWPE, the metal tray distributes the stress uniformly across the distal surface of the tibial component (Fig. 3.5). It is advantageous to cover as much of the resected surface as possible, and to incorporate the cortical rim in the fixation (Townsend et al. 1979; Walker et al. 1981).

The shearing forces generated at the articular surface of the tibial plateau are transmitted to the bone–prosthesis interface. The forces transmitted to the interface are especially noticeable in semiconstrained devices. An anterior lip on the tibial prosthesis increases the compressive and shear stresses and also applies a moment at the anterior portion of the bone–prosthesis interface (Fig. 3.6). If these stresses exceed the yield strength of the bone or of the fixation method used, micromotion will occur, destroying the fixation interface.

Less constrained devices allow more sliding to occur. As the tibial component slides forward relative to the femoral surface, an eccentric load is placed on the interface. Since the contact stress is great due to the nonconformity of the articulating surfaces, the stresses transmitted to the posterior portion of the tibial plateau will be large. If the yield strength of the bone–prosthesis interface is exceeded, loosening will occur.

Surgical alignment for total knee arthroplasty must be precise. A malaligned prosthesis will demonstrate the same biomechanical problems as will an arthritic knee. If the anatomical alignment after a total knee replacement is altered, the resultant load vector through the center of the knee joint may be shifted to the lateral or medial compartment. The shift in the resultant load vector will result in an increase in stress at the bone–prosthesis interface on the respective side of the implant and promote prosthetic loosening. Precise bone resection and proper component sizing is required to restore the anatomical joint line of the knee. A change in joint line position will alter the kinematics of the knee (Matsen et al. 1988). If the intact ligaments are too tight the prosthesis will be subjected to increased contact stress as well as increased stress at the bone–prosthesis interface. These stresses will yield a poor clinical result. If the ligaments are too lax, abnormal sliding motion will occur, resulting in eccentric loading of the tibial component.

Fixation

Component fixation has significant impact on the life expectancy of a total knee prosthesis. The stresses at the bone–prosthesis interface are large and the fixation method must be strong enough to endure the applied forces. Since the mechanical properties of bone may not be altered, fixation methods have been studied to distribute the stress to the bone at a level conducive to bone formation. If the stress is reduced significantly, stress shielding may occur, resulting in bone resorption. Excessive stress, on the other hand, will fatigue bone and result in loosening.

Implant fixation is achieved using cemented, biological ingrowth or press fit mechanisms supplemented by a variety of screws and pegs of varying form and geometry. Traditionally, most arthroplasties have employed cementing techniques. Reports indicate that radiolucencies occur in 25%–40% of the cases (Miller 1989). Fixation of tibial components without cement were performed by Blaha et al. (1982) who utilized flanged polyethylene pegs to hold the prosthesis in place. They reported results that are as good as cemented techniques. Recently, porous ingrowth components have become popular. Bony ingrowth depends on the design of the prostheses, the accuracy of prosthesis fit, and the accuracy of limb alignment. Success of total joint arthroplasty with porous ingrowth requires precise surgical technique and implant components capable of maintaining absolute rigid fixation (Laskin 1988; Miller 1989; Miura et al. 1988).

Bourne et al. (1981) demonstrated that total knee replacement did alter the strain distribution in the proximal tibia. Metal stem designs reduce the strain in the tibia more than plastic stems. Several studies have been developed to measure the amount of micromotion due to different fixation designs. The results indicate that a metal tray device is superior in preventing micromotion at the fixation site (Townsend et al. 1979; Walker et al. 1981). Furthermore, Miura et al. (1988) have shown that the addition of screws with a stem enhance initial tibial fixation.

In the dog model, Manley et al. (1987) found the bone–prosthesis interface of press fit, ingrowth and cemented components all demonstrated more micromotion under the tray than about the fixation pegs or stems.

Bobyn et al. (1982) were able to observe bone ingrowth into porous coated femoral components inserted in dogs. Although they only found fibrous ingrowth into the porous tibial components, clinically this appears to give adequate stability to the implant.

In vivo roentgenographic measurements of micromotion have been performed by Ryd et al. (1986) (see Chap. 14). The results indicate that all prostheses will allow some micromotion to occur. They conclude that absolutely rigid fixation is not required for a clinically successful total joint arthroplasty.

Obviously, there is considerable controversy regarding the amount of fixation and the best method of fixation for successful total knee replacement. Continued research is required to attempt to reduce the problem of component loosening. Only after advances are made regarding materials, articular surface design, development of precise instrumentation and optimal fixation techniques will we be able to expect truly long term fixation of our implants and elimination of loosening as a potential problem.

Summary

The intent of this chapter was to provide an overview of the biomechanics of the normal knee and how biomechanics pertains to total knee arthroplasty. There are many variables involved in the design and implantation of a total joint prosthesis that must be optimized to restore the normal biomechanics of the knee joint.

A compromise between a surface topography that restores stability and one which allows normal kinematics is required. A more conforming device will reduce contact stresses, minimize wear and give added joint stability; however, these improvements will be associated with increased stresses at the bone prosthesis interface. A less conforming prosthesis will result in a greater range of knee motion but will be plagued by increased contact stresses and increased eccentric loading of the tibial plateau. Both of these variables may result in fracture or loosening of the prosthesis. It is evident that for each variable that is optimized another is sacrificed. From the biomechanical stand point, the optimal device is neither semiconstrained nor nonconstrained. A device that straddles the line between the two and which preserves the PCL should provide the best clinical results with the technology available to date.

Component fixation remains controversial. Cemented, noncemented, ingrowth and press fit techniques all have their advantages and disadvantages. Through biomechanical research, the criteria for each method of component fixation will be determined. Long term clinical follow-up studies comparing fixation techniques will become increasingly valuable with time.

Over the last 20 years, significant improvements have been made in total knee arthroplasty. To restore normal joint function, proper implantation is required so as to enable the implant to work in concert with the remaining structures of the joint capsule and musculature. We are at a point where the condylar prostheses have been optimized to their fullest extent. The next major break through in total joint arthroplasty will require new materials and different design concepts. Further research is necessary in the field of prosthetic ligaments which may in the future be incorporated into prosthetic total knees. This concept may resolve the semiconstrained versus nonconstrained controversy, since the normal anatomy of the knee can be recreated, restoring normal kinematics without the problems of instability or constraint of knee motion.

Acknowledgement. This work was supported by the National Institute of Health: grant numbers R01-AR39213 and R01-AR40174.

References

Andriacchi T (1988) Biomechanics and gait analysis in total knee replacement. Orthop Rev 17:470–473

Andriacchi T, Galante J, Fermier R (1982) The influence of total knee replacement design on walking and stair climbing. J Bone Joint Surg (Am) 65:1328–1335

Balazs E, Gibbs D (1970) Chemistry and molecular biology of the intercellular matrix. Academic Press, New York, pp 1241–1253

Barbos M, Benvenuti A (1983) Metallic debris arising from prosthetic abrasion: An investigation of biodegradation of the materials and physiology of bone. Ital J Orthop Traumatol 9:377–386

Bartel D, Burstein A, Santavicca E, Insall J (1982) Performance of the tibial component in total knee replacement. J Bone Joint Surg (Am) 64:1026–1033

Beaupre G, Vasu R, Carter C, Schurman D (1986) Epiphyseal-based designs for tibial plateau components. II. Stress analysis in the sagittal plane. J Biomech 19:663–673

Bennett G, Waine H, Bauer W (1942) Changes in the knee joint at various ages. The Commonwealth Fund, New York

Blaha J, Freeman M, Revell P, Todd R (1982) The fixation of a proximal tibial polyethylene prosthesis without cement. J Bone Joint Surg (Br) 64:326–335

Bobyn J, Cameron H, Abdulla D, Pilliar R, Weatherly C (1982) Biologic fixation and bone modeling with an unconstrained canine total knee prosthesis. Clin Orthop 166:301–312

Bourne R, Finlay J, Cohn N (1981) Principal strain in the human tibia before and after total knee arthroplasty. Trans Orthop Res Soc 6:160

Brostrom L, Gillquist J, Liljedahl S, Lindvall N (1968) Treatment of old ruptures of the anterior cruciate ligament. Lakartidmingen 65:4479–4487

Bullough P, Goodfellow J (1968) The significance of the fine structure of the articular cartilage. J Bone Joint Surg (Br) 50:852–857

Bullough P, Munuera L, Murphy J, Weinstein A (1970) The strength of the menisci as it relates to fine structure. J. Bone Joint Surg (Br) 52:564–570

Calderale P, Scelfo G (1987) A mathematical model of the locomotor apparatus. Eng Med 16:147–161

Cheal E, Hayes W, Lee C, Snyder B, Miller J (1985) Stress analysis of a condylar knee tibial component: Influence of metaphyseal shell properties and cement injection depth. J Orthop Res 3:424–434

Collopy M, Murray M, Gardner G, DiUlio R, Gore D (1977) Kinesiology measurements of functional performance before and after Geometric total knee replacement: One year follow-up of twenty cases. Clin Orthop 126:196–202

Connelly G, Rimnac C, Wright T, Hertzberg R, Manson J (1984) Fatigue crack propagation behavior of ultra high molecular weight polyethylene. J Orthop Res 2:119–125

Fleming B, Stein A, Howe J, Pope M (1987) An in vitro comparative study of total knee arthroplasties. Trans Rehabil Eng Soc N Am 10:256

Fung Y (1981) Bone and cartilage. In: Biomechanics: Mechanical properties of living tissues. Springer-Verlag, New York, pp 383–413

Garg A, Walker P (1986) The effect of the interface on the bone stresses beneath tibial components. J Biomech 19:957–967

Goodfellow J, Bullough P (1967) The pattern of aging of the articular cartilage of the elbow joint. J Bone Joint Surg (Br) 49:175–181

Goodfellow J, O'Connor J (1978) The mechanics of the knee and prosthesis design. J Bone Joint Surg (Br) 60:358–369

Greenwald A, Black J, Matejczyk M (1981) Total knee replacement. In: The AOSS instructional course lectures, 30, pp 301–341

Harrington I (1976) A bioengineering analysis of force actions at the knee in normal and pathological gait. J Biomed Eng 98:167 –172

Harrison M, Scajowicz F, Trueta J (1953) Osteoarthritis of the hip: A study of the nature and evolution of the disease. J Bone Joint Surg (Br) 35:598–626

Hood R, Wright T, Burstein A (1983) Retrieval analysis total knee prostheses: A method and its application to 48 total condylar prostheses. J Biomed Mater Res 17:829–842

Huson A (1974) Biomechanische Probleme des Kniegelenks. Orthopaede 3:119–126

Johnson J, Krug W, Nahon D, Miller J, Ahmed A (1983) An evaluation of the load bearing capability of the cancellous proximal tibia with special interest to the design of knee implants. Trans Orthop Res Soc 8:403

Kapandji I (1970) The knee. In: The physiology of the joints, Vol. 2, Churchill Livingstone, New York, pp 72–135

Kettlekamp D, Chao E (1972) A method for quantitative analysis of medial and lateral compression forces at the knee during standing. Clin Orthop 83:202–213

Kettlekamp D, Jacob A (1972) Tibiofemoral contact area – determination and implications. J Bone Joint Surg (Am) 54:349–356

King R (1966) On the viscosity of synovial fluids. Rheol Acta 1:41–44

Landy M, Walker P (1985) Wear in condylar replacement knees: A ten year follow-up. Trans Orthop Res Soc 10:96

Laskin R (1988) Tricon-M uncemented total knee arthroplasty. A review of 96 knees followed for longer than 2 years. J Arthroplasty 3(1):27–38

Le Veau B (1984) Biomechanics. A summary of perspectives. Phys Ther 64:1812

Lewis J, Galante J (1985) Workshop on the bone–joint implant interface. J Orthop Res 3:380–386

Lewis J, Jaycox D, Wang O (1977) Stress analysis of some features of knee prostheses by finite elements. Trans Orthop Res Soc 2:55

Liljedahl S, Nordstrand A (1969) Injuries to the ligaments of the knee. Injury 1:17–24

Manley M, Stulberg B, Stern L, Watson J, Stulberg S (1987) Direct observation of micromotion at the implant bone interface with cemented and noncemented tibial components. Trans Orthop Res Soc 12:436

Maquet P (1984a) Mechanics of the knee. In: Biomechanics of the knee, 2nd ed. Springer-Verlag, New York, pp 9–74

Maquet P (1984b) The pathomechanics of osteoarthritis of the knee. In: Biomechanics of the knee, 2nd ed. Springer-Verlag, New York, pp 75–131

Mathur P, McDonald J, Ghormley R (1949) A study of the tensile strength of menisci. J Bone Joint Surg (Am) 31:650–654

Matsen FA, Sidles J, Laskin RS, Gabrini M (1988) The effects of joint line position in total knee replacement. Trans of the 54th Annual Meeting of the American Academy of Orthopaedic Surgeons, p 42

Mears D (1979) Mechanical behaviors of real materials. In: Materials in Orthopaedic surgery, 1st ed. Williams & Wilkins, Baltimore, pp 92–106

Mena D, Mansour J, Simon S (1981) Analysis and synthesis of human swing leg motion during gait and its clinical applications. B Biomech 14:823–832

Menschik A (1974) Mechanik des Kniegelenkes: I. Z Orthop 112:481–495

Miegel R, Walker P, Nelson P et al. (1986) A compliant interface for total knee arthroplasty. J Orthop Res 4:486–493

Mikosz R (1985) Mathematical model for the study of forces in the human knee joint during locomotion. University of Illinois, Chicago. Thesis

Mikosz R, Andriacchi T, Andersson G (1988) Analysis of factors influencing the prediction of muscle forces at the knee. J Orthop Res 6:205–214

Miller J (1989) Fixation in total knee arthroplasty. In: Insall J (ed) Surgery of the knee. Churchill Livingstone, New York, pp 717–728

Minns R (1981) Forces at the knee joint: anatomical considerations. J Biomech 14:633–643

Mirra J, Amstutz H, Matos M, Gold R (1976) The pathology of the joint tissues and its clinical relevance in prosthesis failure. Clin Orthop 117:221–240

Mirra J, Marder R, Amstutz H (1982) The pathology of failed total joint arthroplasty. Clin Orthop 170: 175–183

Miura H, Whitesides L, Easley J, Amador D (1988) Effects of screws and sleeve on initial fixation in uncemented total knee tibial component. Pamphlet from the DePaul Biomechanics Laboratories, 12255 DePaul Drive, Bridgeton, MO, 63044

Morrison J (1968) Bioengineering analysis of force actions transmitted by the knee joint. J Biomed Eng 2:164–170

Morrison J (1970a) The function of the knee joint in various activities. B Biomed Eng 4:573–580

Morrison J (1970b) The mechanics of the knee joint during normal walking. J Biomech 3:51–61

Muller W (1938) Kinematics. In: The knee: form, function, and ligament reconstruction. Springer-Verlag, New York, pp 8–28

Nisell R (1985) On the biomechanics of the knee. Acta Orthop Scand 216:4–11

Palmer I (1938) On the injuries to the ligaments of the knee joint. Acta Chir Scand 81 [Suppl] 53

Rittman N, Kettlekamp D, Pryor P, Schwartzkopf G, Hillberry B (19181) Analysis of patterns of knee motion walking for four types of total knee implants. Clin Orthop 155:111–117

Rose R, Crugnola A, Reis M et al. (1979) On the origins of high in vivo wear rates in polyethylene components in total joint prostheses. Clin Orthop 145:277–286

Rostoker W, Chao E, Galante J (1978) The appearance of wear on polyethylene – A comparison of in vivo and in vitro wear surfaces. J Biomed Mater Res 12:317–335

Ryd L, Lindstrand A, Rosenquist R, Selrik G (1986) Tibial component fixation in knee arthroplasty. Clin Orthop 213:141–149

Seedhom B, Dowson D, Wright V, Longton E (1972) A technique for the study of geometry and contact in normal and artificial knee joints. Wear 20:189–199

Seireg A, Arvikar R (1975) The prediction of Musculoskeletal load sharing and joint forces in the lower extremities during walking. J Biomech 8:89–102

Shoemaker S, Markolf K, Finerman G (1982) In vitro stability of the implanted total condylar prosthesis. J Bone Joint Surg (Am) 64:1201–1213

Simon S, Paul I, Mansour J, Munro M, Abernethy P, Radin E

(1981) Peak dynamic force in human gait. J Biomech 14:817–822
Simon S, Trieshmann H, Burdett R, Ewald F, Sledge C (1983) Quantitative gait analysis after total knee arthroplasty for monarticular degenerative arthritis. J Bone Joint Surg (Am) 65: 605–613
Stein A, Fleming B, Howe J, Pope M (1987) Total knee arthroplasty kinematics: An in vivo evaluation of four different designs. J Arthroplasty [Suppl] S31–S36
Thatcher J, Zhou X, Walker P (1987) Inherent laxity in total knee prostheses. J Arthroplasty 2(3):199–206
Townsend P, Diamond R, Wyatt P (1979) Aspects of tibial plateau design: Condyle and stem deflections by micromotion and photo-elastic analysis. Trans Orthop Res Soc 4:251
Treharne R, Young R, Young S (1981) Wear of artificial joint materials III: Simulation of the knee joint using a computer controlled system. Eng Med 10:137–142
Vainionpaa S, Laike E, Kirves P, Tiusanen P (1981) Tibial osteotomy for osteoarthritis of the knee. J Bone Joint Surg (Am) 63:938–946
Vasu R, Carter D, Schurman D, Beaupre G (1986) Epiphyseal-based designs for tibial plateau components. I. Stress analysis in the frontal plane. J Biomech 19:647–662
Walker P (1977a) Friction and wear in artificial joints. In: Human joints and their artificial replacements. Thomas, Illinois, pp 368–422
Walker P (1977b) Lubrication and degeneration. In: Human joints and their artificial replacements. Thomas, Illinois, pp 211–252
Walker P (1989) Requirements for successful total knee replacements. Design considerations. Orthop Clin N Am 20:15–29
Walker P, Hajek J (1972) The load-bearing areas in the knee joint. J Biomech 5:581–589
Walker P, Hsieh H (1977) Conformity in condylar replacement knee prostheses. J Bone Joint Surg (Br) 59:222–228
Walker P, Seitelman D (1978) The interdependence of rotational stiffness and contact stress in condylar replacement knee prostheses. Trans Orthop Res Soc 3:152
Walker P, Zhou X (1987) The dilemma of surface design in total knee replacement. Trans Orthop Res Soc 12:291
Walker P, Reilly D, Ben-Dov M (1980) Load transfer in the upper femur before and after tibial component attachment. Trans Orthop Res Soc 5:16
Walker P, Greene D, Reilly D et al. (1981) Fixation of tibial components of prostheses. J Bone Joint Surg (Am) 63:258–267
Whittle M (1985) Dynamic assessment of knee joint function. Eng Med 15(2):71–75
Wismans J, Veldpaus F, Janssen J, Huson A, Struben P (1980) A three dimensional mathematical model of the knee joint. J Biomech 13:677–685
Wright T, Bartel D (1986) The problem of surface damage in polyethylene total knee components. Clin Orthop 205:67–74
Wright T, Fukubayashi T, Burstein A (1981) The effect of carbon fiber reinforcement on contact area, contact pressure, and time dependent deformation in polyethylene tibial components. J Biomed Mater Res 15:719–730
Wright T, Rimnac C, Faris P, Bansel M (1988) Analysis of surface damage in retrieved carbon fiber reinforced and plain polyethylene tibial components from posterior stabilized tibial components. J Bone Joint Surg (Am) 0:1312–1319

Section II

The Surgical Technique of Total Knee Replacement

Chapter 4

Soft Tissue Techniques in Total Knee Replacement

Richard S. Laskin

Introduction

Adequate surgical exposure is the keystone of any properly performed operation. This dictum is especially true in the performance of a total knee replacement arthroplasty. The wrong incision, in the wrong location, can only lead to improper placement of the implants and decrease the longevity of the arthroplasty.

The incision used for a total knee replacement has to be long enough to safely permit both exposure of the articular surfaces and dislocation the patella without damage to the collateral ligaments or extensor apparatus. Misguided attempts to "minimize" the cosmetic effects of surgery by using small short incisions, invariably lead to poorly performed arthroplasties.

To facilitate localization of key anatomical landmarks, the entire leg should be exposed at surgery and covered with adherent plastic drapes. For our rheumatoid patients, with dermal thinning secondary to chronic corticosteroid use, we first wrap the lower portions of their legs with sterile cast padding prior to placing the plastic drapes. This will prevent inadvertent avulsion of their friable skin.

We identify and mark the tibial tubercle, the anterior crest of the tibia, the patella, the lateral and medial malleoli and the fibular head. All of these landmarks are subcutaneous and are easily palpable. The femoral head lies deep in the groin and is not easily palpable even in the thinnest of patients. Because of this, numerous techniques have been devised over the years clinically to assist the surgeon in locating this landmark. These involve palpation of the anterior superior iliac spine, pubic tubercle, and femoral artery at the level of Poupart's ligament. By appropriate geometric calculations one can then determine the location of the femoral head. Unfortunately such geometry often proves unreliable especially when the reference points are obscured by the surgical drapes and by the pneumatic tourniquet.

We conducted a study (Laskin 1984) in which we attempted to ascertain how easy, or difficult, it really was to localize the femoral head clinically at surgery. In 25 consecutive knee operations we asked the senior surgeon prior to draping the patient, to locate the femoral head with a radio-opaque marker using whatever clinical landmarks he chose. We then took a P/A X-ray of the hip and found that in 68% of the cases, the clinical position was at least 2.5 cm away from the true center of the femoral head. In 20% of the cases the error was as great as 5 cm.

If the femoral head is to be used as a reference point to position the cutting jigs, its position must be ascertained not clinically but radiographically. A marker can be placed on the hip under X-ray guidance. If the marker is large enough, it can be easily palpated under the surgical drapes at operation.

The surgical exposure can conveniently be separated into three steps: making the skin incision, making the capsular incision, and developing the capsular sleeve. With the exception of the posteromedial exposure, any of the skin incisions can be combined with any of the capsular incisions.

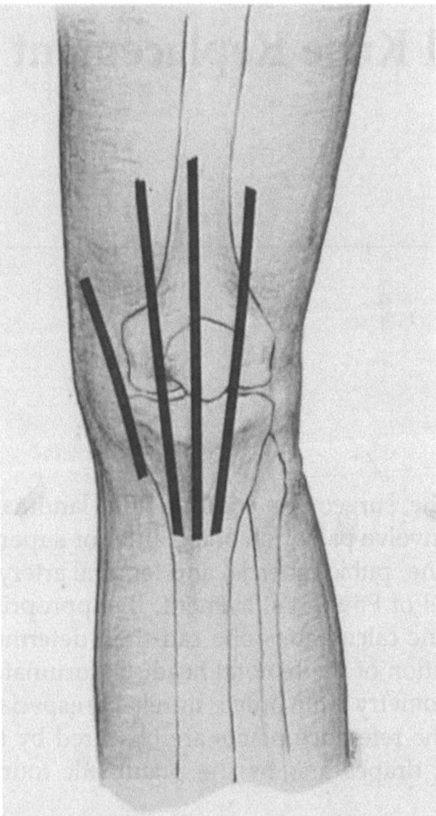

Fig. 4.1. The skin incisions used for total knee replacement. From medial to lateral these are the posteromedial, medial parapatellar, midline, and lateral parapatellar incisions.

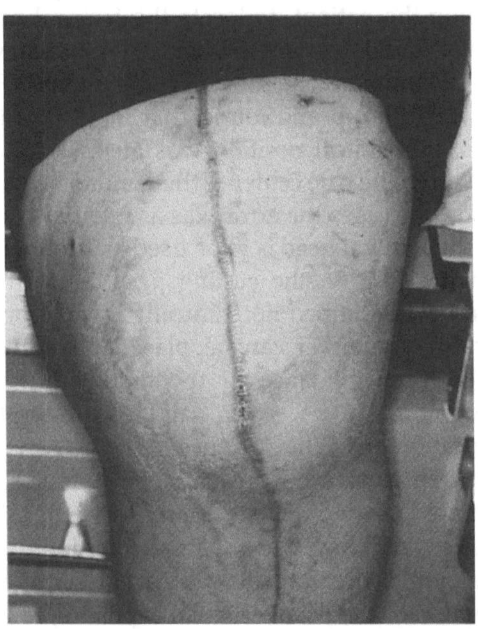

Fig. 4.2. A previous very medial parapatellar incision is unusable for a total knee. A new midline skin incision has been made.

Skin Incisions (Fig. 4.1)

Whatever skin incision is chosen, it should be long enough and extensile enough to enable the knee to be exposed without the necessity of forming skin flaps. The microvascularity of the skin and subcutaneous tissue in older patients requiring a knee replacement is often diminished. Further loss of blood supply occurs in those patients with dermal thinning secondary to chronic steroid use. Any skin flaps which are formed in these patients may necrose with disastrous consequences.

If scars from previous operations are present, an attempt should be made to incorporate them into the surgical incision rather than to leave small skin bridges from parallel incisions. Unfortunately this cannot be done in every case. For example, attempting to use a previous "very medial" parapatellar skin incision may require the formation of a large skin flap to approach the lateral side of the knee (Fig. 4.2). In such cases, there are less potential skin problems if a new incision is made in the midline. Likewise, an old transverse incision, such as that from a high tibial osteotomy, is totally inadequate for total knee replacement and, by necessity, must be crossed with a longitudinal incision. Fortunately, skin necrosis at the intersection rarely occurs (Windsor et al. 1986).

At times the patient may have many healed incisions from prior surgeries on the knee. If possible the most lateral and usable of these incisions should be chosen and re-entered. This will minimize damage to the lymphatic drainage of the skin and subcutaneous tissue over the knee.

The Midline Skin Incision

The midline skin incision (Tooms 1987) begins 6 cm proximal to the superior pole of the patella in the midline of the thigh. It continues distally crossing the center of the subcutaneous border of the patella and then extends distally over the patellar ligament and tibial tubercle. It ends approximately 2 cm distal to the tubercle. The incision should be straight and carried directly down to the deep tissues without forming any skin flaps.

This is an excellent incision which enables visualization of all the capsular structures anteriorly. It is the standard total knee incision that we have used for all our total knee replacements since 1984.

The Medial Parapatellar Skin Incision

The medial parapatellar incision begins 6 cm proximal and 3 cm medial to the patella and curves gently down to a point just below the tibial tubercle (Laskin 1978). This modification of the original Von Langenbeck (Crenshaw 1980) incision gives excellent exposure to both the medial and lateral aspects of the joint. We had used it for almost ten years before changing to the straight midline incision. There were two reasons for this change. The first was that the medial parapatellar incision almost invariably resulted in transection of the infrapatellar branch of the saphenous nerve. The resulting numbness, and at times pain from neuroma formation, impaired the otherwise good results of the knee replacement. The second reason was that if a lateral retinacular release was required (as in the patient with a laterally subluxing patella) we had to make a large skin flap in order to visualize the area for the release. On two occasions this led to skin necrosis.

The Lateral Parapatellar Skin Incision

The lateral parapatellar incision is a mirror image of the medial parapatellar incision. Most often, it is combined with a lateral capsular incision and used in cases of preoperative lateral patellar subluxation. This skin incision should not be used with a medial capsular incision, since it will result in a very large skin flap.

The Posteromedial Skin Incision

The medial incision begins at the tibial tubercle. It then courses proximally and posteromedially just behind the adductor tubercle and then straight proximally for another 7 cm. It is most often used in combination with a medial capsular incision (v.i.).

Capsular Incisions (Fig. 4.3)

The Midline Capsular Incision

The midline capsular approach is initiated at the apex of the quadriceps tendon immediately adjacent to its juncture with the vastus medialis. The incision is carried distally leaving some fibers of the rectus tendon attached to the vastus medialis. This will open the synovium in the area of the suprapatellar pouch. The incision is then carried over the medial quarter of the patella, through the anterior capsule and fat pad distal to the patella and completed on the tibia, one centimeter medial to the patella ligament insertion. The quadriceps retinacular expansion

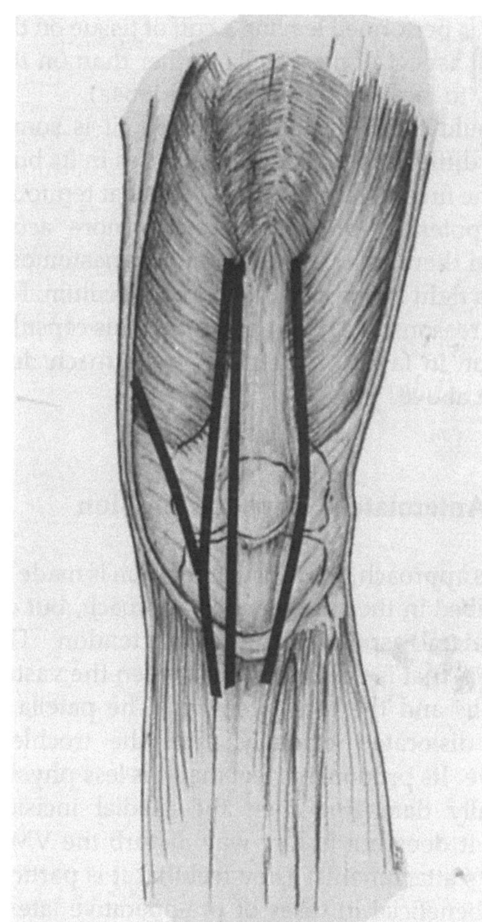

Fig. 4.3. The capsular incisions used for total knee replacement. From medial to lateral they are posteromedial, medial parapatellar, midline and lateral parapatellar incisions.

is sharply elevated off the patella medially and the synovium and fat pad are split.

This incision was originally described by Insall (1984a) for patients undergoing surgery for lateral subluxation of the patella. The incision results in a strong cuff of fibrous tissue and prepatellar retinaculum remaining attached to the vastus medialis obliquus muscle (VMO); this fibrous cuff facilitates suture placement and secure closure at the end of the operation. At present, this capsular incision, combined with the midline skin incision is routinely used at our institution.

The Anteromedial Capsular Incision

Proximally, the anteromedial capsular incision of Von Langenbeck is similar to the midline approach. The parapatellar arthrotomy differs in that it is performed leaving a cuff of tissue on the medial aspect of the patella, rather than on the VMO, to facilitate closure (Insall 1984a).

Should the VMO be attenuated, it is sometimes difficult to place secure sutures in its bulk and the final closure may be somewhat tenuous. This potential problem becomes more acute should there be any tension on the anastomosis from a tight lateral parapatellar retinaculum. For these reasons, we have abandoned this capsular incision in favor of the midline approach described above.

The Anterolateral Capsular Incision

In this approach, the capsular incision is made as described in the anteromedial approach, but on the lateral aspect of the rectus tendon. The interval that is developed is between the vastus lateralis and the rectus femoris. The patella is then dislocated medially from the trochlear groove. Its proponents feel that it is less physiologically damaging then the medial incision since it does not in any way disturb the VMO and its attachments. They feel that it is particularly beneficial in cases of pre-operative lateral patellar subluxation. Despite these potential benefits it is often quite difficult to displace the patella medially for exposure, especially in a muscular patient, and avulsion of the patellar ligament insertion may occur. This therefore severely limits the usefulness of the approach.

The Posteromedial Capsular Incision

To perform a medial capsular approach to the knee one has first to identify the posterior edge of the vastus medialis muscle. The muscle is then bluntly elevated from the adductor magnus tendon and aponeurosis, and separated from the medial intermuscular septum. This separation can be continued proximally to the point where the femoral artery passes through the adductor hiatus. Although in theory this exposure does not detach the VMO from any of its patellar insertion, it does require that the entire bulk of the vastus medialis muscle be retracted laterally, a difficult task in all but the thinnest of patients. We presently use it only in those few cases undergoing isolated medial compartment resurfacing arthroplasty.

Exposure of the Articular Surfaces

In order to visualize the articular surfaces completely, the patella must be everted from the trochlear groove laterally and rotated on its axis. Furthermore, the soft tissues inserting onto the proximal tibial metaphysis medially and laterally must be reflected so that the tibia can be easily subluxed forward.

In order to evert the patella, the medial one quarter of the patellar ligament should be sharply elevated from the tibial tubercle. Insall (1984a) has suggested including a small portion of the medial expansion of the ligament so as to maximize the thickness of this tissue, especially in the thin rheumatoid patient. Patellar osteophytes, especially on the lateral border, should also be removed after which the patella can be easily turned so that its articular surface faces forward.

At times, the surgeon may encounter situations in which it is extremely difficult to evert the patella without placing undue tension on the patellar ligament attachment. For example, a previous high tibial osteotomy usually results in a shortened distance between the femoral con-

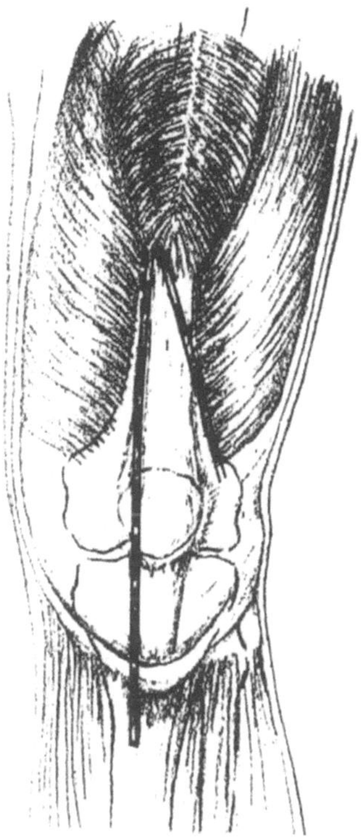

a

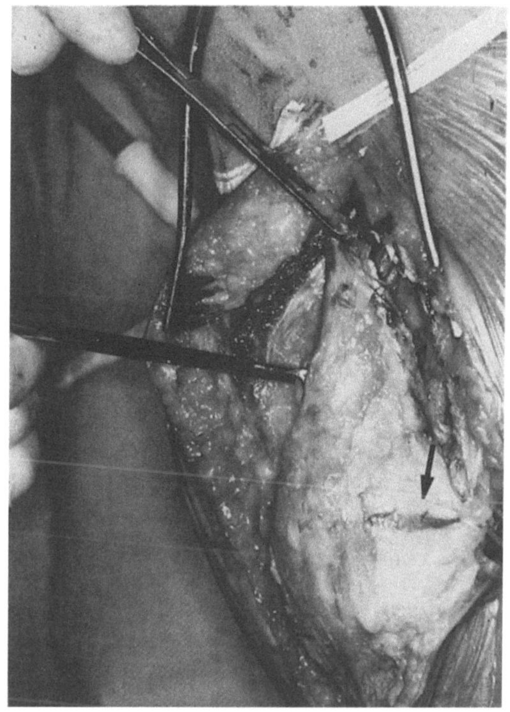

b

Fig. 4.4a, b. The Coones–Adams proximal quadriceps release. **a** The incision begins at the apex of the rectus tendon and inclines inferiorly and laterally. **b** The release stops just proximal to the level of the lateral superior genicular artery (transverse solid line and arrow).

dyles and the tibial tubercle. This severely limits the mobility of the patella laterally. Likewise a patient undergoing a revision total knee replacement often has dense scar tissue that extends between the patella, the patellar ligament, and the lateral femoral condyle and tibial plateau. It is crucial in situations such as these that the patellar ligament not be avulsed! At present there is *no* surgical procedure that can adequately compensate for a patellar ligament avulsion.

In order to prevent undue tension on the ligament while permitting wide exposure in such knees we have used a modified Coones–Adams proximal release as described by Scott (1988). The standard anteromedial or midline capsular incision is first made. At its apex a second capsular incision is begun, angling 45° distally and laterally across the quadriceps tendon, the vastus lateralis and upper portion of the iliotibial tract. This incision should stop short of the superior lateral genicular artery (Fig. 4.4a,b). The patella, its ligament, and the vastus lateralis can then be easily displaced laterally and the knee widely exposed.

Some authors (Dolin 1983; Boiardo and Dorr 1986; Wolff et al. 1989) have suggested that as an alternative to the proximal modified Coones–Adams release, the extensor mechanism should be released distally by removal of the tibial tubercle and the attached patellar ligament. Although this does indeed give wide exposure of the knee, it can severely compromise the vascular supply to the extensor mechanism, and therefore should not be routinely used lest all the previous maneuvers fail. One author reported a complication rate of 20%–25% using this approach to the knee.

To expose the medial tibial plateau fully, a medial subperiosteal sleeve is developed and elevated to a point just beyond the midcoronal line (Laskin et al. 1984; Vince and Dorr 1987) (Fig 4.5). As the sleeve is elevated, the tibia may be externally rotated to expose the posteromedial corner of the tibia. Any rim osteophytes from the femur and tibia are removed. To complete the visualization of the lateral plateau, lateral rim osteophytes are removed and the inferior and lateral portions of the infrapatellar fat pad are excised. It is not necessary to remove the entire

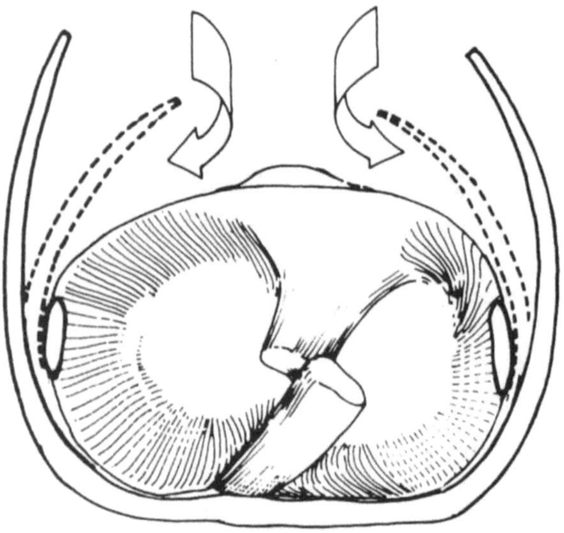

Fig. 4.5. Soft tissue sleeve elevation medial and lateral from the proximal tibia.

fat pad to obtain such visualization. Any remnant of the anterior cruciate ligament should now be removed.

At this point if the knee is flexed to about 100°, the tibia can be easily subluxed forward in front of the femoral condyles. If necessary, a blunt Homan retractor can be placed posteriorly against the tibia to assist in the anterior subluxation. All the articular surfaces can now be easily visualized. It is not necessary to resect the posterior cruciate ligament in order to obtain this excellent exposure of the knee.

Soft Tissue Balance

The soft tissues about the knee form a circumferential sleeve interrupted only partially anteriorly by the presence of the patella. In many patients who require a total knee replacement there is a contracture of portions of this soft tissue sleeve. This results in fixed varus, valgus or flexion deformities. The type of deformity depends upon the portion of this sleeve that is contracted. It is essential that these fixed deformities be corrected so that the reconstructed knee can be brought into proper position and alignment. Failure to do so leads to asymmetrical loads on the implants and their interfaces with either cement or bone, and eventual prosthetic loosening. This process of correcting fixed deformities, so that the leg can be brought into proper neutral alignment of 7° tibiofemoral valgus is known as ligament balancing.

It is not possible to make a *definitive* assessment of the soft tissue deformity or contracture pre-operatively since pain and muscle spasm often mask the true condition. Pre-operative impressions are often found to be erroneous and have to be corrected once the patient is anesthetized.

We routinely evaluate ligament balance at three points during surgery. The first of these occurs after the patient has been anesthetized but before the leg is draped. At that point, we attempt to bring the leg into full extension and into overall neutral tibiofemoral alignment. Although we cannot make any exact measurements at this time, the evaluation can give us a general feeling as to whether or not any significant contracture is present. The next time we check for fixed deformity is after we resect the distal femur. At this point we use distracters as well as alignment guides to give a more exact impression of how much contracture remains and what soft tissue releases we will have to perform. The final check of ligament balance is performed after the proximal tibia is resected. By this time all the peripheral rim osteophytes have been removed so that their tethering effect on the capsule is eliminated. We re-extend the knee and tense the capsular sleeve with two laminar spreaders one final time. Any "fine tuning" of the capsular and soft tissue releases is then performed. Using this sequence of evaluation and re-evaluation, we can avoid the pitfall of under or overreleasing the soft tissues. Freeman (1980) and Insall (1984b) have described similar soft tissue evaluations using tensors or similar instruments to provide the distraction for the same purpose that we have used the laminar spreaders.

Fixed Varus

A fixed varus deformity is the commonest malalignment problem encountered during a total knee replacement. The deformity is caused by a medial contracture and by an associated lateral soft tissue stretching. The lateral component is usually very mild, especially when compared to that which can occur on the medial side in the presence of a severe fixed valgus deformity. The radiographic appearance of lateral joint line widening is the result of this lateral stretching combined with a lateralrotatory subluxation of the tibia on the femur (Fig. 4.6 a,b).

The correction of a fixed varus deformity should progress in discrete steps in order to prevent overcorrection (Dorr 1985). The first step is to remove any remaining osteophytes from the femur or tibia, especially those located posteromedially under the semimembranosis tendon. If the varus deformity persists, we next extend the subperiosteal dissection of the medial capsular sleeve beyond the midcoronal plane to the level of the posteromedial corner of the tibia. Externally rotating the tibia at this point will expose the posteromedial corner and facilitate the dissection.

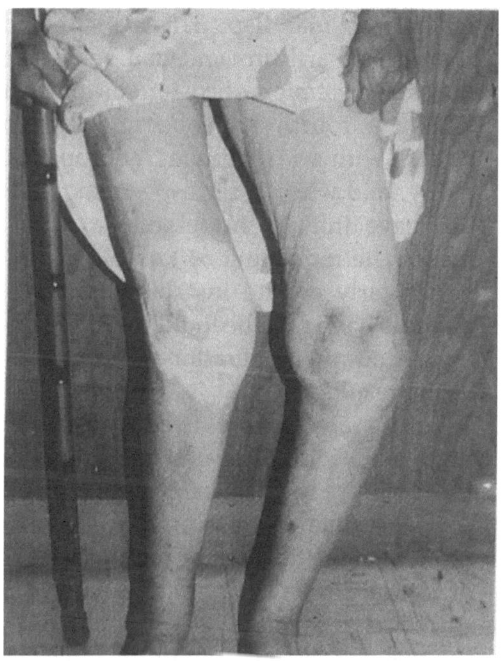
a

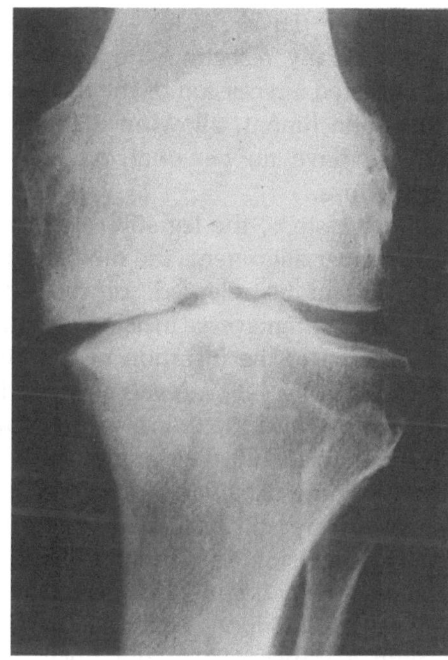
b

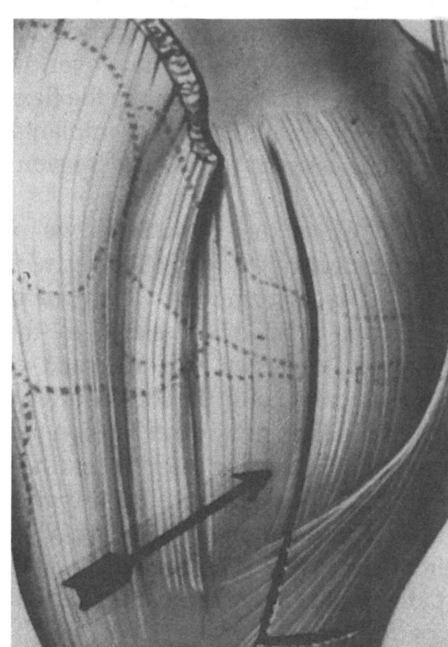
c

Fig. 4.6a–c. Patient with fixed varus deformity of her left knee. **a** The left knee fixed varus measured 20°. **b** X-rays of the patient. There is lateral tibial subluxation and mild lateral joint space widening associated with medial narrowing and some loss of bone from the medial tibial plateau. **c** Medial capsular recession.

Should a varus contracture still persist, we next release the posterior cruciate ligament from its attachment on the tibia. This step will concomitantly release the most posterior portion of the medial capsule. Although for the nondeformed knee, we usually prefer to save the posterior cruciate ligament, we routinely resect it for such cases of severe varus deformity. Attempts to retain it despite a persistent varus contracture will lead to an inability to fully correct the deformity and to a decreased range of motion of the knee (Laskin et al. 1988). As an alternative to actually resecting the ligament, Ritter has suggested a recession of the ligament from its tibial attachment, allowing it to slide proximally. We have no personal experience with this procedure.

If after all these steps, the leg still cannot be brought into proper alignment, the medial capsular sleeve should be released, or recessed (Insall et al. 1979). A transverse incision is made in the sleeve distal to the insertion of the pes anserinus tendons (Fig. 4.6c). A valgus stress is applied to the knee and the entire medial flap allowed to slide proximally. This maneuver will correct any remaining fixed varus deformity.

Some surgeons are still hesitant to perform such a medial recession fearing that marked knee instability will occur. This erroneous impression is based upon equating medial recession with a transection of the tibial collateral ligament at the joint line level, a procedure that indeed will cause marked knee instability. Capsular recession, however, will not cause valgus instability as long as the flexion and extension spaces are filled with implants of the proper thickness so as to maintain tension on the sleeve.

In order to prove this hypothesis we performed a retrospective study of 68 knees with a severe fixed varus deformity in which we performed a medial capsular recession. In these cases the capsular sleeve was recessed and allowed to slide proximally; the soft tissues were balanced and brought into proper tension using tibial components of varying thicknesses (Laskin and Schob 1987). Postoperatively the patients were neither braced nor otherwise immobilized, and their physical therapy program paralleled that in patients in whom a capsular recession was not performed.

Varus-valgus instability occurred in only 4 of the 68 knees. In one case, this instability was due to a technical error and was noted immediately postoperatively. It was corrected by re-operation and insertion of a thicker implant. In a second case the instability developed 3 months later. A tear in the midportion of the tibial collateral ligament was identified at re-operation. This was repaired and augmented with a transfer of the semitendinosus. A third knee required revision due to attenuation and stretching of the medial capsular flap. This patient had severe rheumatoid arthritis and had been taking high doses of systemic corticosteroids for many years. Finally a fourth knee became unstable in a patient with an underlying neuropathic arthropathy, and who, in retrospect, should probably not have initially undergone a knee replacement. The remaining 64 knees did not develop either early or late instability. Many of these patients have now been followed for over seven years since their operation with no deterioration in the results.

With many severe fixed varus deformities there will be an associated lateral subluxation of the tibia on the femur. This subluxation is a combination of lateral shift as well as an external rotation of the tibia on the femur and is the result of contracture of the popliteus muscle. It can be corrected by tenotomy of the popliteus tendon in the posterolateral corner of the knee.

After release of a fixed varus deformity the soft tissue "space" which remains must be adequately filled with implants of sufficient thickness in order to obtain stability. As a general rule, the greater the amount of soft tissue release that was required the thicker the components necessary to obtain stability. In our evaluation of patients underdoing capsular recession we found that the most commonly used thickness of tibial components required were 12–15 mm in thickness while in a comparable series of knees without capsular recession the commonest components used were 6–8 mm in thickness.

Although we have discussed medial soft tissue releases as the optimal method to correct a fixed varus deformity, similar results might be obtained, at least in theory, by lateral soft tissue reefing procedures. We have no personal experience with such procedures.

Fixed Valgus

A fixed valgus deformity is caused by a lateral soft tissue contracture and an associated medial soft tissue stretching (Fig. 4.7a). As opposed to that seen in varus contractures, the stretching on the convex side of the deformity in valgus knees may be very extensive. Furthermore, many fixed valgus deformities are complicated by a lateral subluxation of the patella.

The correction of a fixed valgus deformity should, like its varus counterpart, progress in stages. The first stage consists of removing any peripheral osteophytes from the lateral tibial plateau and lateral femoral condyle as well as elevating all the capsular tissues from the anterolateral portion of the tibial plateau. This may require removal of the remainder of the fat pad so as to expose the lateral tibial rim. At the same time, any adhesions between the iliotibial band and the lateral tibial plateau should be excised, retaining only its tendinous attachment to Gerdy's tubercle.

If the deformity persists, the iliotibial band, the lateral collateral ligament, and the popliteus tendon may have to be released. We usually release the iliotibial band first, although Hungerford (Hungerford et al. 1983) begins his release with the collateral ligament and popliteus tendon (Fig. 4.7b).

The iliotibial band can be safely released from inside the joint. With the knee flexed, and a varus stress applied, the band can be palpated through the synovium and tenotomized using a cautery. We have not noted any clinical postoperative difference if the tenotomy is made in a simple transverse manner or in a Z-plasty fashion as described by Hungerford.

Should a valgus contracture still remain we next perform a tenotomy of the popliteus tendon and the lateral collateral ligament. We had initially suggested that the biceps femoris tendon be tenotomized as well; however, we have abandoned this procedure since it resulted in the peroneal nerve being the only remaining stabilizing structure laterally.

The peroneal nerve is at risk when treating any fixed valgus deformity. If the soft tissues are undercorrected and an attempt at forced manual correction is made, the nerve may be stretched. Likewise, if the knee is inadvertently overcorrected by too great a lateral soft tissue release the nerve may likewise be stretched. Even with proper ligament balancing, the local edema attendant with surgery on the lateral side of the knee joint may cause some compression to the nerve (Rose et al. 1982). We routinely expose the nerve and free it from its sheath behind the fibular neck if any lateral release greater than an iliotibial band tenotomy is required.

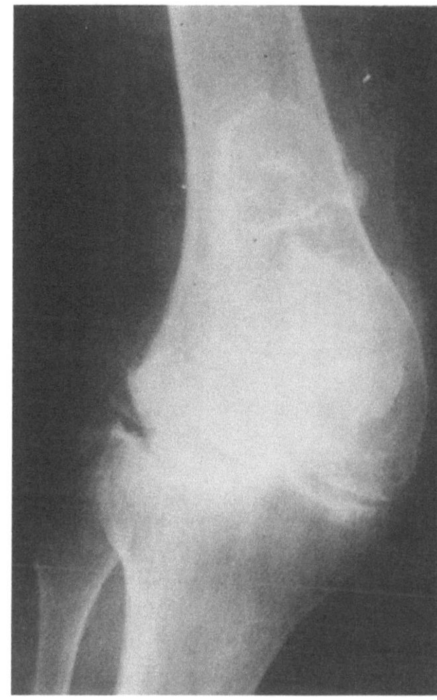
a

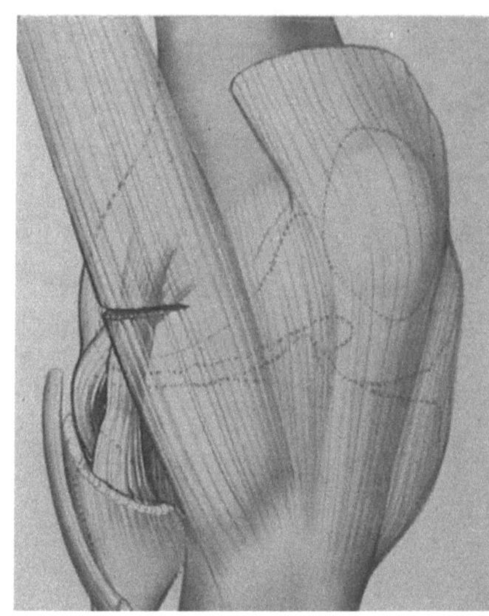
b

Fig. 4.7a, b. Fixed valgus deformity of the knee. **a** X-rays of the patient with a 20° fixed valgus deformity of her right knee. **b** Lateral release for a fixed valgus deformity.

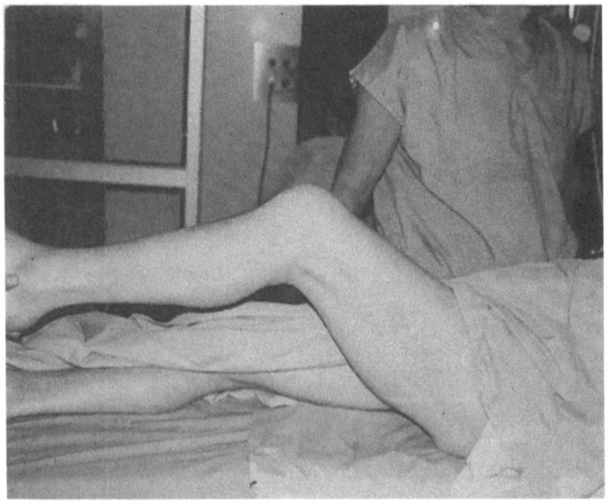

Fig. 4.8. Patient with a fixed flexion deformity of 45°.

Since many severe fixed valgus deformities are associated with marked medial soft tissue stretching, the resultant "soft tissue spaces" after ligament release are large. This requires the use of an extremely thick tibial component in order to obtain knee stability. As an alternative solution, Krackow (Hungerford et al. 1983) has suggested performing only a partial lateral release and combining it with a medial advancement. A medial capsular flap is developed in a way analogous to that formed in patients with a fixed varus deformity. After the flap is released distally it is advanced and then fixed to bone with one or two staples. It should be emphasized that this procedure should be used only for very marked valgus deformities with severe medial stretching. The normal postoperative total knee protocol may then have to be modified lest the reattached medial capsule avulse during the early healing period.

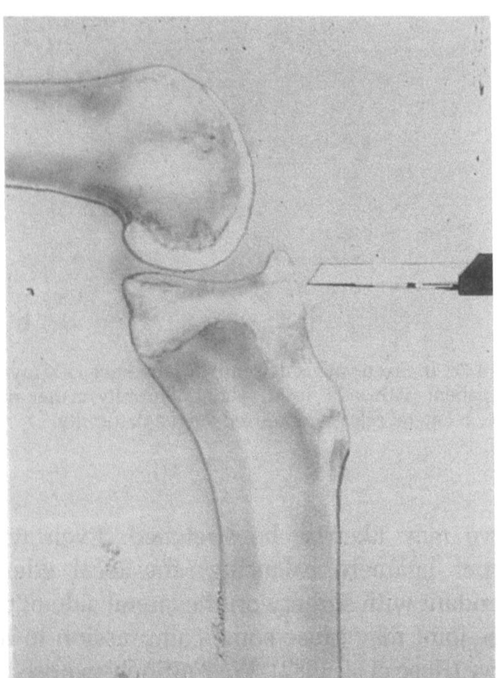

Fig. 4.9. Most patients with a fixed flexion deformity have an anterior tibial osteophyte.

Fixed Flexion (Fig. 4.8)

The term fixed flexion indicates an inability passively to extend the knee fully. It should not be confused with extensor lag, which refers to an inability actively to extend the knee to the level of passive extension.

The commonest cause of a fixed flexion deformity is an anterior tibial osteophyte. This osteophyte abuts against the intercondylar bone of the femur and blocks full extension (Fig. 4.9). In a study we performed in 1986, we were able to identify such an anterior osteophyte in 96% of our knees that had a fixed flexion deformity. Indeed, for those knees with flexion deformities less than 10°, this osteophyte was often the only cause of the block to full extension. If such is the case, correction is easily obtainable when the routine proximal tibial resection is performed, since this will always remove this osteophyte.

For blocks to full extension >10–15° there is usually both an anterior osteophyte and a soft tissue contracture. For these knees both resection of the osteophyte and soft tissue releases are required. These releases may include resection of the posterior cruciate ligament, posterior capsulectomy, and elevation of the gastrocnemius tendons from the posterior femur. For severe flexion contractures (over 45°) it may be necessary to resect an extra amount of distal femur so as essentially to shorten the knee.

The initial step in attempting to correct a flexion deformity >10–15° is to elevate the capsule to the level of the posteromedial and posterolateral corners. If full extension is still not possible, the posterior cruciate ligament should be transected at either attachment site and then excised. Should this be required, the surgeon should seriously consider using a posterior stabilized implant for the arthroplasty. Although one can still obtain anteroposterior stability using a nonposterior stabilized implant in this situation, this will be obtainable only through ensuring an extremely tight fit in flexion. This, in itself, may lead to some limitation of flexion of the knee.

Should this still not be sufficient to allow full extension we next elevate the medial and lateral heads of the gastrocnemius muscle from their insertion on the distal posterior femur. The insertions can easily be located if the knee is flexed to beyond 120°.

For any remaining flexion deformity, we next transect the posterior capsule. The knee should be flexed as much as possible to relax the tension on the capsule and to allow the popliteal vessels and posterior tibial nerve to "fall away" from the capsule posteriorly. A hemostat can be passed behind the posterior capsule from medial to laterally and the capsule safely transected (Fig. 4.10).

Despite all these soft tissue releases there will still remain a few knees in which full extension is not possible. Usually these knees have had flexion contractures >45° pre-operatively. We have found this to be a common problem in both our hemophiliac patients as well as in those patients who have been nonambulatory for more than 6 months prior to surgery. In these situations, the final step is resection of an additional amount of distal femoral bone to enlarge the extension space. This displaces the femoral component proximally and functionally will result in some initial laxity and weakening in the quadriceps musculature. Almost 85% of the knees in which we have had to perform femoral shortening have resulted in an extensor lag which required 3–6 months to be overcome.

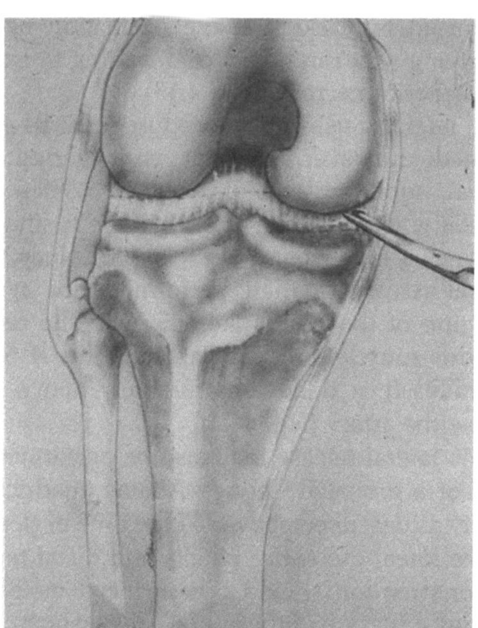

Fig 4.10. Posterior capsular release in patient with severe fixed flexion deformity.

Recurvatum

Recurvatum deformities of the knee are usually associated with distal femoral or proximal bony collapse and severe stretching of the posterior capsule (Fig 4.11a,b). Although we have usually found the posterior cruciate ligament to be grossly intact, it is extremely stretched and therefore probably funtionally incompetent.

To correct a recurvatum deformity we resect the posterior cruciate ligament, make the standard bone resections (as described in the next chapter) and then fill the resulting space with thick enough implants to tense the capsule. We normally use a posterior stabilized implant in this situation as well. Osteotomy of the tibial tubercle and distal advancement would seem, at first glance, to theoretically be a surgical option to correct recurvatum; in actuality such a procedure does not work in the total knee patient because it severely compromises the vascular supply of the quadriceps mechanism.

Lateral Patellar Subluxation

Lateral patellar subluxation is often associated with a fixed valgus deformity. In some patients the patella may actually be dislocated, and have been displaced from the trochlear groove for many years prior to the patient undergoing knee replacement.

Most surgeons are familiar with the lateral release procedures performed to correct patellar maltracking as it occurs in the young adult patient. In such situations, the lateral parapatellar retinaculum is widely incised just lateral to its insertion on the patella. This procedure, whether performed through an arthroscope or during an

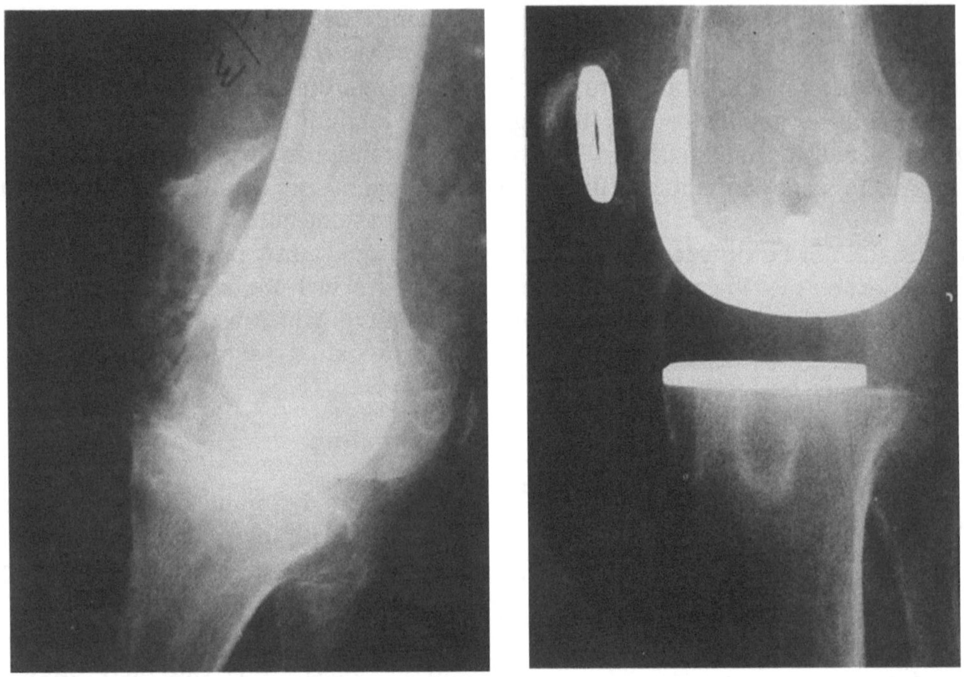

Fig. 4.11. Patient with a recurvatum deformity of the knee and advanced osteoarthritis. **a** Pre-operative X-ray. **b** Post-operative X-ray demonstrating correction of recurvatum deformity and use of a thick tibial component for stability.

open operation, almost always results in transection of superior and inferior lateral genicular arteries (Fig. 4.12). Despite this, avascular problems in the patella in this age group are rare.

Such is not the case, however, in the patient undergoing a total knee replacement. Sacrifice of both these arteries, as well as the superior and inferomedial genicular arteries (as always occurs when the capsule of the knee joint is opened

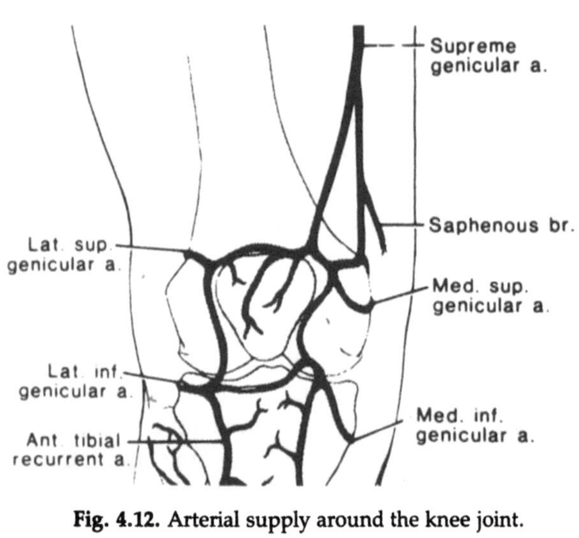

Fig. 4.12. Arterial supply around the knee joint.

medially) may severely devascularize the knee of the older patient. Clayton and Thirupathi (1982) have demonstrated that not only can the circulation to the quadriceps mechanism be compromised but also that the circulation to the overlying skin can be affected leading to extensive anterior necrosis (Fig. 4.13).

A lateral releasing procedure can be performed, however, without endangering the lateral superior genicular artery. When the patella is everted, the artery can be easily palpable as a thick "band" in the soft tissues. The lateral release is then performed not at the junction of the vastus lateralis with the rectus femoris muscle and patella but rather 4–5 cm laterally. It is done longitudinally above and below the artery (Fig. 4.14).

The lateral release may also be performed as part of a proximal Coones–Adams quadricepsplasty as described above. At the time of closure of the knee, the entire patella and distal rectus femoris tendon should be advanced medially, leaving a portion of the lateral capsule open. We perform the release in this manner especially in those cases of chronic frank dislocation of the patella.

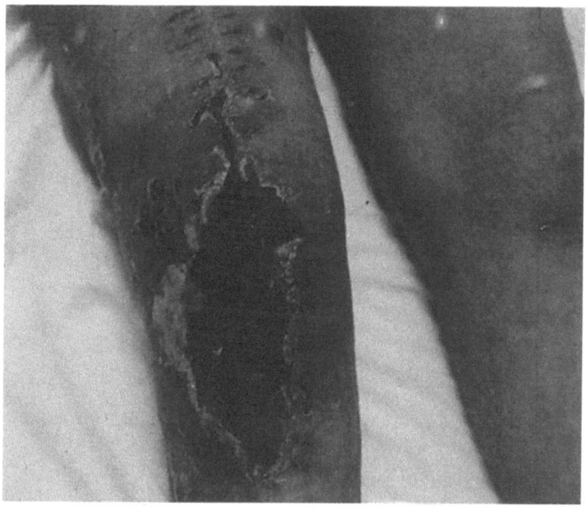

Fig. 4.13. Extensive anterior necrosis secondary to sectioning of both superior and inferior medial and lateral genicular arteries.

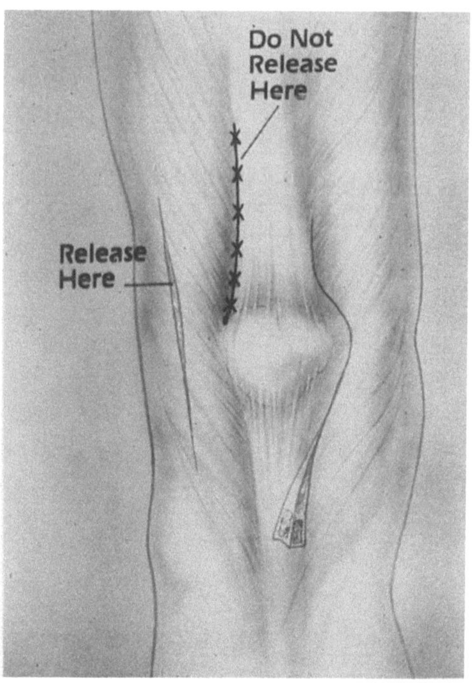

Fig. 4.14. Proper position for lateral release in a patient during total knee replacement.

References

Boiardo RA, Dorr LD (1986) Surgical approaches for total knee replacement arthroplasty. Contemp Orthop 12(3):60–68

Clayton ML, Thirupathi R (1982) Patellar complications after total condylar arthroplasty. Clin Orthop 170:152–155

Crenshaw AH (1980) Surgical approaches. In: Crenshaw AH (ed) Cambell's operative orthopaedics. CV Mosby, St. Louis, p 42

Dolin MG (1983) Osteotomy of the tibial tubercle in total knee replacement. A technical note. J Bone Joint Surg (Am) 65:704–706

Dorr LD (1985) Technique of correction of varus deformity. In: Ranawat CS (ed) Total condylar knee arthroplasty technique, results and complications. Springer-Verlag, Berlin Heidelberg New York, pp 41–51

Freeman MAR (1980) Arthritis of the knee. Springer-Verlag, Berlin Heidelberg New York.

Hungerford D, Krackow K, Kenna R (1983) Total knee arthroplasty: A comprehensive approach. Williams and Wilkins, New York

Insall JN (1984a) Total knee replacement. In: Insall JN (ed) Surgery of the knee. Churchill Livingstone, New York, pp 587–695

Insall JN (1984b) Surgical approaches to the knee. In: Insall JN (ed) Surgery of the knee. Churchill Livingstone, New York, pp 41–54

Insall JN, Scott WN, Ranawat CS (1979) The total condylar knee prosthesis. A report of two hundred and twenty cases. J Bone Joint Surg (Am) 61:173–182

Laskin RS (1978) Modular total knee replacement arthroplasty. A review of eighty-nine patients. J Bone Joint Surg (Am) 58:766–773

Laskin RS (1984) Alignment of total knee components. Orthopedics 7:62–72

Laskin RS, Schob CJ (1987) Medial capsular recession for severe varus deformities. J Arthroplasty 2:313–316

Laskin RS, Denham RA, Apley AG (1984) Replacement of the knee. Springer-Verlag, Berlin Heidelberg New York, pp 139–174

Laskin RS, Rieger M, Schob C, and Turen C (1988) The posterior-stabilized total knee prosthesis in the knee with a severe fixed deformity. Am J Knee Surgery 1:199–203

Rose HA, Hood RW, Otis JC, Ranawat CS, Insall JN (1982) Peroneal nerve palsy following total knee arthroplasty. J Bone Joint Surg (Am) 64:347–351

Scott RD (1988) Revision total knee arthroplasty. Clin Orthop 226:65–77

Tooms RE (1987) Arthroplasty of ankle and knee. In: Crenshaw AH (ed) Campbell's operative orthopaedics, 7th edn. CV Mosby, St. Louis, pp 1152–1202

Vince KG, Dorr LD (1987) Surgical technique of total knee arthroplasty: principles and controversy. Techn Orthop 1:69–82

Windsor R, Insall JN, Vince KG (1986) Total knee arthroplasty after high tibial osteotomy. Presented at the 53rd Annual Meeting of the American Academy of Orthopaedic Surgeons, New Orleans, LA

Wolff AM, Hungerford V, Krackow K et al. (1989) Tibial tubercle osteotomy in total knee replacement. J Bone Joint Surg (Br) 71:848–852

Chapter 5

Bone Resection Techniques in Total Knee Replacement

Richard S. Laskin

Introduction

There are five basic bone resections required to perform any tricompartmental total knee replacement. These are the distal femoral resection, the proximal tibial resection, the anterior femoral resection, the posterior femoral resection, and the patellar resection. Supplemental cuts may be required for a particular implant to accommodate for chamfers in the femoral component, for intercondylar prominences (especially in posterior stabilized implants), and for fixation stems or pegs.

Basic Concepts

Surgical Instruments

Total knee replacement is an extremely "position-sensitive" operation; malposition or malalignment of the components will lead to poor results (Ewald et al. 1984, 1985; Laskin and Schob 1987; Moreland 1988). For example, the incidence of bone cement radiolucencies has been shown to be directly related to the malposition of the tibial component – the incidence being the highest with components left in varus (Lotke and Ecker 1977; Dorr et al. 1985; Laskin 1989). The necessity for accurate implant placement becomes even more critical if the arthroplasty is performed cement free (Laskin 1987; Rand and Bryan 1985). The best and only way to insure that the implants are correctly placed and aligned is to use properly designed instruments. The operation must not be done "free-hand"!

Any total knee instrument set consists of both alignment jigs or rods, and cutting blocks. One should be able to align the jigs with anatomical landmarks which are easily visible, palpable or locatable, with or without X-rays (Townley 1985). There should be a method to affix these jigs and blocks to their respective bones so that they will not be displaced or dislodged by the vibrating saw blade. Finally, the instruments must be simple to understand and use.

Both cutting blocks and cutting slots have been advocated as being most accurate for resecting bone (Dorr and Boirdo 1986) (Figs. 5.1, 5.2). A cutting block allows the surgeon easily to track the progress of the saw blade under direct vision. A theoretical drawback is that the blade may deviate from the surface of the block. To avoid this we presently use a surgical peanut to hold the blade securely against the block during cutting. This technique is especially important when the underlying bone is hard. We find cutting blocks to be most applicable when we resect the distal femur, proximal tibia, and anterior femur. Slots have the advantage of guiding the blade in those areas where direct visualization is not possible. For this reason, we use a cutting slot for resection of the posterior femoral condyle. Recently, instruments using the principle of the double fulcrum have become available (Fig. 5.3). These appear to combine the features

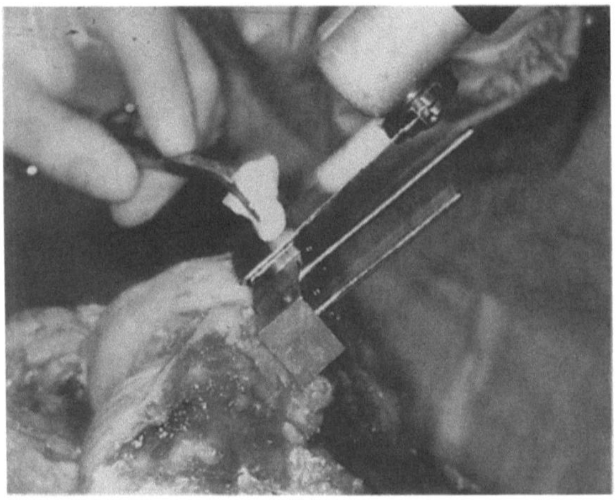

Fig. 5.1. A surgical peanut is used to approximate the saw blade to the cutting block.

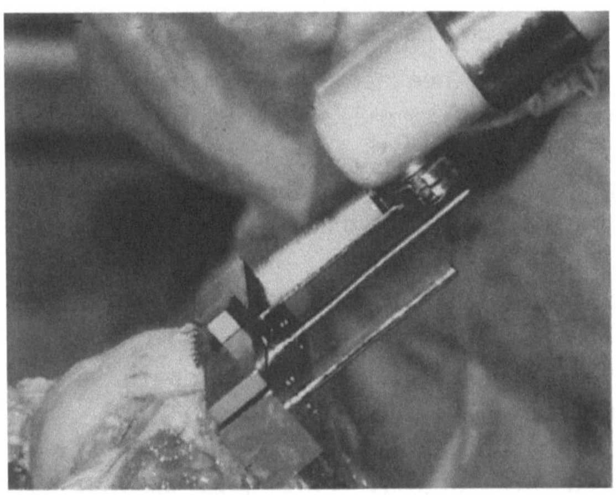

Fig. 5.2. A cutting slot can be used to guide the bone resection if a saw blade of the proper thickness is chosen.

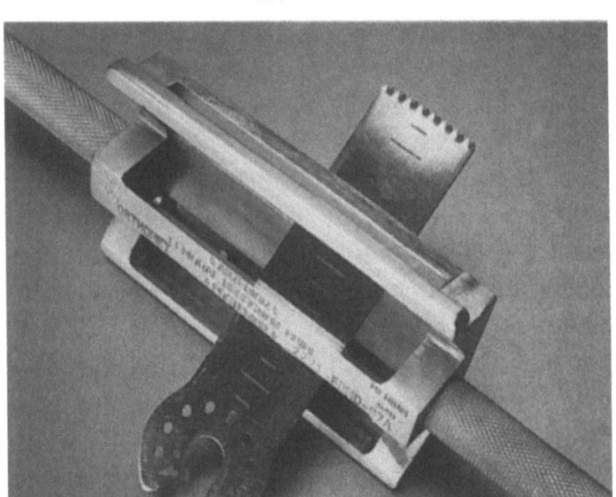

Fig. 5.3. Double fulcrum cutting block.

of both cutting blocks and cutting slots in one instrument.

The choice of the saw blade itself is also important. Blades with thick cross-cut teeth are most effective in cutting hard sclerotic bone, although they generate more kerf (residue) than fine-tooth blades. Fine-tooth blades will result in a smoother cut, with minimal kerf; however, they may bind in sclerotic bone. Blades that are very thick may not fit through a cutting slot, while blades that are very thin and long may whip and result in uneven cut surfaces.

The Flexion and Extension Spaces

The extension space is the gap that is formed after the distal femur and proximal tibia are resected. Its size can be determined by distracting the knee so that the collateral ligaments are tensed with the knee fully extended (Fig. 5.4). The flexion space is the gap that is formed after the posterior femur and the proximal tibia are

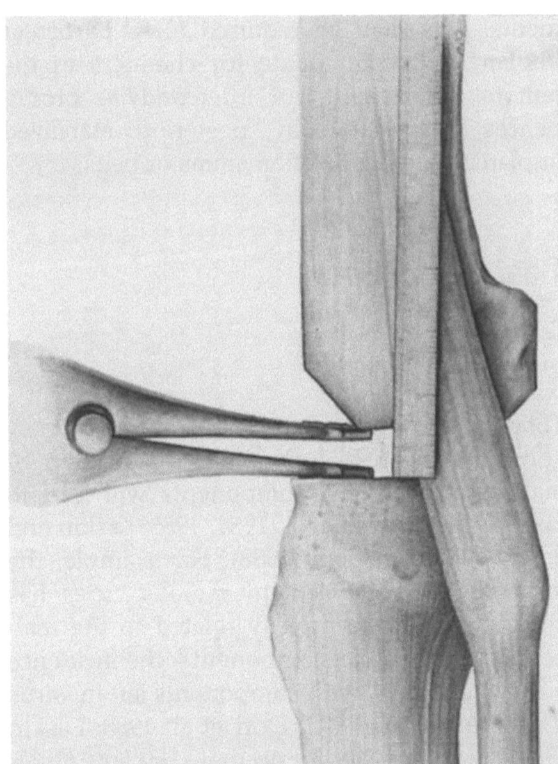

Fig. 5.4. An extension space exists between the cut surface of the distal femur and that of the proximal tibia with the knee fully extended and the collateral ligaments tensed.

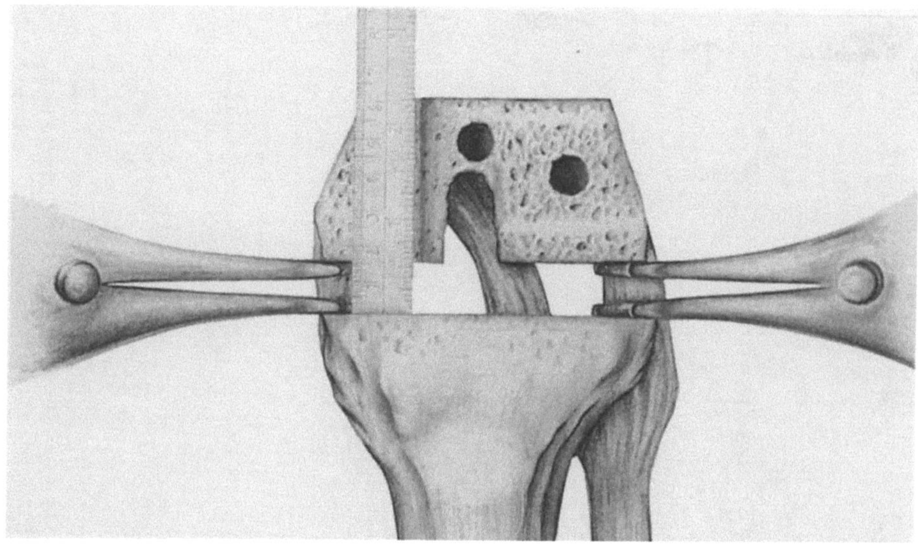

Fig. 5.5. A flexion space exists between the cut surface of the posterior femur and that of the distal femur with the knee flexed to 90° and the collateral ligaments tensed.

resected. Its size can be determined by distracting the knee so that the ligaments are tensed with the knee in 90° of flexion (Fig. 5.5). If the knee is to be stable after a knee replacement, it is important that both the flexion and extension spaces be properly filled with implants of the proper size, shape and thickness. The methods of doing this will be discussed subsequently.

Joint Line Position (Fig. 5.6a,b,c)

The surgeon should create the flexion and extension spaces at the proper spatial orientation in the leg so that the joint line position (the level at which the prosthetic femoral condyle touches the prosthetic tibial plateau) is maintained at a normal position for the limb. This normalization of the joint line is crucial in order to optimize the kinematics of the collateral and posterior cruciate ligaments. In a combined study using both a computer simulation and a retrospective clinical evaluation, Matsen, Sidles, Gabrini and I have (1988) demonstrated marked alterations in joint stability and motion in the presence of abnormal joint line positions. We investigated the following situations in the study.

1. *Raising the joint line.* By raising the joint line and then filling the extension space properly, the knee would be stable in extension as well as in 90° of flexion. However, as the knee flexed up to 90°, the collateral ligaments became increasingly and progressively tighter. In the clinical portion of our investigation, we found that those patients with an elevated joint line had a statistically significant lower total flexion arc as compared to patients with a joint line at a normal position. If, in an attempt to obviate this tightness in flexion, the femoral component was displaced anteriorly (thereby increasing the flexion space), the knee regained the ability to flex easily beyond 90° but at the cost of marked flexion laxity. This situation may have occurred clinically when the surgeon elected to remove only a very small amount of the tibial plateau surface, smaller in thickness than the thinnest tibial component available. Actually some investigators had suggested this type of "minimal resection" in order to maximize the good subchondral bone stock of the tibia. Unfortunately the amount of removed tibial bone was smaller than the thinnest tibial component, and a compensatory larger resection of the distal femur was required in order to seat the implants and obtain full knee extension. This led to a raised prosthetic joint line.

2. *Lowering of the joint line.* When the joint line was abnormally lowered and the extension space filled properly, the knee was stable in

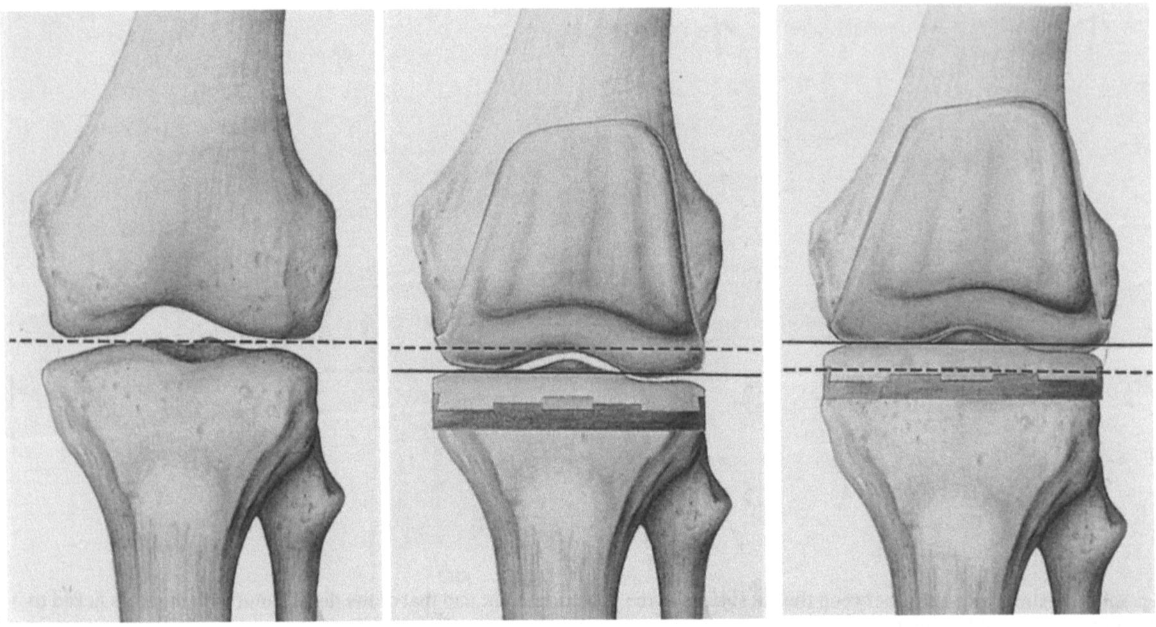

Fig. 5.6.a–c Spatial position of the joint line. **a** The normal joint line is indicated by the dotted line. **b** The joint line has been abnormally elevated (solid line) due to underresection of the proximal tibia and overresection of the distal femur. **c** The joint line has been abnormally lowered (solid line) due to overresection of the proximal tibia and underresection of the distal femur.

extension but became progressively lax as it was flexed. Such a clinical situation might occur if the surgeon removed a large segment of tibial bone stock in an attempt to cut under an asymmetrical tibial defect. To compensate and obtain stability in extension, less femoral bone would be removed than the thickness of the femoral component. As a result the joint line would be displaced distally.

We found that the degree of abnormality in both joint stability and motion was directly related to the type and amount of displacement of the joint line. It was obvious, as a result of this study, that the joint line had to be properly positioned. Logistically we found that this could most easily be done by first resecting the distal femur and removing an amount of bone equal in size to the thickness of the femoral component being used. In a similar study Whitesides and Summers using cadaveric knees came to the same conclusion.

In theory, the sequence of each of the bone cuts may be varied without affecting the final outcome. Most often, the sequence of resections is dependent more upon the instrumentation available and the surgeon's past experience than on any specific biomechanical or anatomical factors. Over the years I have varied the sequence of the bony resections at times because of special problems with exposure, or because of new instruments that were available. I would like to recommend, however, that the following sequence, beginning with the distal femur, be considered as most logical and appropriate.

The Distal Femoral Resection

In the knee with severe arthritis, the distal femoral articular surface configuration is usually well preserved and less variable than that of the proximal tibia. Furthermore, exposure of the distal femur is relatively easy even in the face of soft tissue contractures. For these two reasons, we feel that the distal femoral surface should be identified and resected first and used as the guide for the level of the prosthetic joint line (Laskin and Rieger 1989).

In the coronal plane, the normal femoral condylar surface is oriented perpendicular to the line of leg alignment (defined as a line joining the center of the femoral head and the center of the ankle joint). The condylar surface is likewise oriented at 97° to the anatomical axis of the femur (a line drawn down the center of the

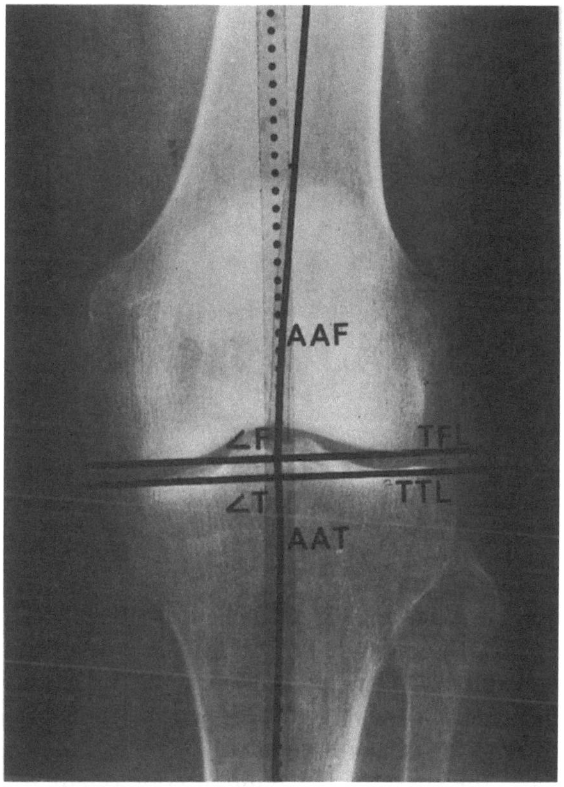

Fig. 5.7. The anatomical axis of the femur (AAF) extends down the center of the intramedullary canal. It intersects the transfemoral line (TFL) forming an angle F which normally measures 97° medially.

intramedullary canal of the distal half of the femur) (Fig. 5.7). In theory, either of these two axes could be used as a reference for making the distal femoral resection.

From a practical point of view, we have had difficulty using the line of leg alignment as a reference because we cannot accurately find one of its end points, the center of the femoral head. Despite the "textbook" descriptions of locating the femoral head using the anterior superior iliac spine, the pubic tubercle, the femoral pulse, etc. its position can often not be accurately ascertained during the operation since the bony landmarks are obscured by the surgical drapes and the tourniquet (Laskin 1984). Radiographic evaluation preoperatively or intraoperatively can obviate this problem but is logistically cumbersome.

Since the line of leg alignment is unreliable to use, the question remains as to whether the anatomical axis of the femur is a better reference guide. We feel that it is. There had been some concern as to whether this axis is consistent enough and whether the angle of declination between it and the condylar transfemoral line (the AAF/TFL Angle) was the same for all patients. Hungerford et al. (1983) reported that the angle was approximately 5°–7° in tall thin patients, but could be as high as 11° in short obese patients. Denham (1984), on the other hand, found that the AAF/TFL was 7° ± 2° in almost all patients regardless of the body habitus. A prospective study in our center of 50 patients prior to total knee arthroplasty corroborated Denham's view. We therefore use the femoral anatomical axis as our guide during knee replacement and orient the femoral cut at 95° to this axis. The reason for choosing this angle will be explained subsequently.

The position of the anatomical axis of the femur can be ascertained either from palpation of the shaft of the bone or by using its intramedullary canal as a reference. In our center, we prefer the latter. We have demonstrated (Laskin 1984) that accurate alignment can be obtained without intraoperative X-rays by using an intramedullary reference rod 8 mm thick and 25 cm long. A rod with these dimensions will snugly fit in almost all femurs without toggle. For the occasional patient with a marked curvature to the femur (i.e. from a previous fracture or from Paget's disease) we cannot use an intramedullary reference rod, and then, by necessity must rely on line of leg alignment (Fig. 5.8). We then rely upon pre-operative radiographic markers and use intraoperative radiographs for their identification (Fig. 5.9a,b)

The entrance hole for the intramedullary rod should be placed just anterior to the insertion of the posterior cruciate ligament in the intercondylar notch and just medial to the midline of the notch itself. It is essential that the hole be large enough so that the rod will not bind on entry or be abnormally deflected. Rand (1988) has recommended using an intramedullary reference rod which is hollow and to which suction may be applied. This would theoretically help prevent embolization of marrow contents into vascular channels during the insertion of the rod (Fig. 5.10).

After inserting the intramedullary reference rod, we affix a cutting block to it set at 95° in the coronal plane and 90° in the sagittal plane. Our cutting block is positioned in a proximal/distal

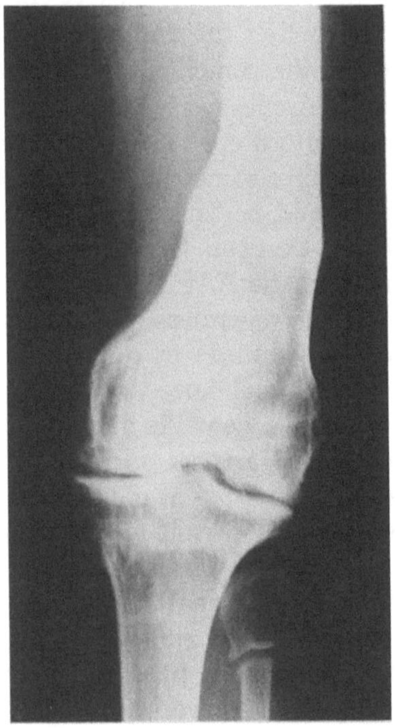

Fig. 5.8. Patient with old malunited fracture of the distal femur. It is not possible to use an intramedullary reference guide in a situation such as this.

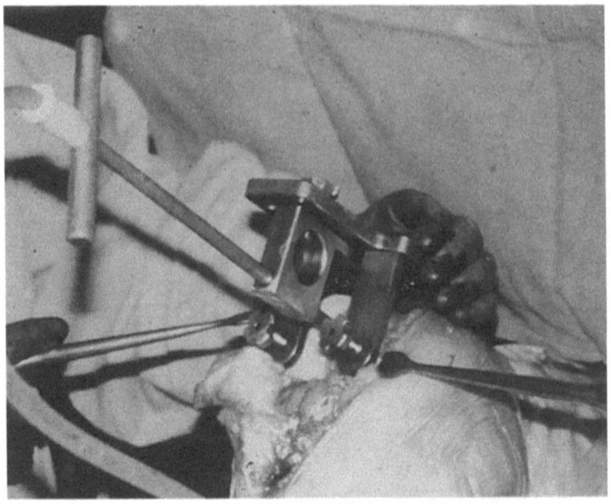

Fig. 5.10. Aspiration of a hollow femoral intramedullary guide in order to prevent possible pressurization of the marrow contents.

direction by two paddles which abut the most distal portion of the femoral condyles. The distance between the paddles and the surface of the cutting block equals the distal thickness of the femoral component. If there is cartilage and bone loss on the concave side of an angular knee deformity (i.e. on the medial side of a varus knee) we advance the block until the paddle touches the condyle on the convex side of the deformity. The block is pinned to the femur and the femoral condyles are resected. By removing an amount of bone equal in thickness to the distal thickness of the femoral component we assure that joint line will be maintained at its proper height (Fig. 5.11).

The bone at the intercondylar notch and at the posterior corners of the femoral condyles is usually very sclerotic so that special care must be taken to ensure that the blade does not deviate from the cutting block in those areas (Fig. 5.12). It is important as well to protect and retract the

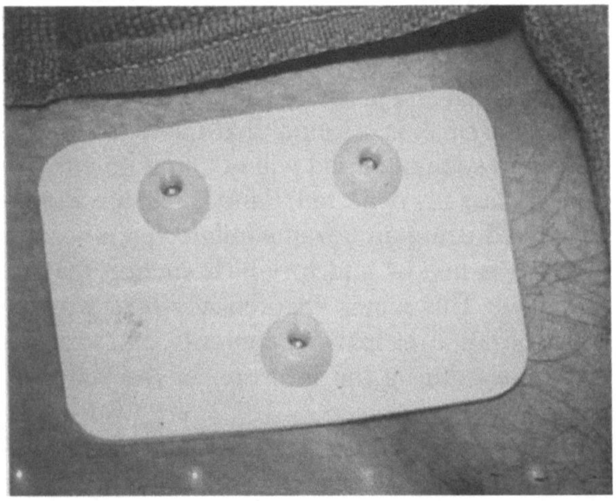

a

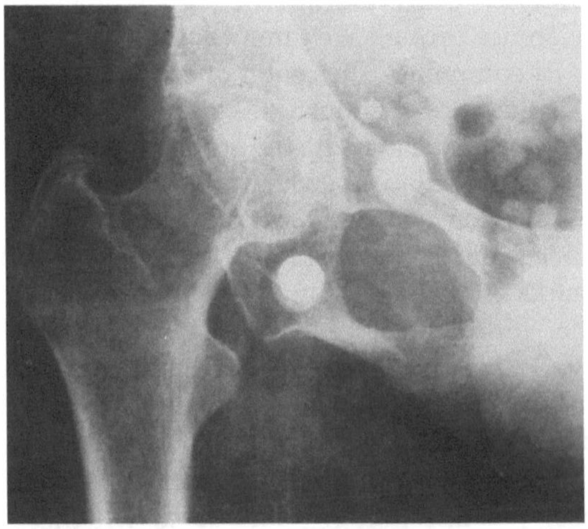

b

Fig. 5.9.a,b. Radiographic marker to locate the femoral head. **a** Placement of pad in groin. **b** X-ray showing reference markers.

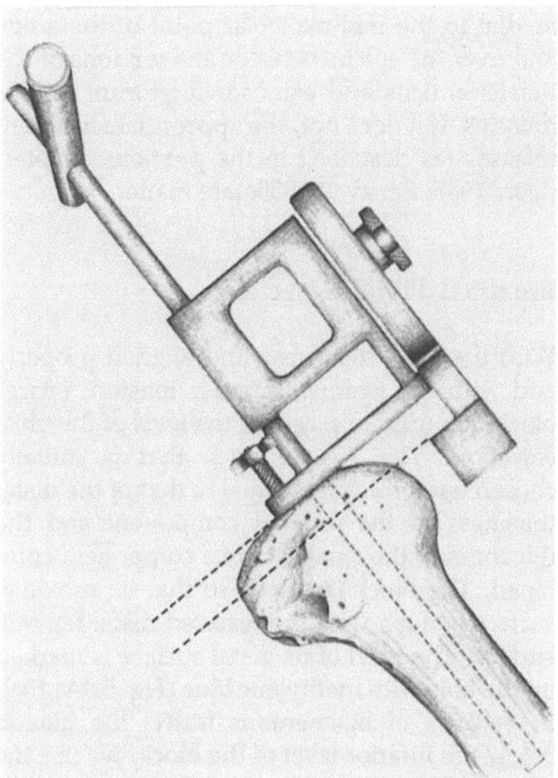

Fig. 5.11. Paddles on femoral cutting guide assure that amount of bone resected equals the distal thickness of femoral component. This positions the joint line properly.

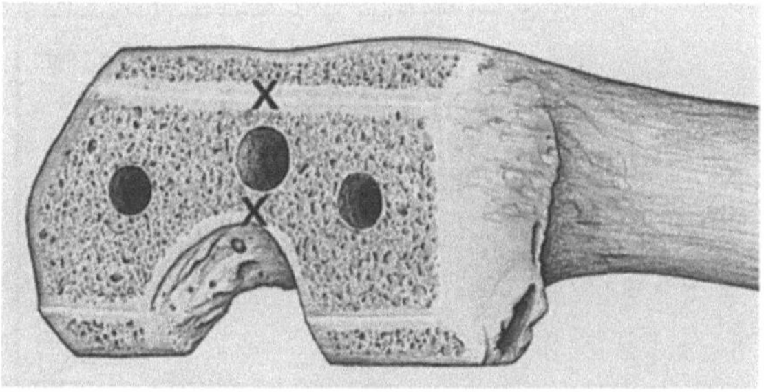

Fig. 5.12. Normal areas of sclerotic bone in the distal femur.

collateral ligaments so that they are not inadvertently damaged during the resection.

Ligament Balancing

We make our first assessment of ligament balance after we have resected the distal femur. Using an appropriate jig, an alignment rod is placed perpendicular to the distal femoral resection line. The joint space medially and laterally is then tensed using two laminar spreaders (Fig. 5.13). If the ligaments are balanced, the end rod should now lie directly

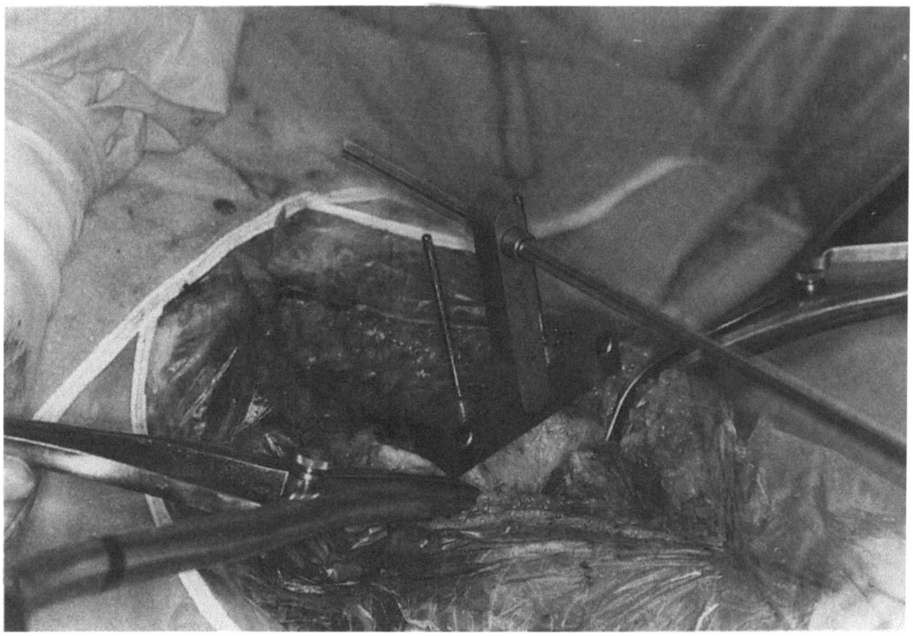

Fig. 5.13. Ligaments tensed. Tibial alignment rod extends down to ankle joint.

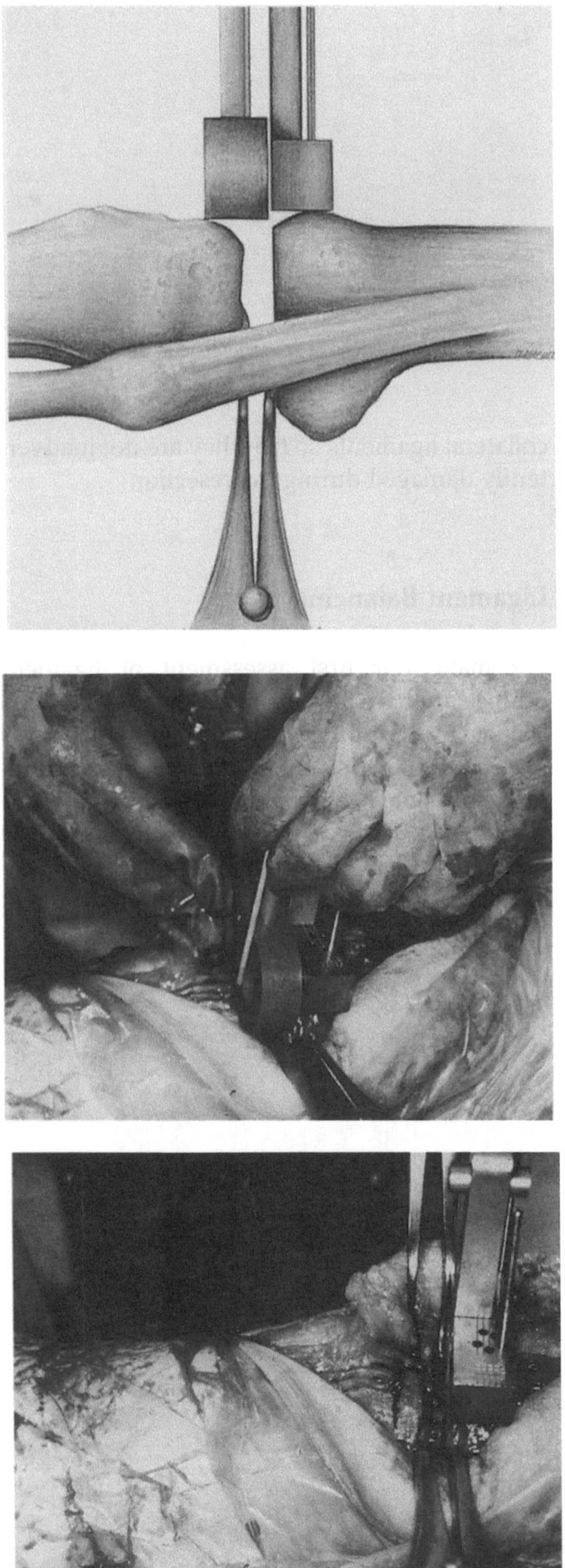

a
b
c

Fig. 5.14a–c Level for resection of the proximal tibia. **a** Ligaments distracted, spacer block placed at level of cut surface of femur. **b** Inferior border of spacer block marked. **c** Methylene blue line notes level for tibial resection.

over the center of the tibial plafond, slightly medial to the mid-malleolar point of the ankle and over the sulcus between the tendons of the tibialis anticus and extensor digitorum longus muscles. If it does not, the appropriate ligament releases (as described in the previous chapter) (Dorr 1985; Ranawat 1985a)are made.

Proximal Tibial Resection

With the knee distracted and aligned properly and with the ligaments under tension, spacer blocks are used to ascertain the level of the tibial resection. The spacer block that is initially chosen has a thickness equal to that of the distal thickness of the femoral component and the thickness of the smallest tibial component combined. The block is placed so that its proximal surface is flush with the resected distal femoral surface. The level of its distal surface is marked on the tibia with methylene blue (Fig. 5.14a,b,c). If, because of ligamentous laxity, the tibia is below the inferior level of the block, we use the next thicker spacer block in the system. This technique will assure that the extension space will be accurately and completely filled by the implants available in our component set. Since the thickness of both femoral and tibial components for various prostheses differ it is important that spacer blocks specific to that prosthesis be used. Furthermore it is extremely important to make sure that the knee is distracted so as to tense the capsular sleeve before marking the tibia. Failure to do so will result in the mark being placed too far distally, ultimately leading to overresection of the proximal tibia (Fig. 5.15).

In the frontal plane, a line joining the surface of both tibial plateaus (the TTL) is oriented at 88° to the anatomical-mechanical axis of the tibia (Fig. 5.16). The relationship of this TTL and the joint surface to the plane of the ground varies, however, dependent upon numerous factors. As an example, the orientation of this line changes when the patient progresses from one-legged stance to two-legged stance. Its orientation likewise is dependent upon any fixed adduction or abduction of the hip joint (Dorr 1985; Hungerford et al. 1983).

Hungerford et al. (1983) have suggested that the proximal tibia be resected at 88° to reproduce the normal anatomical anatomy. That would

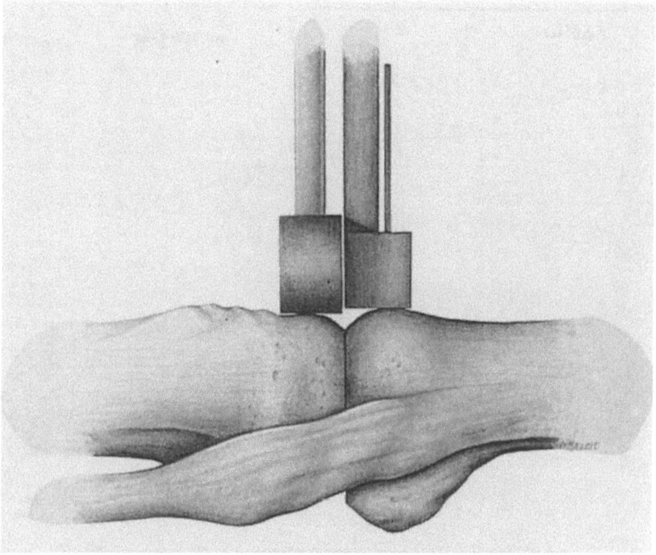

Fig. 5.15. Ligaments not distracted results in resection line being too low.

seem proper until one realizes that all bony resections are accurate only to within ±2°. This being the case, there is a chance that the surgeon attempting to place the component at 88° might inadvertently place the component at 86°. This amount of varus of the component would increase the stress on the medial plateau and could cause early tibial component loosening. To obviate this potential problem Insall (1984b) and others have suggested that the tibial resection be made at a 90° angle in the frontal plane. With the variation in cutting accuracy noted above taken into consideration the components will usually be inserted at "the safe" orientation of between 92° and 88°. One should remember, however, that by making the resection at 90°, the surgeon is actually externally rotating the lower border of the extension and flexion spaces. In theory, one should also externally rotate the upper border of the extension and flexion space (namely the distal femoral cut and the posterior femoral cuts respectively) by 2°. Functionally this appears to be more crucial in the flexion space and somewhat less important in the extension space. We do however, make allowance for this external rotation of the proximal tibia by resecting the distal femur at 95° (rather than 97°) and the posterior femur in 2° external rotation from neutral.

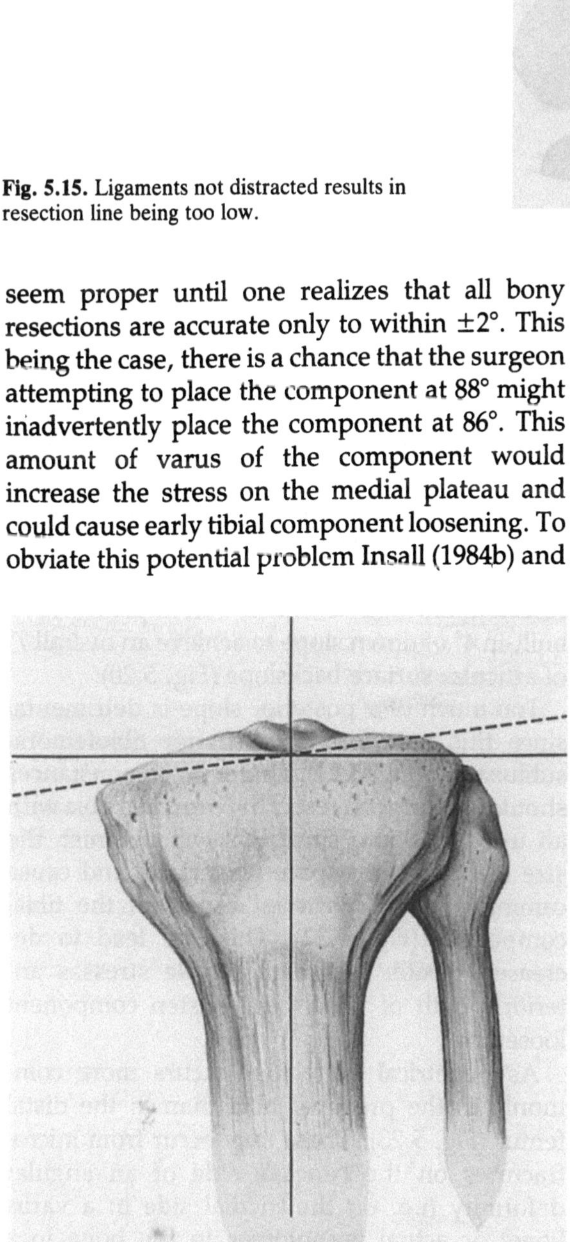

Fig. 5.16. Articular surface of normal tibia is oriented at 88° to anatomical axis of the bone in the P/A plane.

In the lateral plane, the "normal" tibial plateau has a posterior slope of 6–10° (Fig. 5.17). It is this slope that assists the femur to roll back on the tibia as the knee is flexed. Posterior sloping of the prosthetic tibial surface may be accomplished in one of two ways. If the implant has a thickness equal anteriorly and posteriorly, then the tibia should be resected with a downward slope of approximately 6–10°. If the articular surface of the tibial implant has a built-in slope of 6–10° then the tibia may be resected at 90° (Fig. 5.18). For those with intermediate prosthetic articular slopes, an intermediate amount of pos-

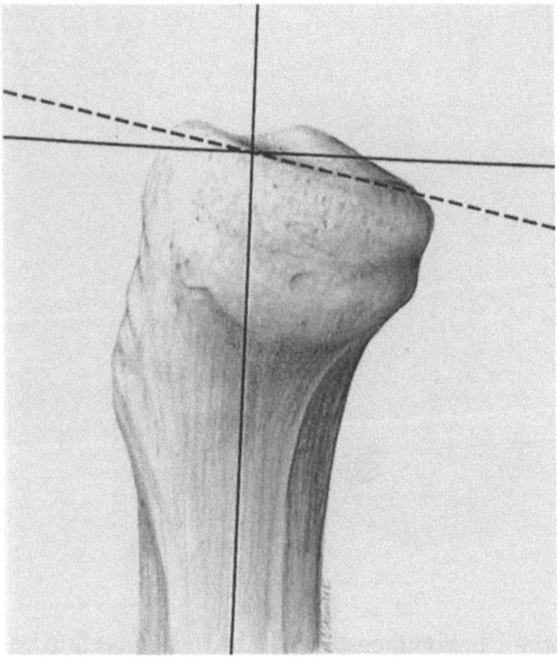

Fig. 5.17. Articular surface of the normal tibia normally slopes posteriorly 6–10°.

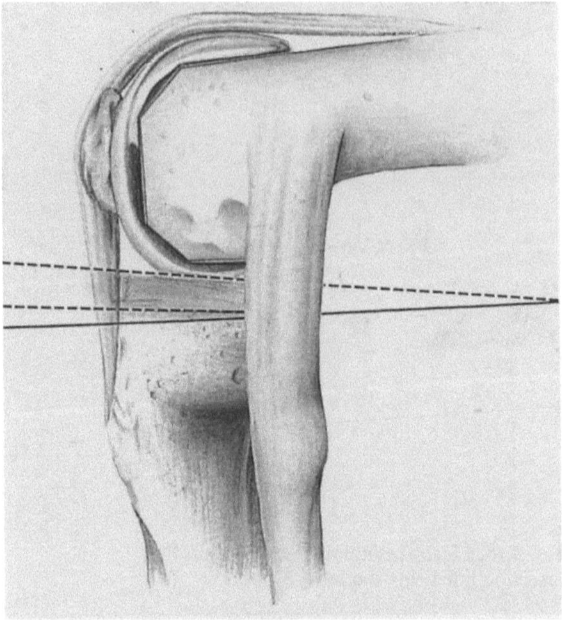

Fig. 5.19 Tibia is resected with slight backslope. Backslope of prosthetic joint results from this and some sloping of the surface of the implant itself.

terior sloping of the resection line must be made (Fig. 5.19). In theory, all three techniques should ultimately achieve the same final outcome. Hoffman et al. (1987) and Sneppen et al. (1981) have shown, however, that the quality of the anterior cancellous bone decreases rapidly as one progresses downward below the joint surface. They felt that one should therefore try to maximize preservation of this anterior bone in an attempt to prevent tibial component subsidence. Bearing all these factors in mind we presently slope the resection line back 3° and use an implant with a built-in 4° of down slope to achieve an overall 7° of articular surface backslope (Fig. 5.20).

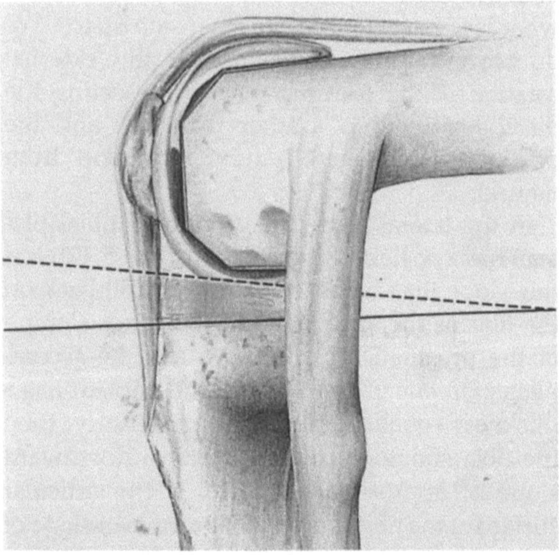

Fig. 5.18. Tibia is resected at 90°. Backslope of prosthetic joint results from backslope completely in the tibial component.

Too much of a posterior slope is detrimental since this may lead to posterior tibiofemoral subluxation (Fig. 5.21). Under no circumstances should the surgeon resect the proximal tibia with an upward slope, since this will diminish the size of the flexion space posteriorly and cause camming of the posterior aspect of the tibial component (Fig. 5.22). This will lead to decreased flexion and high tensile stresses anteriorly both of which will hasten component loosening.

Asymmetrical bone loss occurs more commonly in the proximal tibia than in the distal femur (Fig. 5.23). These may occur from microfractures on the concave side of an angular deformity (i.e. on the medial side in a varus knee) or actual granulomas in the bone in a patient with rheumatoid arthritis. For small defects (less that 2–3 mm in depth) the resection line can be made just below the lowest point on

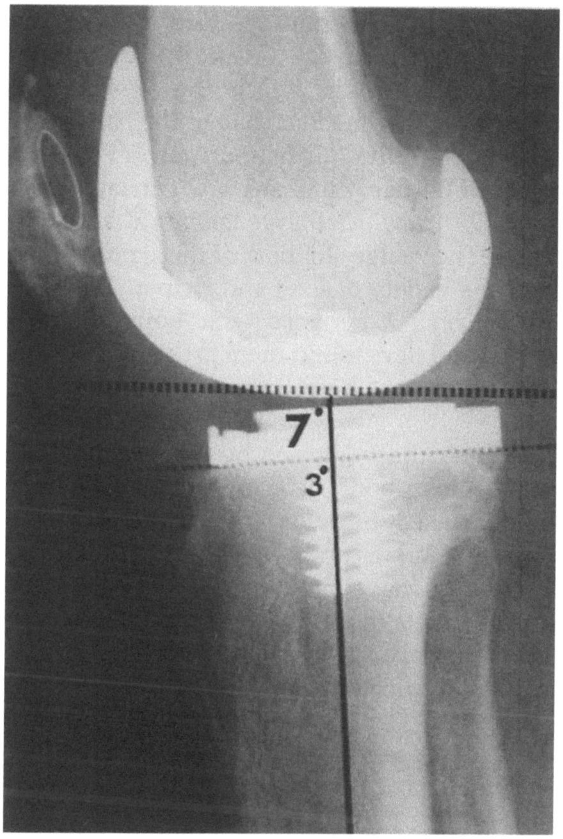

Fig. 5.20. Genesis tibial component lateral X-ray. Overall 7° of backslope results from a 3° posterior cut on the tibia, and a 4° intrinsic backslope in the surface of the implant.

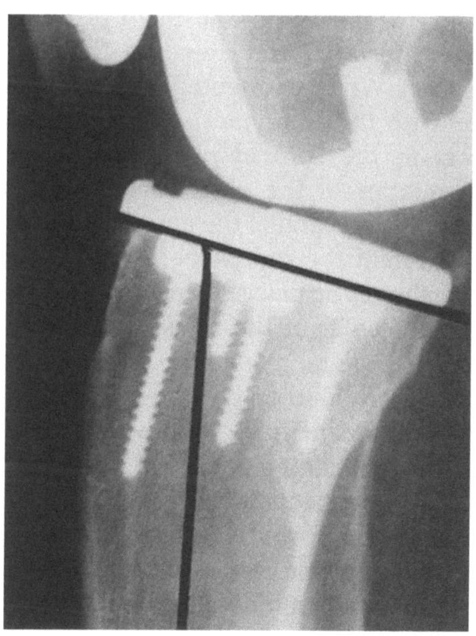

Fig. 5.21. Inappropriate posterior resection of the proximal tibia has led to severe recurvatum deformity of the knee.

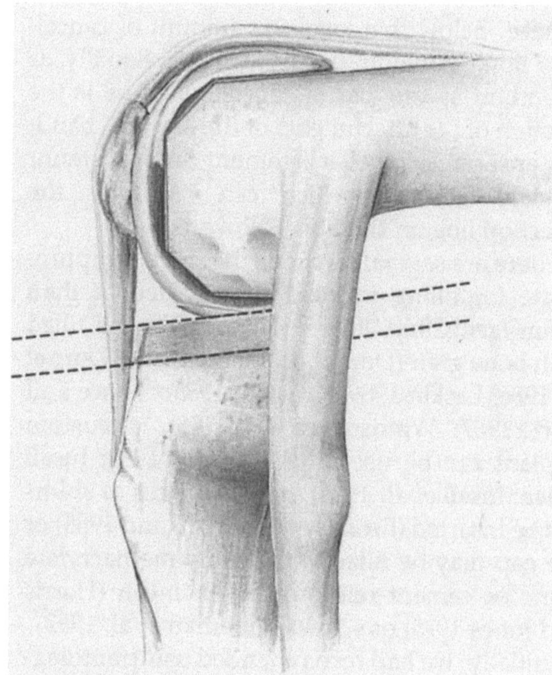

Fig. 5.22. Upsloping of the tibial resection surface results in a smaller space posteriorly and camming of the implant.

the defect. An appropriately large sized tibial implant will then be required.

For defects greater than 3 mm this technique cannot be used. Structurally (and biomechanically) the bone in the subchondral area is the strongest. There is a 25% decrease in both the strength and volume of cancellous bone from

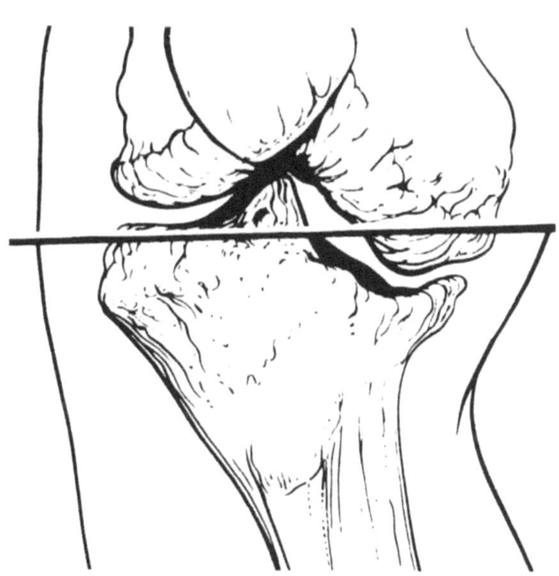

Fig. 5.23. Asymmetrical bone loss from the proximal tibia.

that point down to about 10 mm below the joint surface. Below that level the amount of cancellous bone remaining is minuscule. Equally as important as the loss of cancellous bone is the ablation of the attachments of the iliotibial band, pes anserinus, patellar ligament, and posterior cruciate ligament which can occur as the resection line on the tibia is lowered.

There are several methods that may be appropriate for filling in bone defects deeper than 3 mm (see Chap. 15). The defect can be filled with bone graft (Dorr and Ranawat 1983; Dorr et al. 1986; Laskin 1989; Ranawat 1985b; Vince and Dorr 1987; Windsor et al. 1986), a custom implant can be used (Bartel et al. 1982; Insall 1984a; Insall et al. 1985), metal wedges or shims can be inserted (Brooks et al. 1984; Rand 1988) or the gap may be filled with methylmethacrylate alone or cement reinforced with mesh (Harris and Jones 1975) or screws (Freeman et al. 1982).

Initially, we had recommended using autologous bone graft (taken from the resected distal femoral condyles) to fill large defects encountered during total knee replacement, having had good short term results (Laskin et al. 1986). In 1989, however, we re-evaluated our data and reported a long term follow-up of 26 patients who had undergone this procedure (Laskin 1990). We found that our success rate was only 67%. We had 15% in which there were complete radiolucencies between the graft and the host bone and 18% in which the graft had fragmented and collapsed. A needle biopsy had been performed one year after surgery in nine of the grafts which radiographically appeared to have been successful. We found lacunae devoid of viable osteocytes in five cases. Similar problems with large fragment bone grafting have been reported by Harris (1988) in his reconstruction of hip joints at the time of joint replacement. In view of this high incidence of failure, we are no longer recommending the use of large fragment grafts for these patients and are now reevaluating metal shims or wedges as an alternative.

We can always order a custom implant designed to specifically fill a large defect in the bone. Unfortunately, the logistical and monetary problems associated with custom implants make their use on a large scale basis impractical. Some of the newer total knee prostheses make provisions for the attachment of wedges or shims to the implants, enabling the surgeon to fabricate a "custom prosthesis" at the time of surgery. Two such examples are the Genesis prosthesis (Richards Medical Company, Memphis, Tenn.) in which the wedges are affixed by methylmethacrylate to the base prosthesis and the Insall-Burstein Posterior Stabilized II Knee (Zimmer-USA, Warsaw, Ind.) (Insall 1989) in which the wedges are attached by screws. The wedges for both of these prostheses come in a variety of sizes and shapes. We have had personal experience with both of these systems and have found them to be applicable to a myriad of bone defect patterns found at surgery.

Methylmethacrylate can be used to fill small well-circumscribed defects. Acrylic cement cannot be used, however, for peripheral defects in which there is no bony confinement of the cement. We have not found the addition of screws or metal mesh to the cement to increase its mechanical properties and therefore do not use them on a routine basis.

There are two types of alignment guides which can be used to guide the resection of the proximal tibia: extramedullary and intramedullary:

1. *Extramedullary Guides* (Fig. 5.24a–d). Properly to place an extramedullary tibial guide-rod the distal end must be positioned over the center of the articular surface of the tibia, and the proximal end in the center of the tibial plateau (approximately 0.5 cm lateral to the anterior tibial spine). When so oriented, the guide will be aligned with the anatomical-mechanical axis of the tibia in the coronal plane and cross the medial quarter of the tibial tubercle. In most cases it will also parallel the anterior crest of the tibia. To orient the rod properly in the sagittal plane, it should be placed so as to parallel a line joining the center of the fibular head with the center of the lateral malleolus. The appropriate tibial resection can then be made by referencing from this alignment guide in both P/A and lateral planes. Malpositioning of the rod can occur if its distal end is erroneously placed in the center of the intermalleolar space (that is one half the distance between the medial and lateral malleoli) rather than in the center of the tibial plafond; this will orient its end too far laterally and result in a varus tibial resection proximally. A similar problem can occur if the proximal portion of the

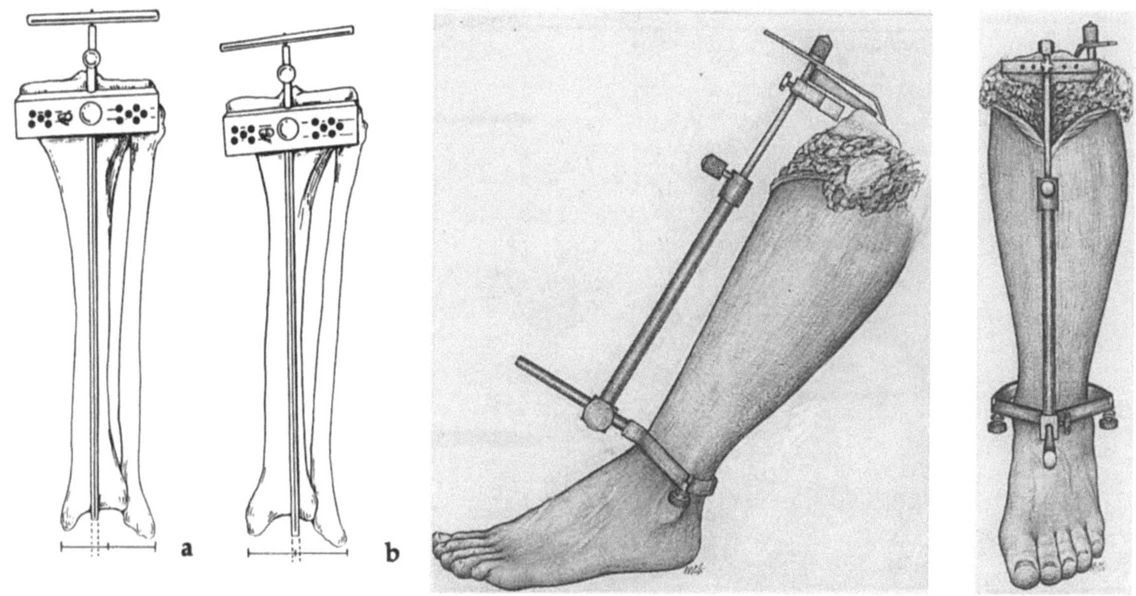

Fig. 5.24a–d. Extramedullary tibial alignment rod and cutting jig. **a** End of rod should be aligned with center of tibial plafond. This is slightly medial to the mid-malleolar point. **b** Alignment with the mid-malleolar point results in a varus orientation of the cutting block. **c** Extramedullary alignment rod and ankle clamp in place (P/A). **d** Lateral view of extramedullary alignment rod.

rod is placed medial to the center of the tibial plateau.

2. *Intramedullary Guides* (Fig. 5.25a–c). Properly to place an intramedullary guide-rod, a hole must be made in the approximate center of the tibial plateau surface; the guide-rod is then inserted down the tibial shaft to the level of the old epiphyseal growth plate of the distal tibia. In a clinical study of both above knee amputation specimens and patients undergoing total knee replacement we were able to show that the exact entrance point on the plateau was not crucial, as long as it was anterior to the midline and generally equidistant from the medial and lateral cortical margins (Laskin and Turtel 1989). Since the tibia has a complex curve in both the coronal and sagittal planes, a rod as thick as the isthmus will not pass completely down the bone. Through geometrical and clinical analysis we determined that a guide rod 8 mm in diameter could be easily inserted through an 11 mm hole in the tibial plateau and passed down to the ankle so as to obtain sufficient purchase in the shaft to yield reproducible and accurate results. The anterior outrigger of the guide-rod is oriented so that it crosses the medial quarter of the tibial tubercle. Although, there can be some problem with seating of an intramedullary guide if the tibia is severely bent in either plane (such as in a patient with Paget's disease or one with a malunited fracture), we have found this problem to occur in less that 1% of cases.

Once the alignment rod has been properly placed, the tibial resection block is affixed to it and lowered to the mark that had been previously made using the external spacer block.

A joint line sensor is placed in the cutting block to determine exactly how much bone will be removed by resecting the tibia at this level. If it is obvious that cutting the tibia at the level where the most proximal reference line was made (that is the line corresponding to the thinnest tibial component) will result in leaving a bone defect, the surgeon must decide whether to lower the cutting block to the next reference line (that is for the next thickest component) or use a metal wedge, bone graft, or cement filler as described above. In no case should the amount of resection be greater that 8–10 mm for the reasons elucidated previously. We prefer a cutting block for the resection of the tibia. We begin the cut medially and then extend laterally as far as possible without injuring the patellar ligament. In some cases we will split the articular surface with a sagittal cut, remove the medial half, and then use the medial cut surface as the

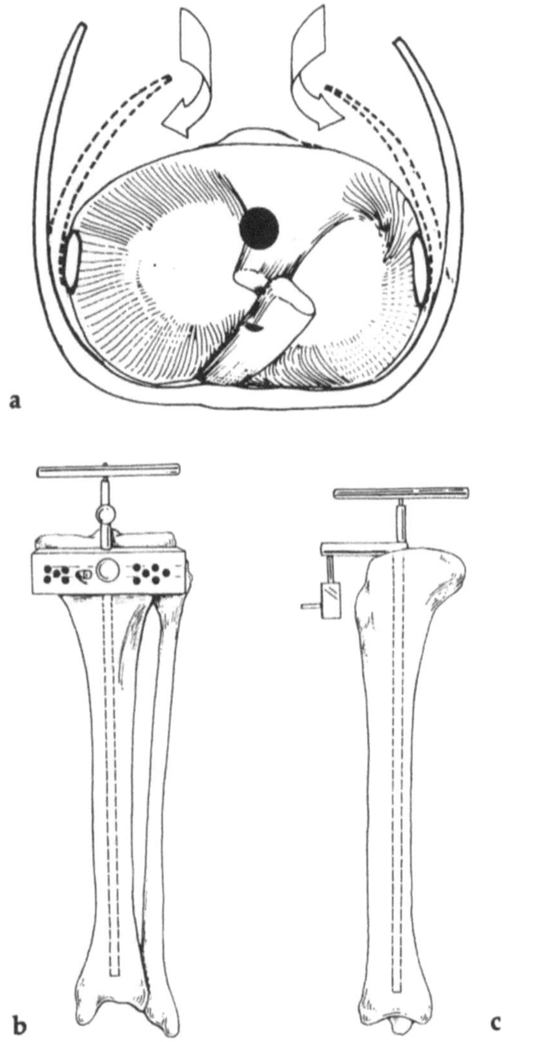

Fig. 5.25a–c. Intramedullary tibial alignment rod and cutting jig. **a** Point of entrance for rod is slightly anterior to the midline. **b** Rod extends down to the level of the old distal tibial epiphyseal plate (P/A). **c** Rod and cutting block in place.

base for resecting laterally. After the proximal tibia has been resected we again tense the knee with the laminar spreaders and recheck that the alignment of the limb is proper. If the spacer block is now reinserted the ligaments should be tense medially and laterally.

Anterior and Posterior Femoral Resections

In order not to displace artificially the joint line anteriorly or posteriorly, the amount of posterior femoral condylar bone that is removed should equal in thickness the posterior condylar dimension of the implant being used (Fig. 5.26). In order to maintain the quadriceps lever arm at a normal length, the amount of anterior femur resected should equal the thickness of the prosthetic trochlear flange. Unfortunately to accomplish both of these aims would require an infinite number of femoral component sizes, each differing slightly in its internal anteroposterior dimension. As a logistical compromise, most total knee designs will maintain the proper posterior femoral condylar size, but allow only a discrete number of prostheses. The amount of anterior femoral bone resected will therefore at times be too little, and at other times be just right. It must never be too much; the anterior femoral cortex must never be notched! A notch in the anterior femoral cortex can set up a stress riser in the femur with the potential for fracture (Fig. 5.27) (Merkel and Johnson 1986). An anterior sensor assures that the femur will never be cut below the level of the anterior cortex (Fig. 5.28). If the femoral component has a posterior thickness equal to its distal thickness, and if the instruments allow for removal of an amount of bone equal in thickness to the thickness of the

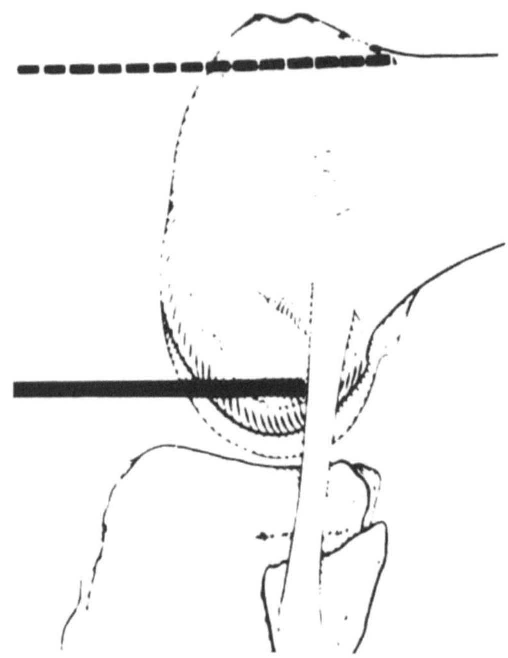

Fig. 5.26. Optimal levels of resection of the anterior and posterior femur.

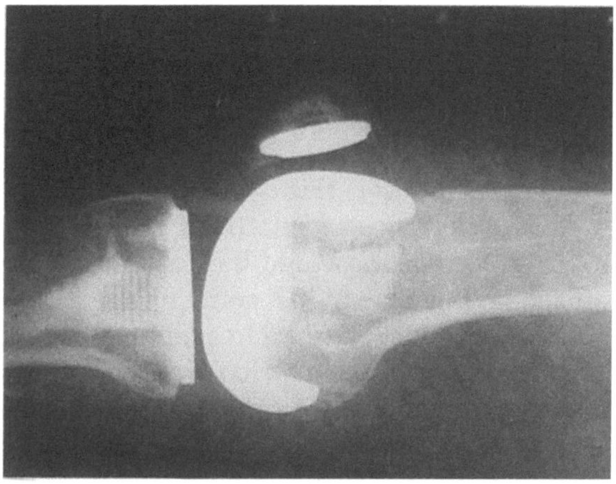

Fig. 5.27 Anterior femur inadvertently notched.

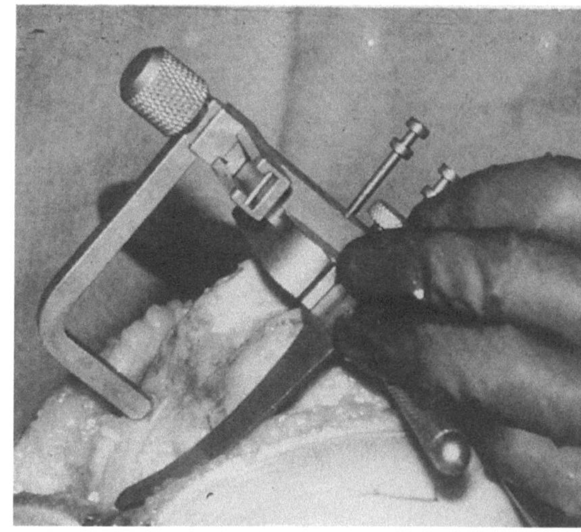

Fig. 5.28. Anterior sensor to prevent anterior cortical notching.

component, then equalization of the flexion and extension spaces is assured.

Rotatory alignment of the anteroposterior cutting jig is normally based upon the orientation of the posterior femoral condyles since they are normally well preserved even in a severely arthritic knee. In the uncommon situation where the condyles are markedly eroded (such as in a patient with severe osteonecrosis), the orientation of the transepicondylar line can be used as a rotatory reference.

If the tibia has been resected at 88° to its anatomical-mechanical axis, then equal amounts of bone should be resected from each posterior condyle. If however, the tibia has been resected at 90° (that is externally rotated by 2°) then the anterior and posterior femoral cuts should likewise be externally rotated by 2° (that is slightly more bone removed from the medial than the lateral femoral condyle). Only by this latter method can the flexion space be made rectangular (Fig. 5.29a–c).

There is a secondary benefit that accrues from slightly externally rotating the femoral component. The trochlear surface of the implant is placed slightly more laterally and this helps

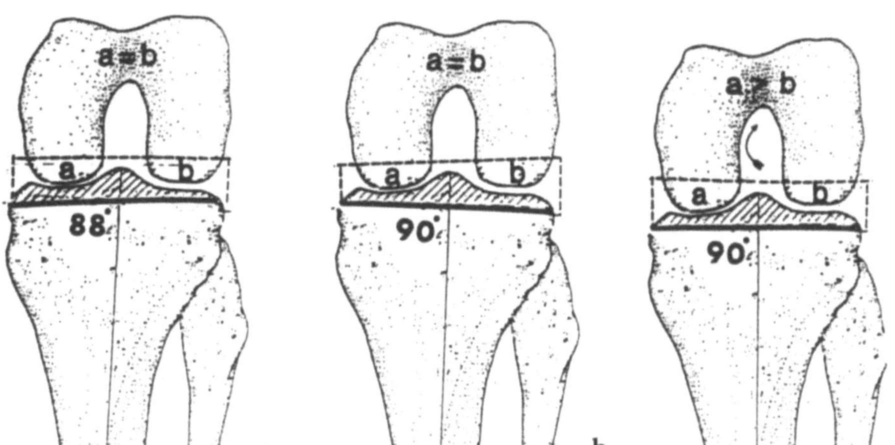

Fig. 5.29a–c. Rotatory orientation of the distal femoral cuts. **a** If the proximal tibia is resected at 88° (slight external rotation), then removing equal amounts of bone from both posterior femoral condyles results in a rectangular flexion space. **b** If the proximal tibia is resected at 90° (slight external rotation), then removing equal amounts of bone from both femoral condyles results in a trapezoidal flexion space. (Incorrect). **c** The proper resect of the distal femur in this case is slight external rotation of 2° so that slightly more bone is removed medially than laterally.

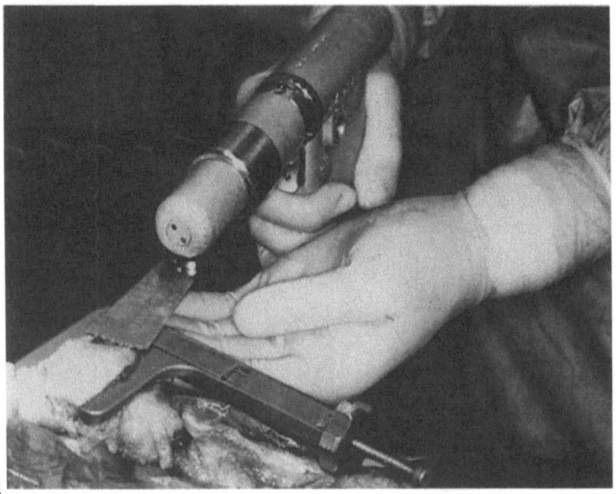

a

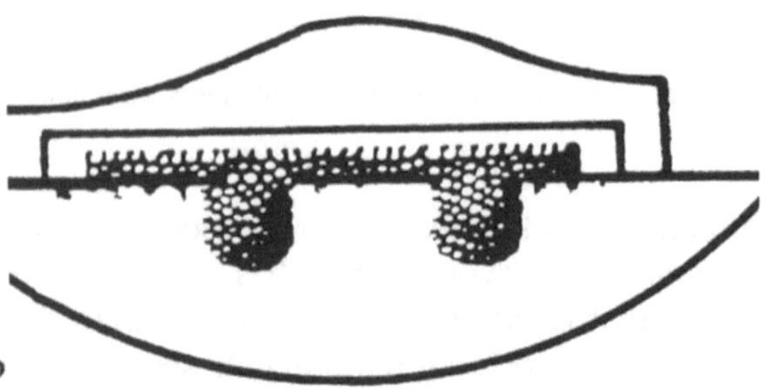

b

Fig. 5.30a,b. Onset technique for the patellar implant. **a** The patella is cut over a patellar hold. **b** The implant is onset on the cut surface of the patella.

insure proper patellar tracking. Under no circumstance should the femoral component be internally rotated. Doing this will displace the prosthetic trochlear surface away from the patella and predispose to post-operative patello-femoral dislocation.

Patellar Resection

When I first began performing tricompartmental knee replacement, I found the most difficult technical part to be preparation of the patella for its implant. Within the last few years, however, instruments have become available to allow the patellar resection to be easily made.

Prior to resecting the patella any rim osteophytes or surrounding synovial overgrowth (especially in the rheumatoid patient) should be removed so that the exact dimensions of the bone can be determined. The location of the insertion of the patellar ligament should likewise be noted.

There are two basic techniques for patellar resection, the onset technique and the inset technique:

1. *Onset Technique* (Fig. 5.30a,b). With this method, the articular surface of the patella is resected to a flat base and the patellar implant affixed on this base. When resecting the patellar surface care must be taken to avoid inadvertent cutting of either the patellar ligament or the quadriceps tendon. The cut should be flat and should not remove "too much bone" lest a fracture of the patella develop. Rand (1988) and Insall (1989) have described the use of a patellar cutting clamp which grasps the bone and then acts as a cutting platform for the resection, avoiding the errors of a free hand cut. After the patella is resected the appropriate hole(s) for the studs of the implant are made.
2. *Inset Technique* (Fig. 5.31a–c). In this technique the patella is held by a cylindrical patellar clamp through which a channel is reamed into the bone; the patellar implant is then inset into this channel. This is a simple technique which provides a recess for both the implant and its fixation stud at the same time. It was initially described by Gschwend (1978) and has been modified by Cameron and myself (Laskin 1984) and by Gomez et al. (1988).

With either of the two techniques enough patellar bone must be removed so that the composite of the bone and implant is not too thick since this may lead to extreme tightness and a limitation of flexion. Resection of too much bone on the other hand can result in a thin and mechanically weak patella which is prone to fracture. We presently use a depth gauge to measure the thickness of the patella pre-operatively and strive to regain this thickness after insertion of the implant.

The prosthetic patellar implant should be aligned with the geometric center of the patella (not with the central ridge, which is slightly medial to the geometric center). Obviously a patellar implant with facets must be aligned properly so as to match the trochlear flange of the femoral component. The use of a spherical patella obviates the necessity for such rotatory orientation. In actuality, the work of Greenwald et al. (1982) and Cameron (see Chap. 13) has

a
b
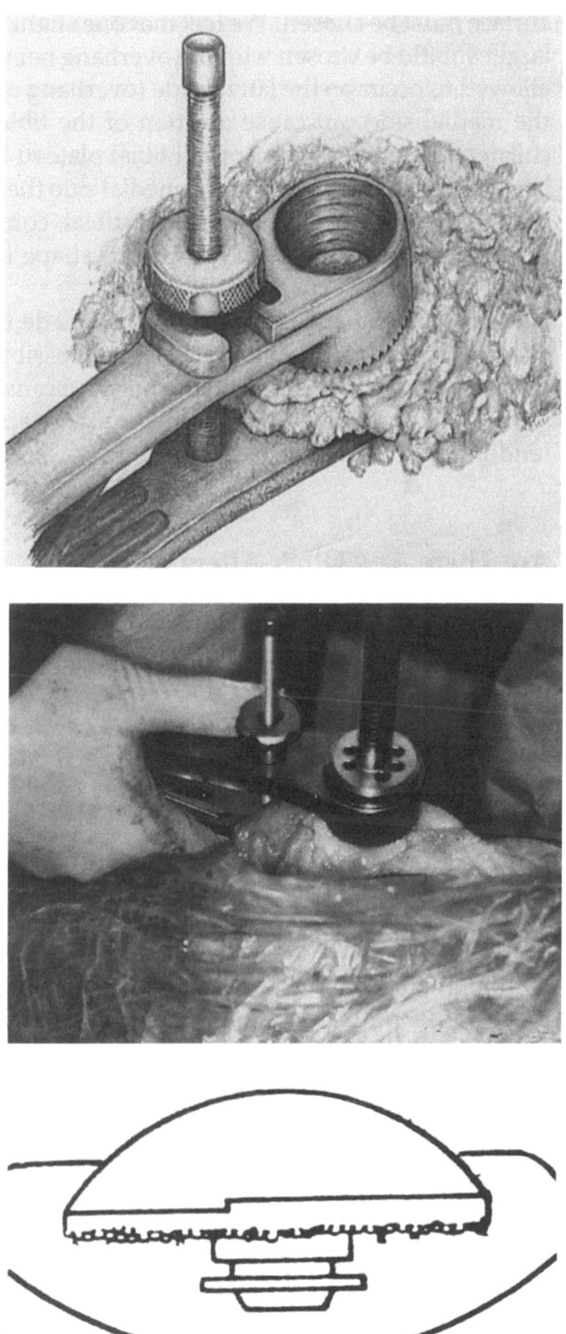
c

Fig. 5.31a–c. Inset technique for the patellar implant. **a** Patellar clamp and reamer guide. **b** Reaming through the clamp/guide. **c** The implant is inset into the bone of the patella.

shown that the concept of using a faceted patellar implant to decrease stress on the implant or to help in patellar tracking is probably without basis.

Chamfer Cuts

The size and orientation of the chamfer cuts for the distal femur vary from prosthesis to prosthesis. No firm guidelines can be given for making this cut other than to say it is crucial that one use the instruments specific to the femoral component being used.

Recess Holes for the Implants

Recess holes must be made in each of the bones to accommodate any fixation studs or pegs on the respective implant. The size, shape, and location of these recess holes will vary from prosthesis to prosthesis. Likewise for posterior stabilized implants a central box must be removed from the intercondylar notch to accommodate the center portion of the femoral component.

Equalization of the Flexion and Extension Spaces (Fig. 5.32)

Occasionally, after balancing the ligaments and resecting the bony surfaces the resultant flexion space may be larger than the extension space. Most commonly this occurs after release of a large fixed varus or valgus contracture. If such a situation exists then the thickness of implant

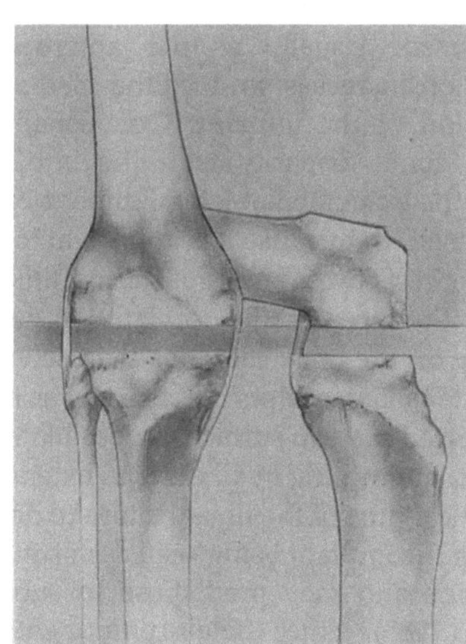

Fig. 5.32. The flexion and extension spaces.

that is required for flexion stability will be too thick in extension and the knee will not fully extend. To correct this, it is necessary to resect an additional amount of distal femur to equalize the spaces. One should not increase the size of the extension space by a resection of more proximal tibia since this will concomitantly increase the flexion space as well, perpetuating the problem. Increasing the extension space unfortunately also slightly raises the joint line so that the benefits and risks of the procedure for the individual patient must be balanced before a choice is made to resect more bone.

Occasionally, the flexion space may be smaller than the extension space. This may happen if too much distal femur was resected (almost always, this is a surgical error in the use of the distal femoral cutting jig). The correction of this problem consists of either resecting more posterior femur (and here you are limited by the actual size of the posterior femur and the presence of the posterior femoral cortex), or by adding bone graft or wedges to the distal femur to decrease the extension space. Neither solution is optimal and therefore prevention of the problem is the best cure.

Choosing Implants of the Proper Size

The size of the femoral component to be used for any individual knee is determined by the anteroposterior height of the femoral condyles and by the dimension of the anteriorposterior cutting block used. Usually as the anteroposterior dimension increases so does the medial-lateral dimension of the implant. Occasionally there will be some disparity with the implant not having the exact medial-lateral dimension of the femur itself. In this case it is important to choose the prosthesis by its anteroposterior dimensions and to then center the implant as nearly as possible on the bony condyles themselves.

For the tibia it is important to cover as much of the resected plateau surface as possible with the implant, attempting in all cases to extend out to the cortical rims of the tibia. Failure to do so will result in the implant being seated on soft cancellous bone and may predispose to subsidence (Laskin 1988). Since tibial components come only in certain discrete sizes, there may be situations in which an implant slightly smaller, or one slightly larger, than the actual bony surface must be chosen. We feel that one slightly larger should be chosen with the overhang being allowed to occur on the lateral side (overhang on the medial side can cause attrition of the tibial collateral ligament). The normal tibial plateau is irregular in shape, larger on the medial side than on the lateral side. We feel that tibial components should attempt to mirror this shape in order to maximize coverage.

For the patella an attempt should be made to cover as much of the bony surface as possible without any overhang. Overhang here can cause attrition of the patellar ligament or quadriceps tendon.

Are There Any Other Alternatives?

We have described the sequence which we presently use for performing a total knee replacement in which we:

1. Resect the distal femur
2. Balance the ligaments and the level of tibial resection
3. Resect the posterior and anterior portions of the distal femur
4. Prepare the patellar surface

Although this sequence seems to us to make most sense other techniques have been described. Insall (1984b) has recommended resecting the proximal tibia first, followed by the posterior femur. He distracts the knee in flexion and measures the flexion space. He then extends the knee, again distracts it, and makes a distal femoral resection so that the extension space equals the flexion space. This sequence of bony cuts often results in the joint line being either elevated or depressed. Although this has very little effect when one uses a prosthesis that requires sacrifice of the posterior cruciate ligament (such as in the Insall-Berstein Posterior Stabilized prosthesis), it has a deleterious effect when performed in a knee in which the posterior cruciate ligament is retained.

Other surgeons have suggested removing the posterior femoral condyles first in an attempt to gain exposure for cutting proximal tibia. This technique again leads to a variation in the proper orientation of the tibial resection. We feel that adequate exposure can easily be obtained using the system we have described, if the knee is flexed and the tibia is subluxed forward.

Summary

In summary, experience over the past 17 years has led to a series of "Dos and Don'ts" to guide the total knee surgeon in his surgical technique. They are applicable regardless of what type of implant one is inserting.

DOs (Fig. 5.33)

1. Remove an amount of distal femoral bone equal in thickness to the thickness of the implant being used in that area
2. Correct soft tissue deformities with soft tissue releases
3. Balance the soft tissues so as to align the leg into normal physiological valgus of 7°
4. Place the components in proper position to their respective bones
5. Ensure that all the components track properly (especially the patella) before closing the wound
6. Ensure that the knee is stable in both extension *and* flexion

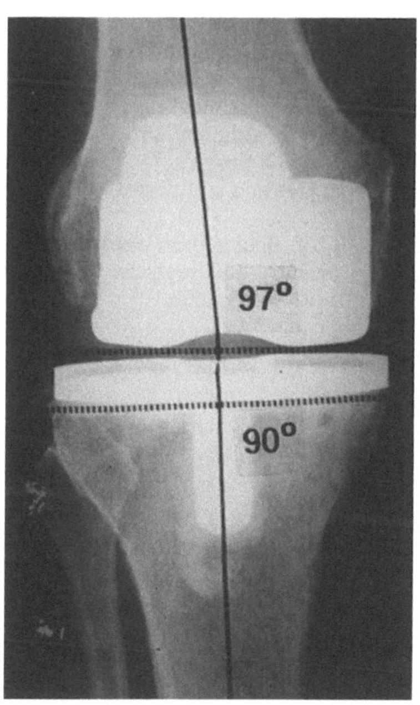

Fig. 5.33. Optimally placed total knee replacement.

DON'Ts

1. Don't place the tibial component in varus
2. Don't slope the tibial cut upward posteriorly
3. Don't notch the anterior surface of the femur
4. Don't internally rotate the femoral component
5. Don't expect that the knee stability will change after surgery. If you cannot obtain full extension with the patient under anesthesia at surgery it will not "loosen up" during the postoperative period. If the knee is unstable at surgery, it will not "tighten up" spontaneously after the operation.
6. Don't make corrections for inequalities of the flexion and extension spaces by resecting the proximal tibia.

References

Bartel DL, Burstein AH, Santavicca EA, Insall JN (1982) Performance of the tibial component in total knee replacement. Conventional and revision designs. J Bone Joint Surg (Am) 64:1026–1033

Brooks PJ, Walker PS, Scott RD (1984) Tibial component fixation in deficient tibial bone stock. Clin Orthop 184:302–308

Denham R (1984) Biomechanics of the knee. In: Laskin RS, Denham R, Apley AG (eds) Replacement of the knee. Springer-Verlag, Berlin Heidelberg New York, pp 52–73

Dorr LD (1985) Technique of correction of varus deformity. In: Ranawat CS (ed) Total condylar knee arthroplasty technique, results and complications. Springer-Verlag, Berlin Heidelberg New York

Dorr LD, Boirdo RA (1986) Technical considerations in total knee arthroplasty. Clin Orthop 205:5–11

Dorr LD, Ranawat CS (1983) Bone grafts for tibial deficits in total knee arthroplasty, In: Dorr LD (ed) Revision of total hip and knee. University Park Press, Baltimore, p 143

Dorr LD, Conaty JP, Schreiber R et al. (1985) Technical factors that influence mechanical loosening of knee arthroplasty. In: Dorr LD (ed) The knee: papers of the first scientific meeting of the Knee Society. University Park Press, Baltimore, pp 121–136

Dorr LD, Ranawat DS, Sculco TP et al. (1986) Bone graft for tibial defects in total knee arthroplasty. Clin Orthop 205:153–165

Ewald FC, Jacobs MA, Miegal RE (1984) Kinematic total knee replacement. J Bone Joint Surg (Am) 66:1032–1040

Ewald FC, Jacobs MA, Walker PS et al. (1985) Accuracy of total knee replacement component position and relation to bone-cement interface reaction. In Dorr LD (ed) The knee: papers of the first scientific meeting of the Knee Society. University Park Press, Baltimore, pp 117–120

Freeman MAR, Bradley GW, Revell PA (1982) Observation

upon the interface between bone and polymethymethacrylate cement. J Bone Joint Surg (Br) 64:489–493
Gomez LSM, Bechtold JE, Gustillo RB (1988) Patellar prosthesis positioning in total knee arthroplasty: a roentgenographic study. Clin Orthop 236:72–81
Greenwald AS, Cepulo AJ, Black JD et al. (1982) Mechanics of patellofemoral replacement. A scientific exhibit at the annual meeting of the Americal Academy of Orthopaedic Surgeons, New Orleans, LA
Gschwend M (1978) The GSB knee: a further possibility, principles, results. Clin Orthop 132:170–176
Harris WH (1988) The results of frozen femoral head allografts in total hip surgery. Proceedings of the Annual Meeting of the American Academy of Orthopaedic Surgeons, Atlanta, Georgia, p 174
Harris WH, Jones W (1975) The use of wire mesh in total hip replacement surgery. Clin Orthop 106:117–120
Hofmann AA, Daniels AU, Wyatt RWB, Bachus K (1987) Clinical and laboratory comparison of the tibial cut for total knee arthroplasty. Orthop Trans p 79
Hungerford D, Krackow K, Kenna R (1983) Total knee arthroplasty: a comprehensive approach. Williams and Wilkins, New York
Insall JN (1984a) Surgical approaches to the knee. In: Insall JN (ed) Surgery of the knee. Churchill Livingstone, New York, pp 41–54
Insall JN (1984b) Total knee replacement. In: Insall JN (ed) Surgery of the knee. Churchill Livingstone, New York, pp 587–695
Insall JN (1989) Insall-Burstein posterior stabilized II surgical technique. Zimmer, USA, Warsawa, Ind.
Insall JN, Binazzi R, Soudry M, Mestriner LA (1985) Total knee arthroplasty. Clin Orthop 192:13–22
Laskin RS (1984) Alignment of total knee components. Orthopedics 7-1:62–72
Laskin RS (1987) Tricon-M uncemented total knee prosthesis. Tech Orthop 1-4:18–30
Laskin RS (1988) Uncemented total knee replacement. J Arthroplasty 3-1:27–38
Laskin RS (1989) Total knee replacement in the presence of large bony defects of the tibia and marked knee instability. Clin Orthop (in press)
Laskin RS (1990) Total condylar knee replacement in rheumatoid arthritis – A ten year follow-up. J Bone Joint Surg (in press)
Laskin RS, Rieger MA (1989) The surgical technique for performing a total knee replacement arthroplasty. Orthop Clin N Am, 20-1:31–48
Laskin RS, Schob CJ (1987) Medial capsular recession for severe varus deformities. J Arthroplasty 2:313–316
Laskin RS, Turtel A (1989) The use of an intrameduallary tibial resection guide in total knee replacement. Am J Knee Surg 2:123–130
Laskin RS, Cameron H, Light R, Schwartz G, Fields R (1986) Correction of tibial bone loss during total knee replacement. A scientific exhibit presented at the 52nd Annual Meeting of the American Academy of Orthopaedic Surgeons, Las Vegas, Nevada
Lennox DW, Cohn BT, Eschenroeder HC (1988) The effects of inaccurate bone cuts on femoral component position in total knee arthroplasty. Orthop 11-2:257–260
Lotke PA, Ecker ML (1977) Influence of positioning of the prosthesis in total knee replacement. J Bone Joint Surg (Am) 59:77–81
Matsen FA, Sidles J, Laskin RS, Gabrini M (1988) The effect of joint line position in total knee replacement. Presented at the 55th Annual Meeting of the American Academy of Orthopaedic Surgeons, Atlanta, Georgia
Merkel KD, Johnson EW (1986) Supracondylar fracture of the femur after total knee arthroplasty. J Bone Joint Surg (Am) 68:29–43
Moreland JR (1988) Mechanisms of failure in total knee arthroplasty. Clin Orthop 226:49–64
Ranawat CS (1985a) Total condylar knee arthroplasty for valgus and combined valgus flexion deformity of the knee. In: Ranawat CS (ed) Total condylar knee arthroplasty: technique, results and complications. Springer-Verlag, Berlin Heidelberg New York
Ranawat CS (1985b) How to compensate for bone loss. In: Ranawat CS (ed) Total condylar knee arthroplasty: technique, results and complications. Springer-Verlag, Berlin Heidelberg New York
Rand J (1988) The Genesis total knee system. Richards Medical Company, Memphis, Tenn
Rand JA, Bryan RS (1985) Alignment in porous coated anatomic total knee arthroplasty. In: Dorr LD (ed) The knee: papers of the first scientific meeting of the Knee Society. University Park Press, Baltimore, pp 111–119
Sculco TP (1985) Technique of correction of flexion contracture during total knee arthroplasty. In: Ranawat CS (ed) Total condylar knee arthroplasty: technique, results and complications. Springer-Verlag, Berlin Heidelberg New York
Sneppen O, Christensen P, Larsen H, Vary PS (1981) Mechanical testing of trabecular bone in knee replacement. Int Orthop 5:251
Townley CD (1985) The anatomic total knee: instrumentation and alignment technique. In: Dorr LD (ed) The knee: papers of the first scientific meeting of the Knee Society. University Park Press, Baltimore, pp 39–54
Vince KG, Door LD (1987) Surgical technique of total knee arthroplasty: principles and controversy. Techn in Orthop 1:69–82
Windsor RE, Insall JN, Sculco TP (1986) Bone grafting of tibial defects in primary and revision total knee arthroplasty. Clin Orthop 205:153–165

Section III

The Results of Total Knee Replacement

Chapter 6

Long-term Results of the Cemented Total Condylar Knee

Giles R. Scuderi, John N. Insall and Russell E. Windsor

Introduction

Cemented total knee arthroplasty has evolved over the decades from simple surface replacements to highly technical designs affording the orthopaedic surgeon the ability to correct deformities of the knee, maintain motion, and relieve pain. The results represent the work of many investigators with different prostheses who have refined the designs, improved surgical technique, and defined the principles of total knee arthroplasty. While other surgeons are advocates of cementless fixation (Hungerford et al. 1987), we continue to be advocates of cement fixation of total knee arthroplasties. Methylmethacrylate provides immediate fixation of prosthetic components to bone and has been widely used in total knee arthroplasty.

Though tibial loosening was the most frequently reported cause of failure in early reports (Insall et al. 1976), it is not accurate to blame it entirely on cement fixation. The early experience with total knee arthroplasty did not appreciate kinematic design, alignment, soft tissue balancing, and precise instrumentation (Vince and Insall 1988). Early prosthetic designs, introduced in the 1950s, were fully constrained, linked arthroplasties which placed high stress on the cement–bone interface (Coventry 1979; Insall 1984). The complications of high rates of loosening and infection were associated with virtually every prosthesis in this class. Other designs in the evolution were surface replacements with an insecure mechanical interlock between component and bone.

Modern total knee arthroplasty evolved over the years to a condylar design surface replacement through the efforts of many investigators (Bargren et al. 1976; Coventry et al. 1973; Ewald et al. 1984; Freeman et al. 1972, 1978; Goldberg and Henderson 1980; Gunston 1971; Hunter et al. 1982; Skolnick et al. 1976). At the Hospital for Special Surgery disappointing results with the unicondylar design led us towards the development of other total knee designs (Insall and Aglietti 1980). Our initial Duocondylar prosthesis had minimal bone resection and allowed for stability to be provided by the ligaments (Ranawat et al. 1976). Tibial component loosening, however, with abundant plastic and cement debris (Sledge et al. 1978) still occurred. Further design changes introduced the Duopatellar prosthesis which had an anterior flange, allowing tricompartmental resurfacing and straight bone cuts (Scott 1982; Thomas et al. 1980). This was the direct forerunner of the Total Condylar knee prosthesis that was introduced in January 1974.

The Total Condylar prosthesis is a semi-anatomic resurfacing implant with three components. The femoral component is symmetrical and consists of two identical runners which are attached by an anterior flange for articulation with the patella. The polyethylene tibial component is one piece with two cup shaped articular surfaces that are separated by a raised inter-

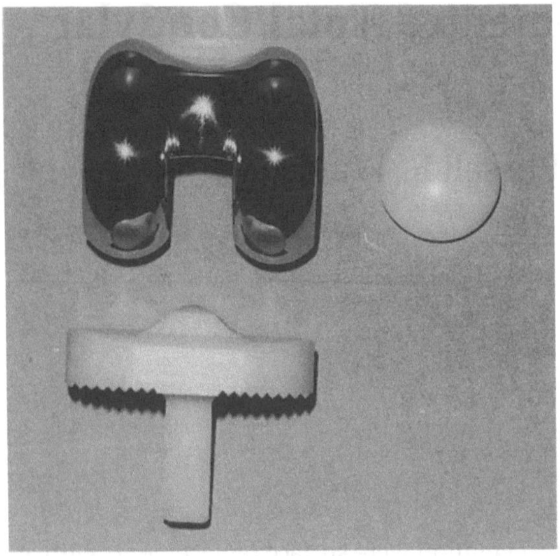

Fig. 6.1. The Total Condylar prosthesis.

condylar eminence to prevent translocation. The all polyethylene patellar button is circular and dome shaped. The implant is semiconstrained and cruciate-sacrificing (Insall and Kelly 1986; Insall et al. 1979, 1983) (Fig. 6.1). The removal of the cruciate ligaments enabled us to correct deformity, facilitated exposure, and in turn improved fixation of the tibial component by increasing the area of the proximal tibia available for coverage.

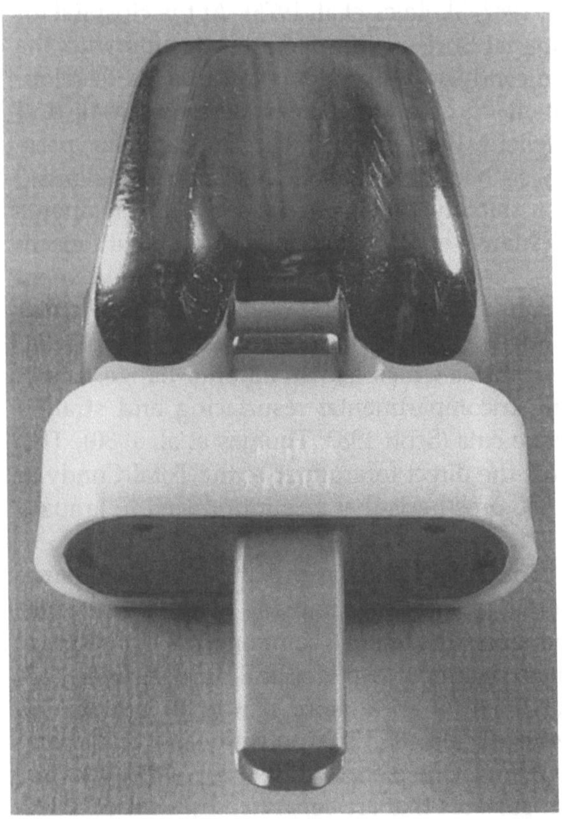

Fig. 6.2. The Insall-Burstein Posterior Stabilized prosthesis.

The Insall-Burstein Posterior Stabilized knee prosthesis (PS) (Fig. 6.2) was introduced in 1978 as a modification of the already successful Total Condylar prosthesis (Insall et al. 1982; Scuderi and Insall 1989). The PS was designed as a posterior cruciate-substituting prosthesis with an intercondylar spine on the tibial component and a transverse cam on the femoral component. In designing this prosthesis the specific aim was to improve stair climbing and range of motion and to prevent posterior subluxation. The interaction between the tibial spine and femoral cam, as well as modification in the center curvature of the prosthesis allowed femoral rollback during flexion. The Posterior Stablized knee prosthesis has an average flexion angle of 115°, a range that has not been surpassed by any posterior cruciate-retaining prosthesis. This in turn allows more normal knee motion. Originally, the Posterior Stabilized tibial component was all polyethylene. A metal backing to the tibial component was added when it was demonstrated that this would transmit the load better to the underlying bone (Bartel et al. 1982)

Surgical Technique

Bone and Soft Tissue Management

The surgical technique has been previously described (Insall et al. 1985; Insall 1981). An anterior midline longitudinal approach allows full exposure of the distal femur and proximal tibia. Soft tissue and ligament releases, to balance the knee in flexion and extension, are performed prior to the bone cuts. It is the intact collateral ligament and not the prosthesis alone which confers stability to the replaced knee. The level of the tibial cut is constant and conservative at a level perpendicular to the long axis of the tibia. The tibial cut should not be lower than 5 mm below the articular surface since tibial cancellous bone weakens as the distance from the joint surface increase (Bartel et al. 1982; Hvid and Hansen 1985).

Resection of the femur follows the tibial resection. The flexion gap produced should be rectangular in shape rather than trapezoidal. This can usually be achieved with adequate soft tissue release. At times, however, it may be necessary to externally rotate the femoral template until it becomes parallel to the cut tibial surface. This results in more bone resection from the posterior medial femoral condyle than the posterior lateral femoral condyle. Up to 20° of rotation is permissible. If it appears that more than 20° of rotation is needed, the medial soft tissue release is probably inadequate. At no time should the femoral template be internally rotated, since this moves the patellofemoral groove of the femoral component medially making it more difficult for the laterally placed patella to capture the groove. Such malrotation of the femoral component may lead to patellar dislocation or subluxation. Once the correct amount of bone is resected and the soft tissue and ligaments are properly balanced, the size of the flexion and extension gaps should be equal.

This ideal limb alignment is 5–10° of valgus. The tibial component should be placed at 90 ± 2° to the long axis of the tibial shaft on both the anteroposterior and lateral radiographs. The ideal placement for the femoral component is 7 ± 2° of valgus angulation on the anteroposterior radiograph and 0–10° of flexion on the lateral view.

To prevent patellar subluxation, or worse, patellar dislocation, care must be paid to patellar tracking at the time of surgery, and when necessary a lateral release or proximal realignment must be done. The lateral retinacular release is performed from the inside out, preserving the lateral superior geniculate artery whenever possible, since sacrificing this vessel has been associated with an increase in patellar ischemia (Scuderi et al. 1987).

The most common cause of patellar dislocation is surgical technique (Merkow et al. 1985). Medial rotation of the femoral implant has been discussed. Internal rotation of the tibial component with respect to the tibia will cause external rotation of the tibia when the knee is reduced, resulting in lateral displacement of the tibial tubercle. This displacement increases the valgus vector and the tendency of the patella to sublux laterally. Correct rotational positioning of the tibial component is best achieved by aligning the intercondylar eminence of the tibial component with the tibial crest in the sagittal plane. Aligning the posterior margin of the tibial component parallel to the posterior margin of the plateau may not position the implant correctly with respect to the insertion of the patellar ligament.

Instrumentation

Instrumentation in total knee arthroplasty has been refined since its early introduction. Most systems use extramedullary tibial guides because of the relative accessibility of the tibia. Intramedullary guides for the femur are popular and have been proven to be accurate provided the femur is not excessively bowed or deformed and the centering hole is properly positioned. A radiograph of the entire femur is needed, so that when the intramedullary guide is used allowances can be made for bowing or deformity. The accuracy of the guide can be affected by the placement of the entry hole in the distal femur, and this can alter the distal femoral cut 2–3° in either direction. The accuracy of the extramedullary femoral guides depends on the precise location of the femoral head. Though this is relatively easy in the thin patient, this can be exceedingly difficult in the obese patient. However, extramedullary guides are beneficial in the presence of femoral shaft deformity, and the ideal system should include the option of intramedullary and extramedullary guides.

Cement Technique

Fixation of methylmethacrylate to the cancellous bony surface is achieved by the irregular configuration of the bony surface and the penetration of the cement into the microstructure of the cancellous bone. Bone preparation is critical in the intrusion of methylmethacrylate into the cancellous bone. Several investigators have studied the optimal depth of cement penetration into the cancellous bone for optimal strength of fixation and viability of bone (Cheal et al. 1985; Krause et al. 1982). Bone viability has been preserved when the methylmethacrylate is no thicker than 1 cm, but 1 cm of cement penetration is not needed for optimal fixation. Two to five millimeters of cement penetration is sufficient for optimal strength of the cement–bone composite (Dorr et al. 1984). This can be easily achieved when the cancellous bony surface is cleansed with the water pik and manually pressurized after the cement is mixed for 3 minutes. The difference in penetration between 1 and 3 minutes is not significant but drops appreciably after 4 minutes (Dorr et al. 1984).

With soft rheumatoid bone, deep cement penetration may occur. On the other hand, with hard sclerotic bone, drill holes at least 6 mm in diameter should be prepared, or else inadequate penetration will occur. Dorr et al. (1984) and Krause et al. (1982) have reported that cement failed within the cement column when the bone was strong, and at the bone–cement interface when the bone was weak.

We presently believe that no more than 1–2 mm of cement penetration into bone is desirable. In recent years infection has been the main cause of failure in total knee arthroplasty. Treatment consists of removal of the implant with all the methylmethacrylate cement, intravenous antibiotics, and second-stage reimplantation after the infection is cured. Excessive penetration of cement into the bone at the time of primary arthroplasty causes excessive loss of bone stock during the bone debridement, compromising reimplantation.

Mechanism of Cement Failure

The results of total knee arthroplasty are closely aligned with surgical technique and are influenced by correct sizing, level of bone resection, level of the joint line, soft tissue balance and, most of all, axial alignment. Based on these determinants there are two schools of thought on the mechanism of loosening. The first believes that micromotion at the bone–cement interface grows ever larger with accompanying loss of bone until the component is grossly loose. The other school argues that the mechanism of failure is due to subsidence, that is, loosening because of bone overload. Overload occurs when the bone itself is very weak and osteoporotic but most often it occurs because of uneven stress. Total knee replacements that loosen do so because of varus malalignment (Windsor et al. 1989). Subsidence has nothing to do with cement fixation or cement technique, although the level of tibial bone resection is important because cancellous bone is weaker farther from the subchondral plate.

Clinical Experience

To the best of our knowledge, the Total Condylar prosthesis is the oldest total knee resurfacing design that has remained unchanged and widely used in its original form. Since 1980 the all polyethylene tibial component has been metal-backed to allow better transfer of load to the underlying subchondral bone. The original review in the first consecutive 220 arthroplasties with the Total Condylar prosthesis reported 137 (62%) excellent; 61 (28%) good; 10 (4.5%) fair and 12 (5.5%) poor results with a follow-up of 3–5 years (Insall et al. 1979). Similar results with longer follow-up, 5–9 years, of the first 100 consecutive replacements also reported 64% excellent, 27% good, 2% fair and 7% poor (Insall et al. 1983). Forty Total Condylar prostheses have been followed for 10 years or more and 35 knees (87.5%) have a satisfactorily functioning arthroplasty (Insall and Kelly 1986). Similar successful results with the Total Condylar prosthesis have been reported by other investigators (Goldberg et al. 1988; Laskin 1981; Ranawat and Boachie-Adjei 1988). In the 15 years since the Total Condylar prosthesis has been used, there have been many modifications to the basic concept leading to the introduction of the Posterior Stabilized prosthesis. Clinical experience and published data demonstrate similar and very satisfactory clinical results.

Since its introduction there was concern that the increase in constraint with the Posterior Stabilized prosthesis might increase stress at the bone–cement interface resulting in a higher rate of loosening. Clinically this has proven not to be the case (Scott et al. 1988; Vince et al. 1988a,b). Stress analysis using finite element methods support these clinical findings that the maximum tensile and compressive stresses under the plateau are no higher in the Posterior Stabilized prosthesis than in a prosthesis of similar geometry without the stabilized cam

(Bartel et al. 1982). The Knee Service at the Hospital for Special Surgery performed 1951 knee arthroplasties between 1974 and 1985. Three hundred and twenty-six were the Total Condylar design and six (1.8%) had tibial loosening. More recently between 1978 and 1985, 1625 Posterior Stabilized prostheses were implanted, and only three (0.18%) had tibial loosening. The difference is probably accounted for by better technique in the later cases and longer follow-up in the Total Condylar series (Insall 1988). Furthermore, since we began implanting metal-backed tibial components, we have not had to revise a knee for tibial loosening.

The relative conformity between the cup-shaped tibial articulation and the curved femoral condyles better distributes the load (Insall 1984, p. 587) and reduces the high stresses of point contact on the polyethylene tibial component. The contact point of the femoral and tibial components in this design is located centrally over each tibial condyle. This contact point does not change appreciably when varus or valgus motion is applied to the knee, avoiding edge loading (Burstein 1984). Retrieval of total condylar tibial components have shown greater damage than acetabular cups from failed total hips (Hood et al. 1981). However, it has not been possible to detect by clinical or radiographic means signs of polyethylene wear, and to date polyethylene wear does not seem to be a clinical problem.

Recently, attention has been directed to restoration of the joint line and patellar height (Laskin and Matson 1987). It is possible to have an ideally aligned knee in which the position of the prosthetic knee joint is different than that of the natural knee. As a result, the optimal length-tension relationship of the quadriceps and hamstrings is not achieved.

Several clinical situations can ococur in which the joint line height is altered from normal. Preoperatively, for instance, if the patient has a patella baja, the joint line is functionally elevated. Even more important, if at surgery the femoral component is placed too far anteriorly or is undersized in the anteroposterior dimension, a large flexion gap will be created. In order to balance the collateral ligaments in extension, more bone would have to be resected from the distal femur. This would result in the necessity of a thicker tibial component, thereby raising the joint line and lowering the patellar height. In the patient with a severe valgus deformity, there may be elongation of the medial collateral ligament. When the elongated medial structures and released lateral structures are balanced, a large extension gap is formed and this too would require a thick tibial component with elevation of the joint line.

Restoration of the joint line is more critical in the posterior cruciate retaining prostheses than in the Posterior Stabilized prostheses (Figgie et al. 1986). In this former group the posterior cruciate ligament has to be properly balanced in order to achieve a good range of motion. In a recent study using the Posterior Stabilized knee, the average joint line elevation was 5.6 mm. This had no clinical correlation with clinical function or patellofemoral performance (Faris et al. 1987). This therefore is one of the advantages in using a Posterior Stabilized prosthesis for total knee replacement.

For a clinical evaluation of the first 118 Posterior Stabilized knees followed for 2–4 years we reported 88% excellent, 9% good or fair and 3% poor results (Insall et al. 1982). More recent follow-up of 96 knees followed 8 years longer revealed 79.2% excellent, 16.7% good and 4.2% poor results. Though there was a slight deterioration of excellent results with time, these results still showed a marked improvement in postoperative function when compared with our results using other prostheses (Vince et al. 1988a,b).

The Posterior Stabilized prosthesis has been successfully applied to various conditions about the osteoarthritic and rheumatoid arthritic knee. For example, the results of knee arthroplasty using the Posterior Stabilized prosthesis in a small series of patients with Charcot and Charcot-like joints has been good to excellent, with a follow-up of 3 years (Soudry et al. 1986). Preoperatively, ligamentous laxity and bone loss created severe instability in these patients. The inherent stability in flexion of the Posterior Stabilized prosthesis was an advantage. In another series with posttraumatic arthritis, the Posterior Stabilized prosthesis had 90% excellent to good results over an average of 4 years (Zelicof et al. 1988). In still another study the Posterior Stabilized prosthesis yielded 86% excellent and good results in osteonecrotic knees with a 4-year follow-up (Stern et al. 1988).

The survivorship method of analysis was applied to 1430 cemented primary total knee arthroplasties performed by the Knee Service between 1974 and 1986 (Scuderi et al. 1989). This included 224 Total Condylar prostheses with a polyethylene tibial component (implanted from 1974 to 1978), 289 Posterior Stabilized prostheses with an all polyethylene tibial component (implanted from 1978 to 1981), and 917 Posterior Stabilized prostheses with a metal-backed tibial component (implanted from 1981 to 1986).

There were twelve failures in the Total Condylar series with an average annual failure rate of 0.65% and a 15 year overall success rate of 90.6%. Failure in the Total Condylar series included three infections, four loose tibial components, two loose femoral and tibial components, two unstable arthroplasties and one femoral supracondylar fracture. There were no reported revisions after 9 years.

The Posterior Stabilized prosthesis with the polyethylene tibia demonstrated six failures with an average annual failure rate of 0.27% and a 10 year overall success rate of 97.3%. Failure included two loose tibial components, three loose femoral components and one tibial stress fracture.

The Posterior Stabilized prosthesis with the metal-backed tibia demonstrated seven failures with an average annual failure rate of 0.19% and a 7 year overall success rate of 98.75%. The failures in the metal-backed Posterior Stabilized group were six infections and one loose femoral component. No metal-backed tibial components were revised for loosening. The incidence of femoral loosening requiring revision was 0.89% in the Total Condylar Group and 0.33% in the combined Posterior Stabilized group.

The overall incidence of infection for all total knee replacements was 0.63%. The overall success was comparable between knees with a diagnosis of osteoarthritis and rheumatoid arthritis. Patient sex, age and percentage of ideal body weight did not influence the overall survival.

Comparing our survivorship data with that from recent studies using the same endpoint for failure revealed similar results. Knutson et al. (1985) reported a 5 year overall survival rate of 100% for tricompartmental prostheses, and in a nationwide multicenter study of 8000 knees, a 6 year overall survival rate of 90% for similar prostheses (Knutson et al. 1986). The results with our implants do appear better than some earlier designs. Though some of these prostheses are outdated, they do allow a long-term experience against which newer designs can be judged. Tew, Waugh and Forster (1985) reported a 6 year overall survival of 72% with 365 replacements using the Freeman, Sheehan and Manchester prostheses (Tew and Waugh 1982). Lewallen, Bryan and Peterson (1984) reported a 10 year overall survival of 66% with the polycentric total knee. The longevity of our three prostheses is much better than the hinged arthroplasties. Grimer, Karpinski and Edwards (1984) reported a 7 year overall survival of 80% and Lettin et al. (1984) an 8 year overall survival of 83% for the Stanmore Hinged Prosthesis. Knutson, Lindstrand and Lidgren (1986) reported a 6 year overall survival of 75% with the Guepar Prosthesis.

The appearance and distribution of radiolucencies do not seem to differ between the Posterior Stabilized and the Total Condylar prostheses. The original experience with the Total Condylar prosthesis demonstrated a 36% incidence of incomplete tibial radiolucent lines at 5 years (Insall and Kelly 1986), whereas radiolucencies were observed in 32% of the Posterior Stabilized prostheses at 2–4 years (Insall et al. 1982). Although there may be concern that the incidence of radiolucent lines would increase with time, this does not seem to be the case. Further longer follow-up of the Total Condylar prostheses at 10 years and the Posterior Stabilized at 8 years demonstrated radiolucencies in only one-third of the cases (Insall and Kelly 1986; Vince et al. 1988a,b).

In conclusion, cemented total knee replacement is a reliable and predictable procedure withstanding the test of time and should be the "gold standard" against which alternate means of fixation are compared. There have been improvements in total knee replacement, but it can be best attributed to improved technique. Presently at the Hospital for Special Surgery the Total Condylar and the Posterior Stabilized prostheses are implanted and both are cruciate excising designs. Both prostheses are reporting similar and very successful results.

Based on the success with the original design of the Posterior Stabilized prosthesis, it has been modified to the Insall-Burstein Posterior

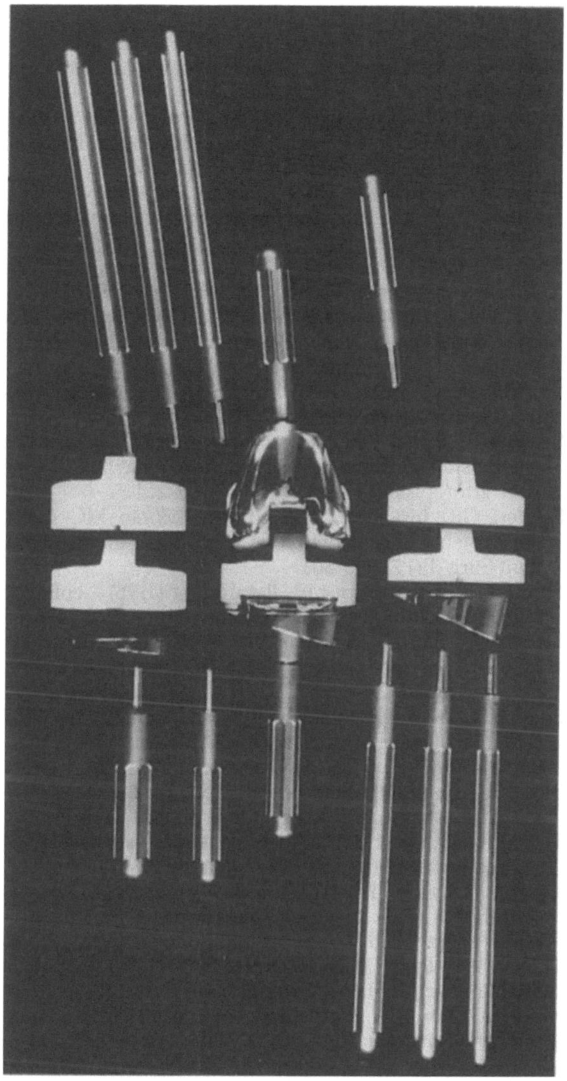

Fig. 6.3. The Insall-Burstein Posterior Stabilized modular II system.

Stabilized II (Fig. 6.3). This is a completely modular system with the ability to modify the prosthesis at the time of surgery, depending on individual needs. Available in this design are optional stems for both the femur and tibia, metal augmentations for the femur and metal wedges for the tibia. Polyethylene tibial inserts of various thicknesses are interchangeable on a metal tibial tray and have the capability of being a standard Posterior Stabilized or Constrained Condylar design. Further changes have included a wider range of component sizes to accommodate the individual patient and deepening the patellar groove on the anterior flange of the femoral component in order to improve patellar tracking.

References

Bargren JH, Freeman MAR, Swanson SAV, Todd RC (1976) ICLH (Freeman/Swanson) arthroplasty in the treatment of arthritic knee. A 2 to 4 year review. Clin Orthop 120:65–75

Bartel DL, Burstein AH, Santavicca EA, Insall JN (1982) Performance of the tibial component in total knee replacement. Conventional and revision designs. J Bone Joint Surg (Am) 64:1026–1033

Burstein AH (1984) Biomechanics of the knee. In: Insall JN (ed) Surgery of the knee. Churchill Livingstone, New York, pp 21–39

Cheal EJ, Hayes WC, Lee CH, Snyder BD, Miller J (1985) Stress analysis of a condylar knee tibial component: Influence of metaphyseal shell properties and cement injection depth. J Orthop Res 3:424–434

Coventry MB (1979) Two-part total knee arthroplasty: Evolution and present status. Clin Orthop 114:29–36

Coventry MB, Upshaw JE, Riley LH, Finerman GAM, Turner RH (1973) Geometric total knee arthroplasty. II. Patient data and complications. Clin Orthop 94:177–184

Dorr LD, Lindberg JP, Claude-Faugere M, Malluche HH (1984) Factors influencing the intrusion of methylmethacrylate into human tibiae. Clin Orthop 183:147–152

Ewald FC, Jacobs MA, Miegel RE et al. (1984) Kinematic total knee replacement. J Bone Joint Surg (Am) 66:1032–1040

Faris PM, Insall JN, Stern SH (1987) Patellar symptoms in the posterior stabilized knee: A critical analysis. Presented at the 69th Annual Meeting of the Alumni Association, The Hospital for Special Surgery, New York

Figgie HE III, Goldberg VM, Heiple KG, Moller HS, Gordon NH (1986) The influence of tibial-patellofemoral location on function of the knee in patients with the posterior stabilized condylar knee prosthesis. J Bone Joint Surg (Am) 68:1035–1040

Freeman MAR, Swanson SAV, Zahir A (1972) Total replacement of knee using metal-polyethylene two-part prosthesis. Proc R Soc Med 65:374–375

Freeman MAR, Todd RC, Bamert P, Day WH (1978) ICLH arthroplasty of the knee: 1968–1977. J Bone Joint Surg (Br) 60:339–344

Goldberg VM, Henderson BT (1980) The Freeman-Swanson ICLH total knee arthroplasty. Complications and problems. J Bone Joint Surg (Am) 62:1338–1344

Goldberg VM, Figgie MP, Figgie HE III, Heiple KG, Sobel M (1988) Use of a total condylar knee prosthesis for treatment of osteoarthritis and rheumatoid arthritis. J Bone Joint Surg (Am) 70:802–811

Grimer RJ, Karpinski MRK, Edwards AN (1984) The long-term results of Stanmore total knee replacements. J Bone Joint Surg (Br) 66:55–62

Gunston FH (1971) Polycentric knee arthroplasty. Prosthetic simulation of normal knee movement. J Bone Joint Surg (Br) 53:272–277

Hood RW, Wright TM, Burstein AH, Insall JN (1981) Retrieval analysis of seventy total condylar knee prostheses. Orthop Trans 5:319

Hungerford DS, Krackow KA, Kenna RV (1987) Two- to-five-year experience with a cementless porous-coated total knee prosthesis. In: Rand JA, Dorr LD (eds) Total arthroplasty of the knee. Proceedings of the Knee Society, 1985–1986. Aspen, Rockville, pp 215–235

Hunter JA, Zoma AA, Scullion JE et al. (1982) The geometric knee replacement in polyarthritis. J Bone Joint Surg (Br) 64:95–98

Hvid I, Hansen SL (1985) Trabecular bone strength patterns at the proximal tibial epiphysis. J Orthop Res 3:464–472

Insall JN (1981) Technique of total knee replacement. In: Instructional course lectures, the American Academy of Orthopaedic Surgeons, vol 30. CV Mosby, St. Louis, pp 324–334

Insall JN (1984) Total knee replacement. In: Insall JN (ed) Surgery of the knee. Churchill Livingstone, New York, pp 587–695

Insall JN (1988) Presidential address to the Knee Society. Choices and compromises in total knee arthroplasty. Clin Orthop 226:43–48

Insall J, Aglietti P (1980) A five to seven-year follow-up of unicondylar arthroplasty. J Bone Joint Surg (Am) 62:1329–1337

Insall JN, Kelly M (1986) The total condylar prosthesis. Clin Orthop 205:43–48

Insall JN, Ranawat CS, Aglietti P, Shine J (1976) A comparison of four models of total knee-replacement prostheses. J Bone Joint Surg (Am) 58:754–765

Insall J, Scott WN, Ranawat CS (1979) The total condylar knee prosthesis. A report of two hundred and twenty cases. J Bone Joint Surg (Am) 61:173–180

Insall JN, Lachiewicz PF, Burstein AH (1982) The posterior stabilized condylar prosthesis: A modification of the total condylar design. J Bone Joint Surg (Am) 64:1317–1320

Insall JN, Hodd RW, Flawn LB, Sullivan DJ (1983) The total condylar knee prosthesis in gonarthrosis. A five to nine-year follow-up of the first one hundred consecutive replacements. J Bone Joint Surg (Am) 65:619–628

Insall JN, Burstein AH, Freeman MAR (1985) Principles and techniques of knee replacement. (Brochures) Zimmer, Warsaw, Indiana; Johnson and Johnson, New Brunswick, New Jersey

Knutson K, Tjornstrand B, Lidgren L (1985) Survival of knee arthroplasties for rheumatoid arthritis. Acta Orthop Scand 56:422–425

Knutson K, Lindstrand A, Lidgren L (1986) Survival of knee arthroplasties. A nationwide multicentre investigation of 8000 cases. J Bone Joint Surg (Br) 68:795–803

Krause WR, Krug W, Eng B, Miller J (1982) Strength of the cement–bone interface. Clin Orthop 163:290–299

Laskin RS (1981) Total condylar knee replacement in rheumatoid arthritis. A review of one hundred and seventeen knees. J Bone Joint Surg (Am) 63:29–35

Laskin RS, Matson F (1987) The influence of joint line position during total knee replacement. Orthop Trans 11:535

Lettin AWF, Kavanagh TG, Craig D, Scales JT (1984) Assessment of the survival and the clinical results of Stanmore total knee replacements. J Bone Joint Surg (Br) 66:355–361

Lewallen DG, Bryan RS, Peterson LFA (1984) Polycentric total knee arthroplasty. A ten-year follow-up study. J Bone Joint Surg (Am) 66:1211–1218

Merkow RL, Soudry M, Insall JN (1985) Patellar dislocation following total knee replacement. J Bone Joint Surg (Am) 67:1321–1327

Ranawat CS, Boachie-Adjei O (1988) Survivorship analysis and results of total condylar knee arthroplasty. Eight- to 11-year follow-up period. Clin Orthop 226:6–13

Ranawat CS, Insall J, Shine J (1976) Duo-condylar knee arthroplasty. Hospital for Special Surgery design. Clin Orthop 120:76–82

Scott RD (1982) Duopatellar total knee replacement: the Brigham experience. Orthop Clin Am 13:89–102

Scott WN, Rubinstein MA, Scuderi G (1988) Results after knee replacement with a posterior cruciate substituting prosthesis. J Bone Joint Surg (Am) 70:1163–1173

Scuderi GR, Insall JN (1989) The posterior stabilized knee prosthesis. Orthop Clin Am 20(1):71–78

Scuderi G, Scharf SC, Meltzer LP, Scott WN (1987) The relationship of lateral releases to patella viability in total knee arthroplasty. J Arthroplasty 2:209–214

Scuderi GR, Insall JN, Windsor RE, Moran MC (1989) Survivorship of cemented total knee replacement. J Bone Joint Surg (Br) 71:798–803

Skolnick MD, Coventry MB, Ilstrup DM (1976) Geometric total knee arthroplasty. J Bone Joint Surg (Am)58:749–753

Sledge CB, Stern P, Thomas WH et al. (1978) Two-year follow-up of the duocondylar total knee replacement. Orthop Trans 2:193

Soudry M, Binazzi R, Johanson NA, Bullough PG, Insall JN (1986) Total knee arthroplasty in Charcot and Charcot-like joints. Clin Orthop 208:199–204

Stern SH, Insall JN, Windsor RE (1988) Total knee arthroplasty in osteonecrotic knees. Orthop Trans 12:722

Tew M, Waugh W (1982) Estimating the survival time of knee replacements. J Bone Joint Surg (Br) 64:579–582

Tew M, Waugh W, Forster IW (1985) Comparing the results of different types of knee replacement. A method proposed and applied. J Bone Joint Surg (Br) 67:775–779

Thomas WH, Ewald FC, Poss R, Sledge CB (1980) Duopatella total knee arthroplasty. Orthop Trans 4:329–330

Vince KG, Insall JN (1988) Long-term results of cemented total knee arthroplasty. Orthop Clin N Am 19:575–580

Vince KG, Kelly MA, Insall JN (1988a) Posterior stabilized and total condylar knee arthroplasties: Comparative long-term survivorship analysis. Presented at the American Academy of Orthopaedic Surgeons Annual Meeting, Atlanta, Georgia

Vince KG, Kelly MA, Insall JN (1988b) The posterior stabilized knee prosthesis: follow-up five to eight years. Orthop Trans 12:157

Windsor RE, Scuderi GR, Insall JN, Moran MC (1989) Mechanisms of failure of the femoral and tibial components in total knee arthroplasty. Presented at the Annual Meeting of the Knee Society, Las Vegas, Nevada

Zelicof SB, Scuderi GR, Vince KG, Urs WK, Insall JN (1988) Total knee arthroplasty in post-traumatic arthroplasty. Orthop Trans 12:54–7

Chapter 7

The Total Condylar Knee Prosthesis

Kelly G. Vince and John N. Insall

Introduction

Few topics in the orthopaedic literature have become more boring or contentious than the recitation of good surgical results, especially when a prosthetic device is involved. Nonetheless, these devices and the operations devised for them must be assessed. This type of clinical research should identify the *principles* of the design and surgical technique to determine whether they should be abandoned, retained or enhanced.

Many aspects of these reconstructions are controversial – does the experience with a prosthesis contribute to the resolution of the controversy or to the stronger entrenchment of both camps? Furthermore, what do the previously published results for a prosthesis actually mean? While studies with long-term follow-up have been held in the highest esteem, just how valid are current results of surgery done according to the practices of over a decade ago. What can we learn by comparing results from different institutions and surgeons? Do they corroborate each other? Are there similar or different shortcomings with each study? In this spirit, we discuss what has been reported to date about the Total Condylar knee prosthesis, from the Hospital for Special Surgery where it was developed and from independent institutions. This prosthesis occupies a significant spot in the history of knee arthroplasty and is still in clinical use.

Knee Arthroplasty before the Total Condylar Prosthesis

Early attempts at arthroplasty date back to the nineteenth century when a variety of interpositional materials were implanted, from pig-bladder (Insall 1984) and fascia lata (Campbell 1931; Miller and Friedman 1952; Speed and Trout 1949) to gold (Jones 1908; Walker 1977) cellophane and nylon (Haberman 1986). Influenced by Smith-Petersen's cup arthroplasties of the hip (Smith-Petersen 1939), Dr Willis Campbell implanted a contoured vitallium plate on the femoral condyles of two patients whose knees were ankylosed following acute pyogenic infectious arthritis. Fixation consisted of two triangular flanges that hooked into the posterior femoral condyles and a screw that was placed in the bone anteriorly. While restoration of motion was poor, and only one articular surface was substituted, this was in concept the first resurfacing knee arthroplasty (Campbell 1940).

Interpositional tibial components, made first of acrylic by MacIntosh (1958, 1966) and then of metal by McKeever (1960) generally improved the function of patients with rheumatoid arthritis, but pain relief, correction of deformity and restoration of stability could not reliably be achieved (Ranawat et al. 1973). Up to this point the problem of fixation had been avoided by "self retention". In McKeever's words, this means the prosthesis "must be so designed and inserted that the normal forces existing in the joint in action hold it in place. Any screw, pin, flange or other retention device that functions as anything more than a guide to alignment or to retention of the prosthesis when the joint is at rest must eventually give way as a result of cyclic stress" (McKeever 1960).

Having worked with Charnley, who was using methylmethacrylate cement for fixation of hip arthroplasties, Gunston returned to Canada and developed the "polycentric knee arthroplasty". It surpassed the interpositional arthroplasties of McKeever and MacIntosh by resurfacing both the tibial and femoral surfaces, using methylmethacrylate fixation. Several important principles of normal knee function were incorporated into the polycentric design. As the name implies, the polycentric allowed the knee to function according to the mechanics of "multiple instant centers of rotation," whereby the center of rotation moves posteriorly as the knee flexes. Axial rotation in full extension, a part of the "screw-home mechanism", was also permitted by the polycentric arthroplasty. At about 10° of flexion, axial rotation in the normal knee ceases and the femur moves over the tibia with a "rocking" motion. This then changes to a "sliding motion" at about 20° of flexion. The hinged arthroplasties, first introduced in the 1950s, only permitted motion around a single, fixed axis. This was the single most important factor leading to their frequent failure and universal abandonment. The Gunston polycentric was a generally sound design, with unconstrained kinematics and methylmethacrylate fixation, but required a demanding surgical technique (Gunston 1971).

The evolutionary continuum of the polycentric arthroplasty, permitting complex natural knee kinematics, is probably best exemplified by the modern unicompartmental arthroplasties. Because of early dissatisfaction with the clinical results of unicompartmental replacement at the Hospital for Special Surgery, however, research there concentrated on the development of a bicondylar type of replacement. The paper reflecting this decision has been criticized for several reasons, especially the inclusion of patients with patellectomies (Insall and Aglietti 1980). This does not detract from the excellent results obtained by others with unicondylar designs, perhaps by using more limited indications for implantation, (limited disease, less deformity, intact patellofemoral joint) (Laskin 1978; Marmor 1985; Scott and Santore 1981).

The other developmental branch of knee arthroplasty, based on the concept of retaining both cruciate ligaments and using a prosthesis in which medial and lateral components were joined, was embodied by the geometric prosthesis. Following several years' experience with the polycentric, the geomedic research group developed a prosthesis in 1971 that had single piece tibial and femoral components. The early history of this device has been recorded by Coventry (1979). Methylmethacrylate fixation was used and the articular geometry of the prosthesis was more conforming than the polycentric had been. Loosening of the tibial component occurred frequently and was attributed in part to a phenomenon that has been described as "kinematic conflict" (Insall 1984), a situation in which the motion permitted by the articular surfaces is at variance with that which the cruciate ligaments dictate. During flexion, the posterior aspects of the prosthesis would bind and impart large forces to the cement and bone. The geometric prosthesis eventually evolved through several stages, designated Mark I through IV and culminating with the Anametric in the later 1970s (Finerman et al. 1979). By that time it resembled many contemporary resurfacing arthroplasties with less conformity and more inherent laxity than the geometric (Markolf et al. 1981).

Freeman and associates in London introduced the ICLH prosthesis in 1970. It was characterized as a "roller in a trough", with the femoral component functioning as the roller. Despite other problems, the design demonstrated the feasibility, and some of the advantages of cruciate ligament excision (Freeman et al. 1972).

In 1972, Charles Townley (1985) designed a resurfacing arthroplasty that was unconstrained and roughly anatomic in its surface geometry. He implanted the device retaining both the anterior and posterior cruciate ligaments. Mallory (1982) later reported a series of these prostheses that were adapted for use with excision of both cruciate ligaments, thus resembling the Total Condylar concept. Experience with the UCI knee arthroplasty lead to the conclusion that problems with tibial component loosening resulted from nonmetal-backed, thin polyethylene that was subject to deformity, breakage and subsidence (Ducheyne et al. 1978; Hamilton 1982).

By the time the Total Condylar was introduced in 1974, the concept of replacing articular cartilage with metal and plastic was a decade old and the advantages of resurfacing both sides of the joint had been established. Methylmethacrylate cement had been used successfully in both the hip and knee, and some of the most important aspects of knee kinematics were recognized. Chrome cobalt had proven biologically compatible (Venable and Stuck 1938), and had satisfactory wear resistance. Sacrifice of both cruciate ligaments facilitated the surgery and stable arthroplasties with this technique had already been performed for several years. Similarly, knee arthroplasty with preservation of cruciate ligaments had also enjoyed early success. In general though, by 1970 a design was needed that could: (a) provide more durable tibial fixation with a simplified surgical procedure, (b) restore stability, (c) correct deformity, and (d) resurface the patello-femoral joint (Insall et al. 1976a). The importance of valgus tibial-femoral alignment was not appreciated until the mid 1970s, (Lotke and Ecker 1977) and soft tissue techniques for correction of deformity had not been developed.

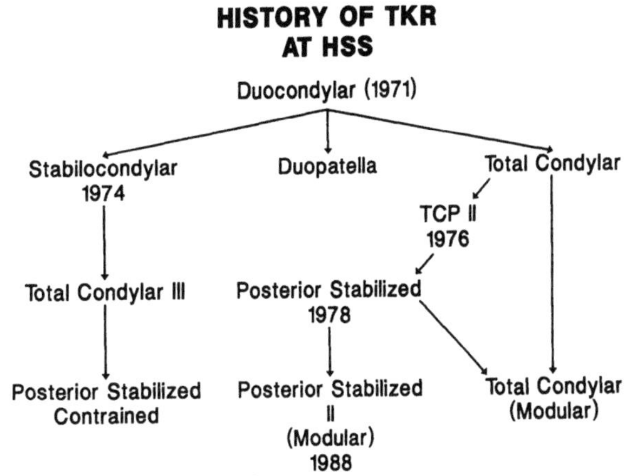

Fig. 7.1. History of total knee replacement at the Hospital for Special Surgery. The duocondylar prosthesis (effectively two unicondylar arthroplasties linked together) led to the Duopatella and the Total Condylar designs. The former retained the posterior cruciate ligament, and the Total Condylar, with a more conforming articulation was implanted after cruciate ligament sacrifice. Both provided for resurfacing of the patellofemoral joint. The Duopatella design was not pursued at the Hospital for Special Surgery, but was developed into the kinematic prosthesis at the Brigham Hospital in Boston.

The TCP II was designed to provide posterior stabilization to the Total Condylar. It became the Insall-Burstein Posterior Stabilized prosthesis in 1978, after substantial modification. The Posterior Stabilized and Total Condylar designs have been introduced in modular formats.

Mechanical substitution for absent collateral ligaments was initially attempted with the stabilocondylar. Refinements of this design resulted in the Total Condylar III and the Constrained Condylar prosthesis.

Design of the Total Condylar at the Hospital for Special Surgery

The Total Condylar was conceived from the outset as part of a system of progressively more constrained implants (Insall et al. 1979b) (Fig. 7.1). The developers of the Total Condylar prosthesis were influenced by the previous designs as has been recounted in excellent historical narratives (Ranawat and Sculco 1985; Walker 1985). The experience at the Hospital for Special Surgery from the mid sixties to mid seventies with unicondylar, duocondylar, geometric and Guepar prostheses was reviewed in a seminal paper (Insall et al. 1976a). Ironically, the Guepar prosthesis gave the best results of all in this early follow-up despite the fact that it was used to reconstruct the most severely affected knees. Soon after, however, the high loosening and infection rate of the Guepar and other linked hinges became apparent (Jones et al. 1979). The duocondylar device was the most kinematically anatomical, but lacked inherent stability (Ranawat et al. 1976). It was essentially two unicondylar devices with bars linking the medial and lateral sides of the tibial and femoral components. The geometric prosthesis was more conforming and thus more stable, but aforementioned problems with "kinematic conflict" were eventually recognized (Insall 1984). Both the duocondylar and geometric prostheses preserved cruciate ligaments, but neither enabled resurfacing of the patellofemoral joint. While no Freeman-Swanson ICLH prostheses had been included in the study, the "four models" manuscript discussed how it would be implanted with an easier technique due to sacrifice of the cruciate ligaments and by making only flat bone cuts (Insall et al. 1976a). This concept was not lost on the developers of the Total Condylar who incorporated these features of the ICLH (Ranawat and Sculco 1985). The absence of stability in the medial-lateral plane, no patellofemoral resurfacing and inadequate tibial component fixation were shortcomings of the ICLH that were improved in the Total Condylar prosthesis.

Walker described two designs that emerged from this period of clinical experience and laboratory investigation: the Duopatella and Total Condylar (Behrens et al. 1974; Hsieh and Walker 1976; Walker 1977, 1985; Walker and Hajeck 1972; Walker and Hsieh 1977; Walker et al. 1976). The former had low, nonconforming geometry and cruciate ligament retention. It was implanted with flat bone cuts and offered the option of resurfacing the patellofemoral joint (Inglis and Lane 1978). The Total Condylar, distinguished by cruciate ligament sacrifice and more conforming geometry, was the product of specific design goals formulated in 1973–74; and stated by Walker (1985):

1. Replacement of all the condylar bearing surfaces to provide defined and reproducible artificial joint surfaces.
2. Straight cuts on the bone to allow accurate component fittings, accurate alignment, and correct tensioning of collateral ligaments and capsular soft tissues in extension and flexion.
3. Femoral-tibial geometry which provided adequate stability in the anteroposterior plane and in rotation by the "uphill principle".
4. Femoral-tibial geometry which was partially conforming to allow some laxity.
5. Sufficient femoral-tibial conformity to provide reasonable areas of contact on the plastic and avoid the high stresses of point contact so that final stability would be provided by a combination of the joint surfaces and soft tissues.
6. Close to anatomic geometry in the frontal and sagittal planes to allow compatibility with remaining ligaments and other soft tissues and to obtain normal muscle lever arms.
7. Enhanced tibial fixation by a one-piece plastic component which covered most of the tibial surface, augmented by a central peg.
8. A central peg on the tibial component which alone could provide complete fixation to shear forces and torques, even if the upper surfaces were not fixed.
9. Cement fixation for taking up areas of lack of fit between the components and the bone, for broad transmission of load to the entire joint surfaces, and for elimination of micromotion.

Kinematics and Mechanical Testing

The term "Total Condylar" thus designated a specific prosthesis that was developed and introduced to clinical practice at the Hospital for Special Surgery in New York in 1974 (Fig. 7.2). The term eventually became a generic designation for an entire class of prostheses that are, generally speaking, semiconstrained knee resurfacing designs. The Total Condylar femoral component is somewhat anatomically shaped when viewed laterally, especially in comparison with other designs of the time. The radius of curvature on the posterior femoral condyle is tighter than anteriorly. Consequently, the distal femoral condyle, which makes contact with the tibial component in extension, is more conforming. This was expected to be more stable and reduce wear. As flexion progresses and the smaller radius curvature comes into contact with the tibia, some rotary and sagittal sliding motions are permitted.

The anterior femoral component has a flange over which the polyethylene patellar dome rides. This design of the dome was derived from the experience with a vitallium patellar arthroplasty at the Hospital for Special Surgery (Aglietti et al. 1975) (Fig. 7.3) and elsewhere (McKeever 1955) for the treatment of patellofemoral arthritis. The dome is symmetric to facilitate rotational positioning at surgery.

The tibial articular surface is cupped to receive the femoral component. An intercondylar eminence provides medial lateral stability as do the tibial spines in a normal knee. With this geometry, considerable force is required to drive the femoral condyles out of the wells in the tibial plastic. The greater the excursion, the more the femoral condyle has to ride uphill and overcome progressively increasing tension in the collateral ligaments. A similar mechanism exists in the

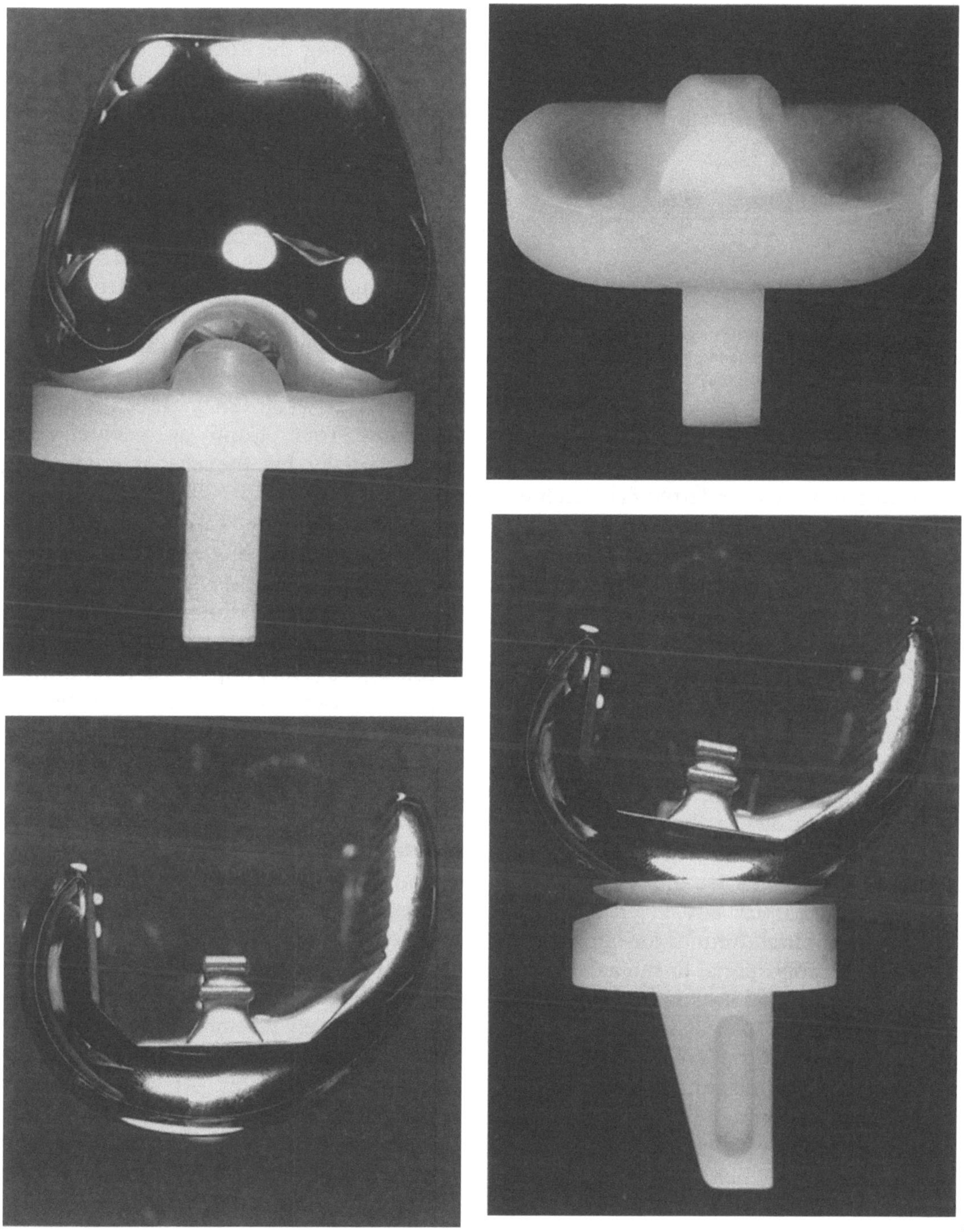

a b c d

Fig. 7.2a–d. The Total Condylar prosthesis. **a** Anterior view articulated prosthesis. The distal end of each femoral condyle is a half circle with a short arc radius. The tibial component has wells on each condyle that conform to the femur. An intercondylar eminence on the tibial component provides medial-lateral stability. **b** Lateral view, femoral component. The radius of curvature on the component is tighter posteriorly, such that the distal articular surface is flatter and the arthroplasty is more stable in extension. The grooved anterior femoral flange is for texturing of the cement mantle. Two fixation lugs are present on the distal femoral articulation. **c** All polyethylene tibial component. The conforming wells on each tibial condyle are the basis for the "uphill mechanism" of stability. As the femoral component is displaced, the collateral ligaments tense and laxity decreases. **d** Lateral view of articulated tibial and femoral components. The conformity between the femoral and tibial articulations is apparent from the seating of the femoral condyle in the tibial wells. This increased conformity with reduced point loading may decrease polyethylene wear. No posterior slope was built into this original design. Relative hyperextension of the components will be necessary for the patient to achieve full extension of the knee joint if the tibial bone cut is sloped posteriorly and the femoral component is implanted with some flexion. A hyperextension stop would increase the risk of loosening.

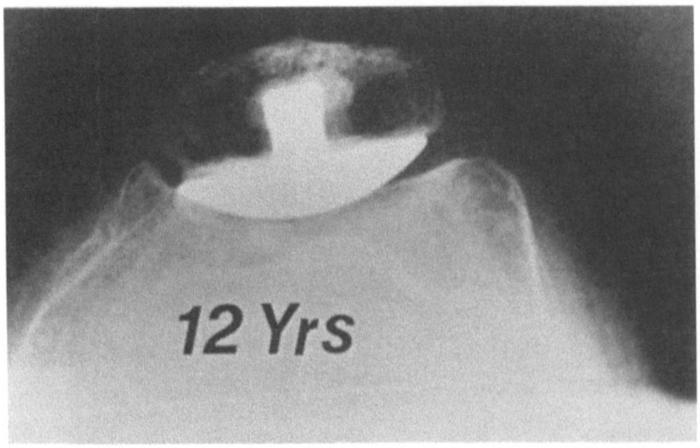

Fig. 7.3. The Hospital for Special Surgery vitallium patellar resurfacing. This prosthesis was abandoned, but the design was rendered in polyethylene for the Total Condylar arthroplasty.

normal knee (Hseih and Walker 1976). In prostheses where the cruciate ligament is preserved, a flatter tibial geometry is preferred (Thatcher et al. 1987) to avoid kinematic conflict (Fig. 7.4). The great theoretical concern about flatter tibial polyethylene is that the components make contact over a much smaller surface area resulting in far greater contact stresses and increased wear. This has not been demonstrated in clinical studies as yet (Insall 1984).

Werner and associates (1978) evaluated the transmission of torque across various knee prostheses in a laboratory setting. They found that next to the Geometric device, the Total Condylar required the most torque to rotate the tibial component relative to the femoral component. They also found that for any given angle of rotation, the transmitted torques for nonhinged prostheses were proportional to the axial load. Their study was based on the concern that more conforming geometry, such as is necessary for the "uphill mechanism" could result in transmitted torques of sufficient magnitude to contribute to component loosening. This theoretical concern would now seem inconsequential for the Total Condylar prosthesis in light of clinical experience (Schurman et al. 1987; Vince and Insall 1988; Vince et al. 1987, 1989). The converse side of this issue is apparent from Wang and Walker's (1974) observation of permanent ligament stretching after repeated testing of cadaver knees for rotatory laxity. While the fear is that greater conformity may lead to failure of component fixation, prostheses with nonconforming geometry transmit correspondingly greater stresses to ligaments that can lead to plastic deformation and joint instability.

Thatcher and colleagues performed in vitro tests of the inherent laxity of several knee prostheses, including the Total Condylar. Stability, expressed as force-displacement curves, was measured while varying amounts of compression were applied across the arthroplasties in a specially constructed simulator. One of the points made by these investigators should be considered axiomatic in the design of knee prostheses: "ideally, the implanted prosthesis should compensate for anatomic structures that are deficient or removed in the procedure, and thus restore what would be the normal laxity characteristics and kinematics for that particular knee" (Thatcher et al. 1987). Thus, the relatively conforming Total Condylar geometry substitutes partially for the absent cruciate ligaments.

A previous study by Walker and Hsieh (1977) had shown the stabilizing effect of compressive loads across prosthetic devices, concluding that large loads rendered the prostheses less lax (more stable) than a normal knee. Shoemaker and colleagues (1982) implanted Total Condylar prostheses in cadaver knees and then mechanically tested laxity. They also demonstrated that knees with a Total Condylar implant displayed significantly greater decreases in anteroposterior and torsional laxity than did intact knees. They attributed this to increased congruency between the articulating components, friction between the metal and plastic and possible indentation of the femoral runners into the polyethylene tibial component. The knees with Total Condylar implants under compressive loads had stability curves that closely resembled the isolated Total Condylar components for small displacements about the neutral point. At large excursions, however, isolated components subluxed while cadaver ligaments imparted constraint to the implanted specimens. This mechanical bench test largely confirmed the "uphill mechanism" inherent in the Total Condylar design by an independent laboratory. This study by Shoemaker and colleagues as well as an earlier one by the same group, also identified the phenomenon of "condylar rock-off". When varus or valgus loads are applied to a knee, the condyle opposite the force is distracted and eventually "rocks-off" (Markolf et al 1981). Compression across the joint, however, raises the magnitude of varus-valgus moment necessary to create rock-off. At a

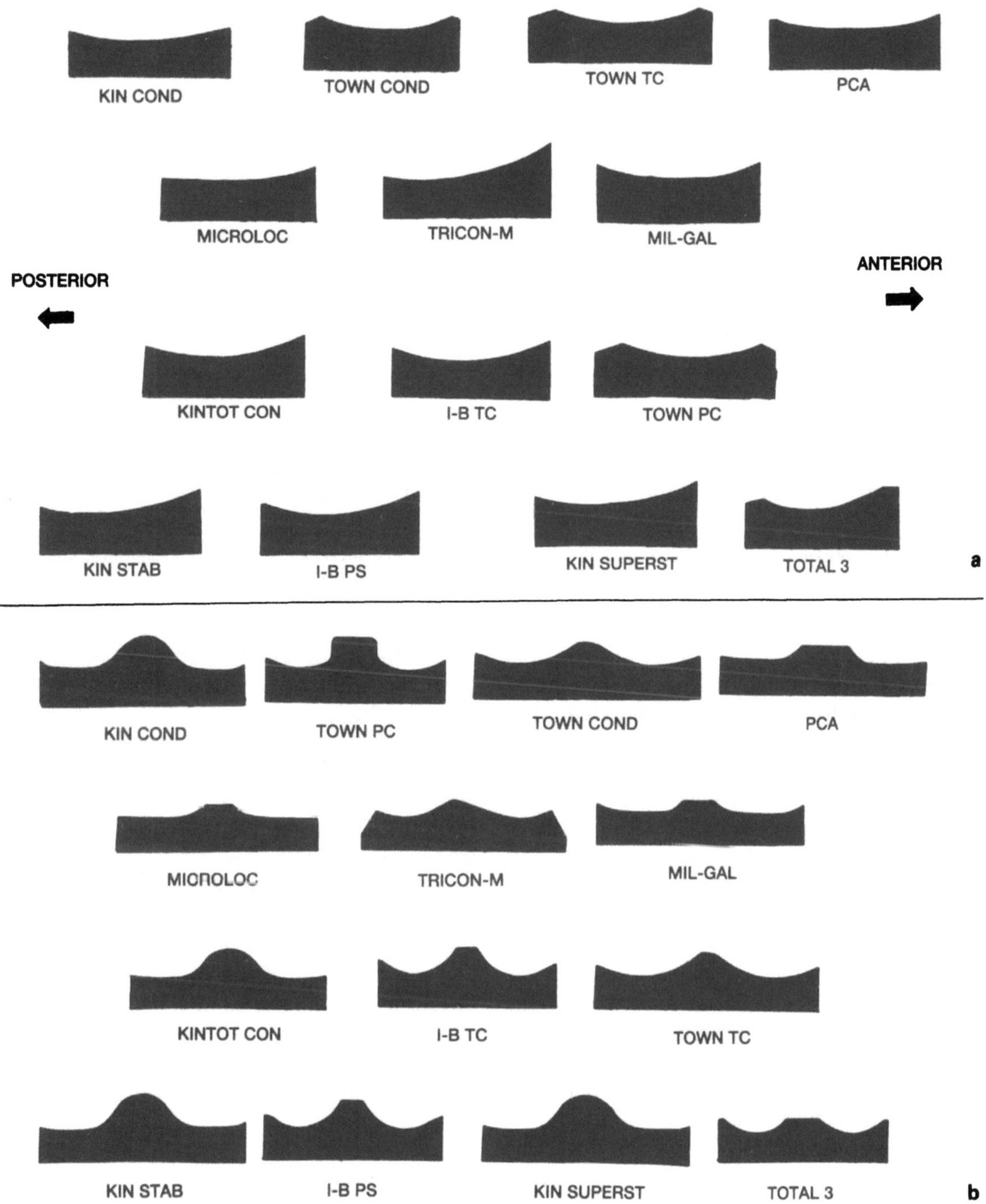

Fig. 7.4.a Sagittal profiles of several knee arthroplasty tibial components. The Insall-Burstein Total Condylar appears in the center of the figure with a generally smaller radius of curvature reflecting more conforming articulation. Cruciate conserving designs have flatter, less conforming geometry e.g. Microloc, PCA, Mil-Gal. **b** Coronal profiles of tibial components. The Insall-Burstein Total Condylar articulation is more conforming than any other design. Having the femoral tibial contact point centralized over the condyle reduces edge loading, but also decreases the moment arm and mechanical efficiency of collateral ligaments in response to varus and valgus stresses. (From Thatcher et al (1987), with permission)

given compressive load, the varus or valgus moment necessary to cause rock-off in knees with a Total Condylar implant was significantly less (20%) in the study by Markolf and colleagues (1981) than that in intact knee specimens. This difference is in large part attributed to the shorter distance between contact points in the prosthetic components as compared with a

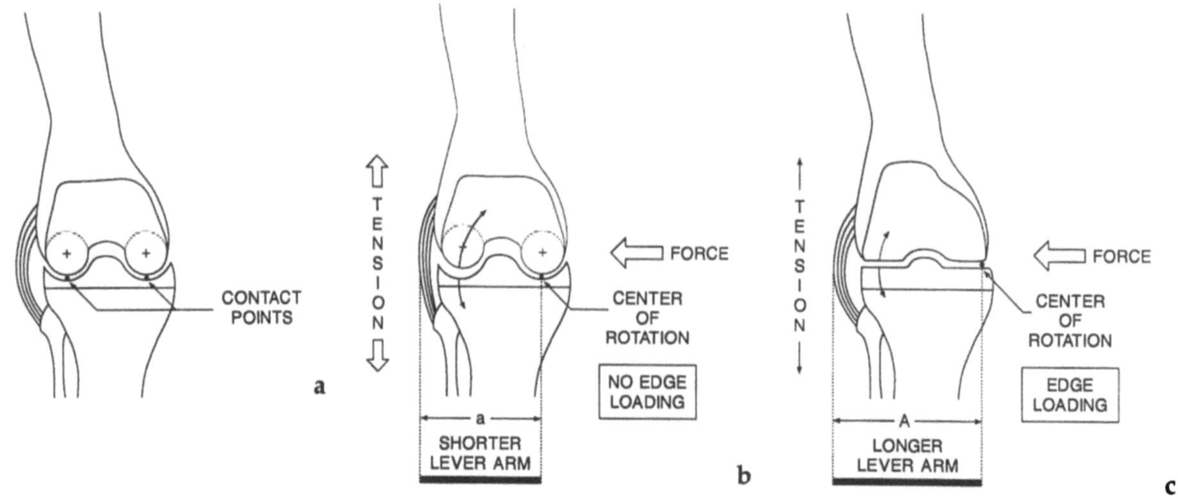

Fig. 7.5. "Rocking off" in response to varus or valgus stress. **a** The femoral condyles of the Total Condylar are circular in the frontal plane and contact a point over the center of each tibial condyle. **b** As a varus force is applied, the medial femoral condyle rotates on the tibia, the lateral compartment is distracted, and tension is applied to the lateral ligaments. Edge loading is avoided, but because of a relatively shorter lever arm "a" a relatively greater tensile force is applied to the collateral ligaments. **c** Edge loading occurs in response to the same stresses with flatter tibial designs. The advantage here is of a greater lever arm A with correspondingly less tension in the collateral ligaments. (Adapted from Burstein (1984).)

normal knee (Fig. 7.5). These investigators pointed out that this may reduce the stabilizing effect of compressive loads. Burstein has devoted considerable attention to this phenomenon, describing the shorter distance between contact points as desirable when compared with "edge loading" that may occur with prosthetic devices where the tibia and femur make contact close to the edge of the tibia (Burstein 1984). Such edge loading would be expected to occur in relatively flat components, (such as the ICLH) (Freeman et al. 1972), to increase load at the periphery of the proximal tibia and to cause bone collapse and prosthetic loosening.

Within the confines of these design principles, there has been some variation in the Total Condylar system between different manufacturers since 1974. Originally available in only one femoral size with three accompanying tibial thicknesses, the prosthesis was soon released in a wider range of sizes. Other changes, both successful and not, were made during more than a decade of clinical use: metal-backed tibial trays (Lewis et al. 1982) (Fig. 7.6), carbon reinforced polyethylene components, and several instrument systems. The carbon impregnated polyethylene, known commercially as "Poly II", did not prove to be advantageous in resisting wear in a retrieval study, and produced carbon fiber wear debris (Wright et al. 1988). Theoretically, any increased durability that might be expected from the addition of carbon fiber is probably offset by the approximate doubling of the modulus of elasticity over plain polyethylene. This could be expected to reduce the area of point of contact and increase local stresses by 35%–40% (Wright and Bartel 1986; Wright et al. 1988). Wear is anticipated ultimately to pose problems for all knee arthroplasties as damage correlates directly with patient weight and duration of implantation (Hood et al. 1981, 1983).

A later version of the prosthesis, called the "Insall-Burstein Total Condylar", differed by a

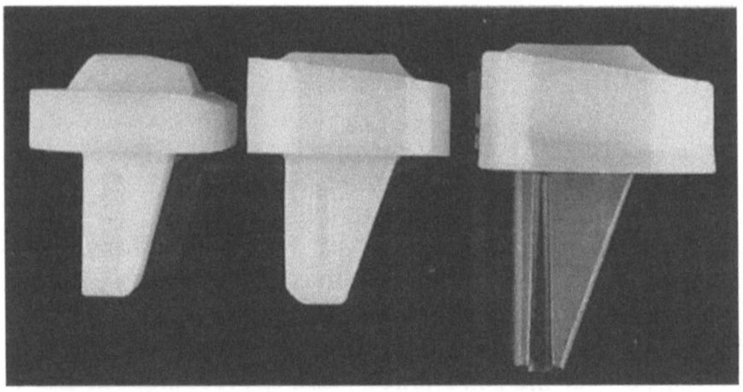

Fig. 7.6. *Left*: Original Total Condylar made entirely of polyethylene with no built-in posterior slope. *Middle*: All polyethylene Insall-Burstein Total Condylar with a built-in posterior slope that resembles normal anatomy, diminishes risk of posterior tibial subluxation and is generally felt to provide greater flexion. *Right*: Metal backing added to the Insall-Burstein Total Condylar.

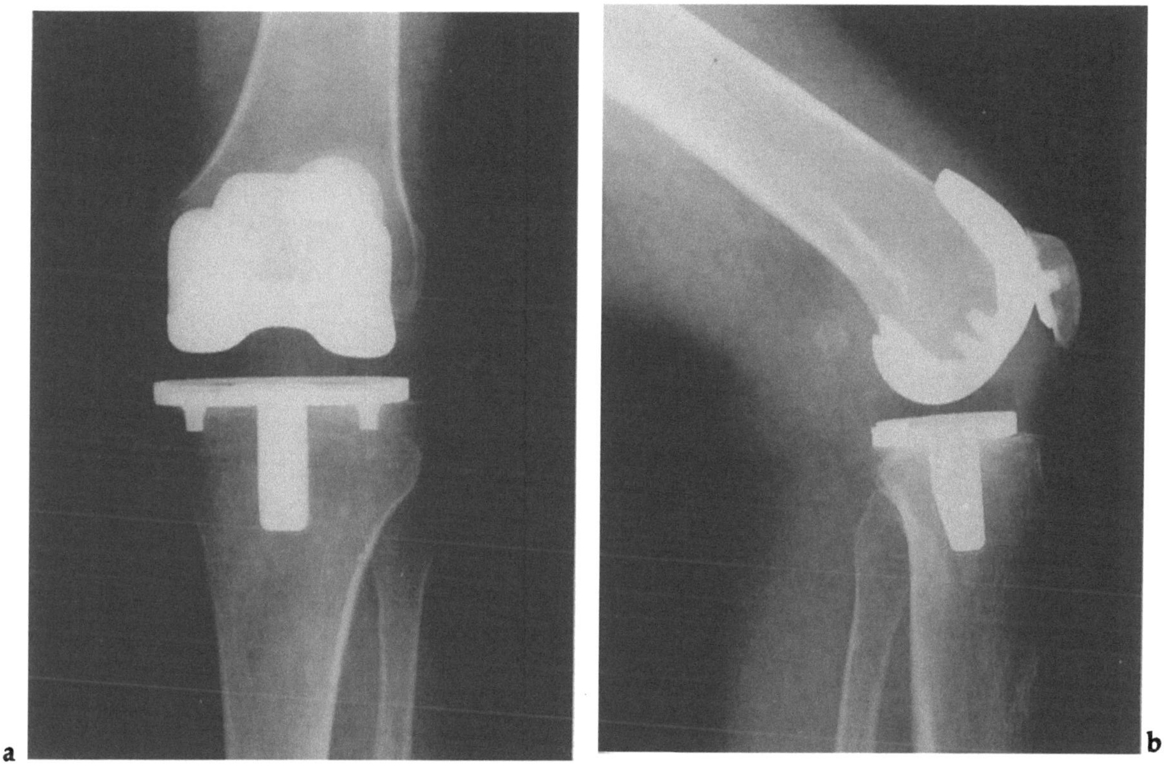

Fig. 7.7. A porous coated prototype of the Total Condylar. Other uncemented versions of the Total Condylar have been brought into production. (Courtesy of L. Dorr.)

posterior slope that was "built-in" to the tibial component (Fig. 7.6). A posterior slope is generally believed to improve flexion and may decrease the risk of posterior tibial dislocation – having the slope built into the prosthesis reduces the risk of inadvertently positioning the component in an anteriorly sloped position. A prototype Total Condylar prosthesis was developed by Ranawat and Dorr (1985) with a porous coating for uncemented application (Fig. 7.7). Development of this option was not pursued by them although one has been made commercially available by others.

Development of Instrumentation

The preliminary clinical report on the Total Condylar, published in 1976, was pre-occupied with surgical technique and the means of accurately positioning the components (Insall et al. 1976b). The surgical goals at the time were to place the tibial component at 90° to the long axis of the tibia in the anteroposterior and lateral planes. The femoral component was said to be ideally placed in 5° of valgus when viewed in the anteroposterior plane and at right angles to the long axis of the shaft in the lateral projection. Five degrees of error on either side of these figures was considered acceptable. Clearly, as we reflect on this degree of accuracy, a 5° error in the placement of both components, could result in an overall 5° of varus tibial-femoral angle – an alignment which is now recognized as unacceptable. In the earliest experience with the Total Condylar, a neutral tibial-femoral angle (representing a varus mechanical axis) was considered appropriate (Insall and Kelly 1985). It was not until 1977 that Lotke and Ecker (1977) – who had both been trained at the Hospital for Special Surgery – emphatically made the point that varus alignment was a major cause of tibial component loosening. There is now general agreement amongst surgeons on the importance of alignment irrespective of other controversies that persist.

The first instrument system for the Total Con-

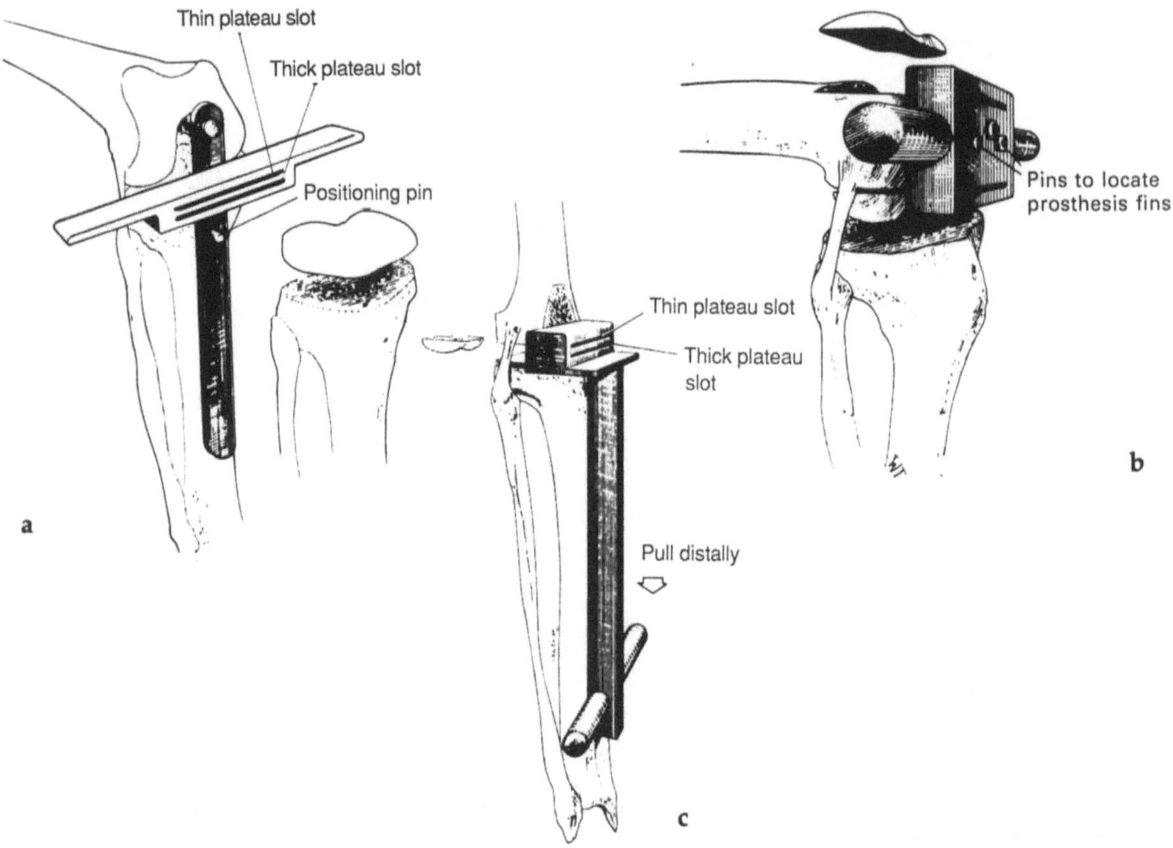

Fig. 7.8. The original Total Condylar instruments shown in the sequence of their use. **a** Original tibial cutter: an extra-medullary device with two captured saw guides. The proximal end of the guide had a fixed pin that was hammered into the distal femur. **b** The femoral shaper. Note that without provision for aligning the anterior cut with the anterior femoral cortex, a notch has been neatly created. **c** The distal femoral cutter functioned as a device for manually determining the angle and level of resection that would give correct ligament tension and knee alignment. (From Insall et al. (1976b), with permission.)

dylar, consisted of three pieces (Insall et al. 1976b) (Fig. 7.8a). There was an extramedullary tibial cutter, consisting of a single bar placed along the long axis of the tibia. A cross-piece provided slotted cutting guides, and the entire jig was secured by a short stem that was inserted into the femoral canal of the flexed knee.

The second instrument in the original system was the "femoral shaper" (Fig. 7.8b). It was held against the distal femur by an intramedullary pin and was used to resect the anterior and posterior femoral condyles. There was no provision for aligning the anterior cut with the anterior femoral cortex, and interestingly, the original drawing clearly shows an anterior femoral notch having neatly been created. Such notches were later recognized as a risk factor for supracondylar femur fractures (Merkel and Johnson 1986). Although intramedullary femoral guides have now become widely accepted for many other knee systems, no such rod was used for the Total Condylar. The rationale for an intramedullary femoral guide is that while the level of distal femoral resection may vary, the desired angle of resection will always bear a constant relationship to the long axis of the femur. As such, the distal femoral cut is made early in the procedure for many current knee systems, and can be revised to a more proximal level if the extension gap is too tight.

The third instrument in the original set was the (distal) "femoral cutter" which had a platform that rested on the resected proximal tibia while the knee was extended. An axial rod attached at right angles to the platform was oriented parallel to the tibia. Handles attached to the distal end of this instrument enabled the surgeon to distract the knee joint and determine the level as well as the angle of distal femoral resection (Fig. 7.8c), while assessing ligament tension. Just prior to using this third instrument, spacer blocks were inserted between the resected proximal tibia and the posterior femoral condyles (after ligament release) to measure the flexion gap. The distal femur was then cut to create an extension gap of equal dimensions, using one of two slots on the femoral cutter; one to accommodate the thick plateau component and the other the thin component. These were the only two tibial component sizes available at the time. In 1976 the concept of matching the dimensions of the flexion and extension gaps was conveyed in two sentences: "A spacer is used . . . to check that the appropriate amount of bone has been removed. The fit should be snug in both flexion and extension" (Insall et al. 1976b). This concept was to receive much more attention in later reports (Insall et al. 1979a).

With time, the instrumentation included guides that helped reduce the risk of "notching" the femur, and a "tensor" (introduced first by Freeman) to integrate the soft tissue releases with accurate bone cuts (Freeman et al. 1972). Ranawat, who continued to implant the Total Condylar prosthesis, after Insall had adopted the Posterior Stabilized design in 1978, described several early refinements to the original instrumentation (Ranawat 1985) and then later developed a set of "precision cutting instruments" (Ranawat and Dorr 1985). The tensor was retained in both of his systems, and was used to confirm the size and tension of both the flexion and extension gaps. While the precision instrument system had several pieces dedicated to improving component position, the sequence of bone cuts followed the original concept of creating a flexion gap and then matching it in extension by resecting an appropriate amount of distal femur. No intramedullary cutting guides were introduced, although one instrument could be placed in the tibial canal to confirm the angulation of the resected proximal tibia.

The tensor now appears to be falling out of favour; most systems have adopted intramedullary femoral cutting guides. There is also a trend towards making the distal femoral cut first, and resecting an amount of bone equal to that which will be replaced by the femoral component. In this way the level of the natural joint line can be preserved. While these newer systems do not regard creation of equal flexion and extension gaps as a priority, the concept of equal gaps must still be respected, as it is essential to the stability and mobility of a knee arthroplasty.

Evolution of Surgical Technique for Correction of Deformity

Many of the soft tissue techniques for correction of angular deformity were inspired by Freeman's ideas on the pathophysiology of deformity (Freeman 1984), and were largely perfected in the early years of Total Condylar use. They have been described in great detail (Dorr 1988; Insall 1984; Laskin 1981; Ranawat 1988; Vince and Dorr 1987).

The first publication to describe soft tissue releases for the Total Condylar prosthesis provided tenuous guidance and included advice that would currently be regarded as incorrect: "fifteen degrees of fixed (varus) deformity can be corrected by asymmetric bone resection without fear of postoperative instability, but greater deformities require (soft tissue releases)" (Insall et al. 1976b). It is now accepted that bone cuts must always be made at the same angle, with the tibia cut at right angles to its long axis, and the distal femur cut at the necessary angle to restore the "normal" or neutral mechanical axis of the limb. Stability must be correspondingly restored by osteophyte removal and/or ligament release. The same 1976 report stated " . . . release of the lateral soft tissue structures for correction of fixed valgus deformities is not recommended because of the risk of peroneal palsy (Insall et al. 1976b). By 1979 very explicit descriptions of soft tissue releases for both varus and valgus deformities included graphic illustrations that emphasized progressive releases for increasingly severe, fixed deformity (Insall et al. 1979a).

Current techniques for medial release are essentially unchanged (Dorr 1988; Insall 1984). Correction of valgus deformity is required less frequently, has been perfected more slowly and still remains somewhat less satisfactory. Following the warning against this procedure in 1976, a detailed description of sequential releases was provided in 1979: (a) iliotibial band about 10 cm above the level of the knee, (b) lateral capsule, lateral collateral ligament and popliteus tendon, and (c) the posterior capsular attachment to the femur (Insall et al. 1979a). This sequence has been modified at times to begin with release of the lateral collateral ligament (Insall 1984). When lateral releases were first described, surgical dissection to isolate the peroneal nerve was recommended as a means of minimizing the hazard of nerve palsy (Insall et al. 1979a; Rose et al. 1982). Isolation of the nerve has not, however, proven to be helpful and has largely been abandoned (Ranawat 1988). The technique of lateral release, including descriptions of some infrequently encountered, but important situations has been described in detail by Ranawat (1988).

Arthroplasty of the valgus knee may result in flexion gaps that cannot easily be equalized, or collateral ligaments that cannot easily be balanced. The latter situation results from the gross attenuation of the medial collateral ligament (MCL) that may occur in profound valgus deformity, the critical importance of this structure to the stability of a knee arthroplasty, and the absence of compensatory medial structures. While the lateral collateral ligament may be transected with impunity in the correction of valgus deformity, the MCL must only be lengthened by sliding its proximal tibial attachment and keeping the entire ligamentous sleeve intact. The MCL is essential in a way that the lateral collateral ligament is not. No resurfacing knee arthroplasty, including the Total Condylar, is feasible in the absence of a funtional MCL. When reconstructing a knee with severe valgus deformity, it is wise to ensure immediate access to a prosthesis such as the Total Condylar III, constrained condylar or kinematic stabilizer if problems develop with unequal gaps or instability (Insall 1984). Severe valgus deformity was a factor associated with all three cases of posterior tibial dislocation in one series of Total Condylar arthroplasties (Goldberg et al. 1988).

If tight medial structures on the concave side of the varus joint are lengthened to *equal* the length of elongated structures on the convex side, then the entire limb could be expected to lengthen. The joint line will migrate proximally relative to the patella if this gap is filled with thicker tibial components. A similar effect occurs if a flexion contracture is corrected by removal of distal femur. This proximal repositioning of the joint line has been shown in a computer simulation to impair flexion due to an effect on collateral ligament function (Laskin and Matsen 1987). Other surgeons have argued that it is the retained posterior cruciate ligament (PCL) which is in fact most susceptible to this effect (Dorr and Boiardo 1986). Designs such as the Total Condylar, which are intended to function without a PCL appear to be less susceptible to the decreased flexion which has been observed when the joint line is re-established in a more proximal location (Vince et al. 1988). A low position of the patella relative to the joint line (patella infera) is, however, undesirable for any prosthesis, leading to poor flexion and persistent pain (Fig. 7.9). Early work with some relatively crude cadaver preparations recommended the use of thicker tibial components as one factor that contributed to favorable location of the tibiofemoral contact in terms of load distribution on the proximal tibia (Moller et al. 1983). This would, however, be at the expense of a lower patellar position.

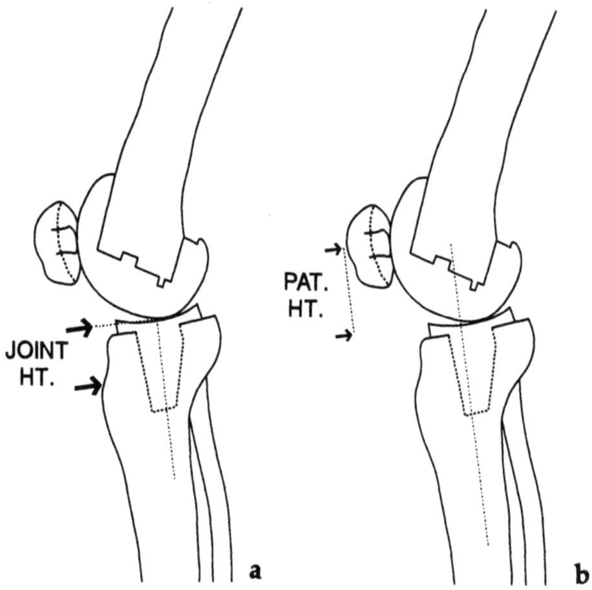

Fig. 7.9. Joint line position. Elevation of the joint line with respect to its preoperative position (**a**) did not produce significant reduction in flexion, whereas a lower position of the patella with respect to the joint line (**b**) can result in pain and restricted flexion. (From Vince et al. (1988).)

Clinical Results of the Total Condylar Prosthesis

The experience with the Total Condylar prosthesis at the Hospital for Special Surgery has been reported at intervals from 1976 to the present (Insall and Kelly 1985; Insall et al. 1979a, 1979b, 1983; Ranawat and Boachie-Adjei 1988a;

Ranawat and Hansraj 1989; Ranawat and Rose 1985; Vince et al. 1987, 1989). Clinical results with this device are also available from independent institutions (Anglietti and Rinonapoli 1981, 1984; Borden et al. 1982; Clayton and Thirupathi 1982; Colwell et al. 1988; Ecker et al. 1987; Eto et al. 1988; Goldberg et al. 1988; Hvid et al. 1987; Hvid and Nielsen 1984; Laskin 1981, 1984, 1990; Nafei et al. 1990; Neilsen et al. 1985; Ritter and Stringer 1979; Schurman et al. 1985; Sneppen et al. 1985; Soudry et al. 1980, 1981, 1986a; Tauber et al. 1986, 1987), including studies by surgeons who received at least part of their training at the Hospital for Special Surgery and studies from Italy, Scandinavia, the Middle East and the Orient (Aglietti and Rinonapoli 1981, 1984; Colwell et al. 1988; Ecker et al. 1987; Goldberg et al. 1988; Ritter and Stringer 1979; Soudry et al. 1980, 1981, 1986b). Methylmethacrylate cement fixation was used in each of these series.

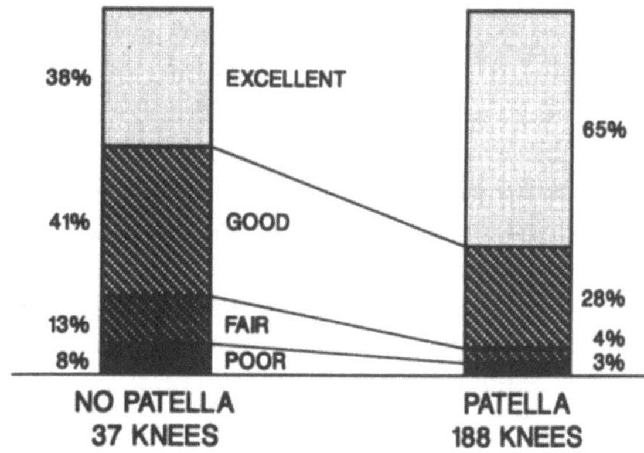

Fig. 7.10. Patellar resurfacing. Some of the original work endorsing universal patellar resurfacing was done with the Total Condylar arthroplasty. The percentage of good and excellent results is diminished if the patella is not resurfaced. The number of patients requiring additional surgery to resurface a painful patella exceeds those with complications of patellar resurfacing. (From Scott et al. (1978).)

From the Hospital for Special Surgery

The Total Condylar prosthesis was the first choice for knee reconstruction of the Knee Service at the Hospital for Special Surgery from 1974 to 1979 when it was supplanted by the Posterior Stabilized prosthesis (Insall 1984). The Total Condylar was used before and after 1979 as the primary arthroplasty for patients with inflammatory arthropathy who attended the "Combined Arthritis Program" of the hospital. The prosthesis is unlikely to become obsolete until another device uniformly demonstrates superior long term results.

The clinical studies of the Total Condylar prosthesis from the Hospital for Special Surgery have not always included the identical cohort of patients. Some studies were restricted to patients with gonarthrosis (Insall et al. 1983) and other studies reported predominantly rheumatoid arthritis patients or exclusively those with juvenile rheumatoid arthritis (Ranawat et al. 1983). The most recent and longest follow-up included only patients who had the Total Condylar implanted for what were, in retrospect, appropriate indications (Vince et al. 1987, 1989) (i.e. no patellectomy, no ankylosis). Patients were originally reported jointly by Insall and Ranawat (Insall et al. 1976b, 1979a), but as their numbers increased the patients overseen by each surgeon were reported separately.

All but one of these reports (Ranawat and Hansraj 1989) have included some of the first patients to receive the Total Condylar prosthesis in 1974. By 1976, when approximately 300 devices had been implanted, the first 116 consecutive cases were reported, with about a two year duration of follow-up (Insall et al. 1976b). In this first study group, 81 patellae had received a polyethylene dome, 33 were not resurfaced and 2 had undergone a previous patellectomy. A later study concluded that further surgery to resurface a painful patella after the initial arthroplasty was a more frequent problem than the need for further surgery as a result of patellar complications (Scott WN et al. 1978) (Fig. 7.10). Examination of the all-polyethylene buttons in 20 components retrieved from Total Condylar type prostheses demonstrated minimal wear from 3 to 62 months (Hood et al. 1981c). Patellar resurfacing soon became standard practice at the Hospital for Special Surgery. Ranawat, (1986) reviewing the patellofemoral joint in 100 Total Condylar knees, found one loose patella and no fractures. He advocates routine resurfacing, while having noted two patellar fractures in Total Condylar arthroplasties that were performed after this 1974 to 1978 series.

Another, later study of 27 Total Condylar arthroplasties from the Knee Service that were implanted with no patellar resurfacing showed only slightly inferior knee scores. However, the patients without a patellar button had more difficulty stair climbing and one-third of them avoided this activity altogether (Soudry et al. 1986a). Universal patellar resurfacing for inflammatory arthropathy was posited by Sledge and Walker (1984) based on the premise that residual articular cartilage is an antigenic stimulus to synovitis and pain. In spite of the acknowledged desirability of resurfacing the patella, this joint remains problematic for the Total Condylar and subsequent designs.

The patients in all these study groups have been relatively uniform. Consistent with the established indications for knee arthroplasty, the mean age of study patients has been in the mid-sixties, with rheumatoid arthritis accounting for younger individuals. Whether the general predominance of women reflects a greater incidence of arthropathy amongst women or a reluctance amongst men (or amongst surgeons for men) to have this type of surgery is not known. It is generally believed that males will fare less well with all types of arthroplasty because of greater weight and activity.

Two aspects of the results of arthroplasty surgery deserve seperate attention: performance and longevity. The former has been expressed as HSS knee scores and the latter in recent years by a statistical method known as "survivorship analysis" (Armitage 1971; Ranawat and Boachie-Adjei 1988a,b; Ranawat and Hansraj 1989; Tew and Waugh 1982; Vince et al. 1987, 1989). Each joint replacement is entered into a survivorship analysis once, as either a success or failure at the time of the most recent assessment. A definition of failure is arbitrarily established from the outset. Some that have been used are:

1. Revision surgery having been performed or recommended (Vince et al. 1987, 1989).
2. The above criteria plus radiographic evidence of global radiolucency or shift of components (Ranawat and Boachie-Adjei 1988a,b; Ranawat and Hansraj 1989).
3. Re-operation for any cause.
4. Failure requiring arthrodesis or permanent resection arthroplasty only, i.e. unrevisable failure (Goodfellow and O'Connor 1986).
5. Return of pain.

The Hospital for Special Surgery reports have used definitions one and two which are similar. Invariably, by the time conditions in situation 2 are apparent, painful symptoms have appeared that indicate revision surgery. Arthroplasties in patients who are lost or die in the course of the study are legitimately included, based on the assumption that these patients are *not* subject to a higher rate of failure or complication than that of the group at large.

Three survivorship analyses of the Total Condylar have been published from the Hospital for Special Surgery (Ranawat and Boachie-Adjei 1988a,b; Ranawat and Hansraj 1989; Vince et al. 1987, 1989). The longest duration study described the original 1974–75 cohort of patients at 10–12 years post surgery (Vince et al. 1987, 1989). The vast majority of patients were accounted for, with only 2% lost to follow-up. The survival curve predicted 93.2% success at 12 years with failure defined as revision having been recommended or performed. A similar study by Ranawat and Boachie-Adjei (1988a,b) of patients who had surgery between March 1974 and December 1977 predicted 88.7% success when failure was defined as circumferential radiolucency and 94.1% if revision surgery was the criterion for failure. Survivorship of Total Condylar prostheses implanted between 1979 and 1980 with generally improved surgical technique and the availability of a complete range of component sizes was 98.9% at 9 years, with a single failure, from sepsis (Ranawat and Hansraj 1989).

The knee scores have been very similar for all HSS reports. Mean preoperative scores have all been in the low to mid-forties, and mean postoperative scores in the low to mid-eighties. Scores of zero have always been assigned to knees that required revision surgery. The lowest mean postoperative scores, as one might expect, were reported with the longest duration follow-up of the original cohort (Ranawat and Boachie-Adjei 1988a,b; Vince et al. 1987, 1989) (Table 7.1). These are the oldest patients assessed, at an age when general debility impairs scores by any system that rates activities such as stair climbing and walking. There is a general shift over time, of patients who originally scored excellent results, into the "good" category because of general functional decline unrelated to the arthroplasty.

Table 7.1. HSS knee scores for Total Condylar prosthesis

	Years		% Knees		
	F/U	Exc	Good	Fair	Poor
Insall/Tria	Min 2	68	23.5	4	4.5
Insall/Scott	3–5	68	24	3	4.5
Insall/Hood	5–9	64	27	2	7
Insall/Vince	10–12	51	37	4	8
Ranawat/Rose	3–8	80	13	4	3
Ranawat/Boachie	9–11	53.3	39	3.8	4.4
Ranawat/Hansraj	2–9	64	35	0	1
Aglietti/Rinona	2–5	62.5	27	8.5	2
Aglietti/Rinona	Min 5	64	21	9	6
Hvid (R.A. only)	4–6	44	43	8	4
Nielsen	0.25–2	55	36.5	6.5	2
Kjaersgaard (OA)	4–6	56	33	7	4
Schurman	8–10	41	36	16	7

While the preliminary 1976 report on the Total Condylar prosthesis provided few results, there had not by that time been any cases of confirmed or suspected loosening of tibial or femoral components (Insall et al. 1976b). The larger cohort reviewed in 1979, included patients with rheumatoid and osteoarthritis. Infection complicated three knees and four had persistent pain that was corrected in two by resurfacing of the patella. The tibia subluxed posteriorly in three knees, that had previously undergone patellectomy. The patellar component loosened in two cases, one of which was removed at the time of revision for tibial instability (Insall et al. 1979a).

An even larger group of 354 Total Condylar I (synonymous with "Total Condylar"), 103 Total Condylar II and 4 Total Condylar III prostheses were reported late in 1979. By then, three Total Condylar prostheses had suffered tibial component loosening and 1 had femoral component loosening that was encountered at the time of revision for a known loose tibial component (Insall et al. 1979b).

A longer follow-up of the first 100 consecutive Total Condylar prostheses implanted for gonarthrosis was reported in 1983 (Insall et al. 1983). Seven knees were regarded as failures. One knee suffered a deep infection and was later arthrodesed, and one had posterior tibial subluxation in flexion. Another arthroplasty, aligned in varus, was painful and had revision surgery to correct alignment. The pain persisted. Of two knees with loosening of the tibial component, one had been aligned in varus. One knee suffered progressive varus instability and was revised eight years later. A final patient had a patellectomy prior to the Total Condylar replacement and then suffered pain post arthroplasty that persisted even after arthrodesis. None of the studies from 1976 to 1983 included a survivorship analysis.

In the 10–12 year follow-up of surgeries performed in 1974 and 1975 (Vince et al. 1987, 1989) patients with preoperative patellectomy or ankylosis were excluded as these conditions are considered inappropriate indications for the Total Condylar prosthesis. The majority of knees had stable bone–cement interfaces after more than a decade of implantation (Vince et al. 1987, 1989) (Fig 7.11a,b). Six failures were recorded: one with varus instability (Fig. 7.12), three with tibial component loosening (Fig. 7.13), one with femoral component loosening (Fig. 7.14) and one with posterior tibial dislocation (Fig. 7.15). The cases of loosening and instability were regarded as shortcomings in surgical technique in the early phase of this prosthesis. The case of femoral loosening was, however, unusual and more difficult to explain. The patient's valgus deformity had been corrected at surgery. A disturbing, progressive resorption of anterior femoral bone occurred over the course of several years and culminated in frank loosening of the unsupported prosthesis (Fig. 7.14). Multiple bacteriologic cultures did not demonstrate infection and the failure was attributed to allergy when skin testing revealed sensitivity to cobalt chloride and cobalt sulfate. There was no way to demonstrate what effect, if any, stress shielding of bone may have played in the failure. Avascularity of the femoral condyles that could theoretically have resulted from extensive soft tissue release was not evaluated. Irrespective of the origins of failure, the case has been unique. Revision to a custom manufactured titanium prosthesis received a good rating at 2 years, without evidence of recurrent problems (Vince et al. 1987, 1989). Comparison of the Total Condylar survival curve with previously published survivorship analyses of a group including Freeman, Sheehan and Manchester arthroplasties shows the improved longevity of the Total Condylar (Tew and Waugh 1982; Vince et al. 1987, 1989) Fig 7.16).

Of Ranawat's original patients, who had surgery between March 1974 and December 1977, four arthroplasties had poor results, including

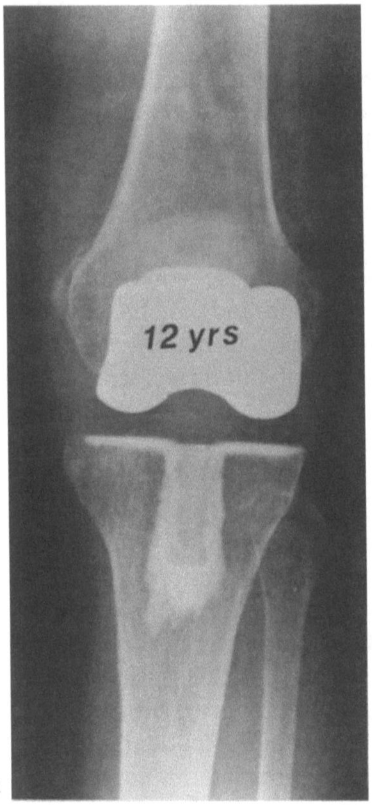

a

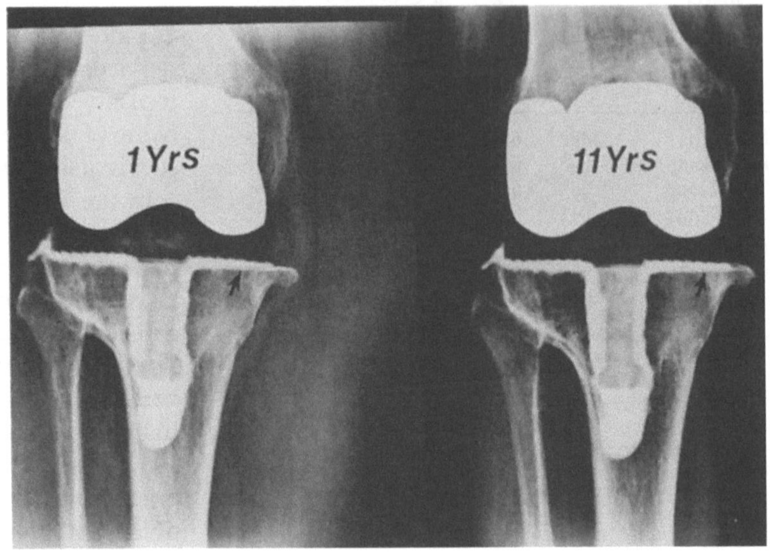

b

Fig. 7.11. a The well-aligned, cemented Total Condylar arthroplasty with an all polyethylene tibial component demonstrates enduring results. At 10–12 years, over 80% of surviving patients enjoyed good to excellent results (Vince et al. (1989). **b** Most radiolucencies that appeared after surgery characteristically remained unchanged during the duration of our study. While circumferential radiolucencies usually indicate loosening, this lucency, unchanged from 1 to 11 years was consistent with an excellent result.

one deep infection, persistent pain in one obese patient with general debility, one tibial component loosening, and one patellar component loosening (Ranawat and Boachie-Adjei 1988a,b).

Ranawat and Hansraj (1989) then published a highly instructive paper reviewing the results of Total Condylar prostheses implanted between 1979 and 1980, when a satisfactory range of component sizes was available and when the basic surgical techniques had been refined. The clinical results from this later cohort are, in some respects, superior. The distribution of 64% excellent and 35% good results reflects general debility due to age and inflammatory arthropathy. The absence of fair results is probably due to better patient selection, reproducible bone cuts and accurate soft tissue surgery. The improved results of surgery performed at this later date shed new light on prior conclusions about the intrinsic properties of the Total Condylar design. Notably, this later study shows mean flexion of 109°, a significant improvement over the 95° that is usually attributed to the Total Condylar prostheses (Ranawat and Hansraj 1989) (Fig. 7.17).

Schneider, (Schneider et al. 1982, 1984; Schneider and Soudry 1986) of the HSS radiology staff, has organized and published extensive information pertinent to imaging knee arthroplasties. This material was collected largely

→

Fig. 7.12.a Pre-operative radiograph of a knee that may have been affected with neuropathic arthropathy. Note the intra-articular debris. **b** Postoperative varus instability requiring revision arthroplasty.

Fig. 7.13.a Radiolucency under the medial plateau apparent at 1 year in conjunction with varus mechanical axis. **b** By 5 years, the medial tibial plateau has subsided, with deformity of the polyethylene component.

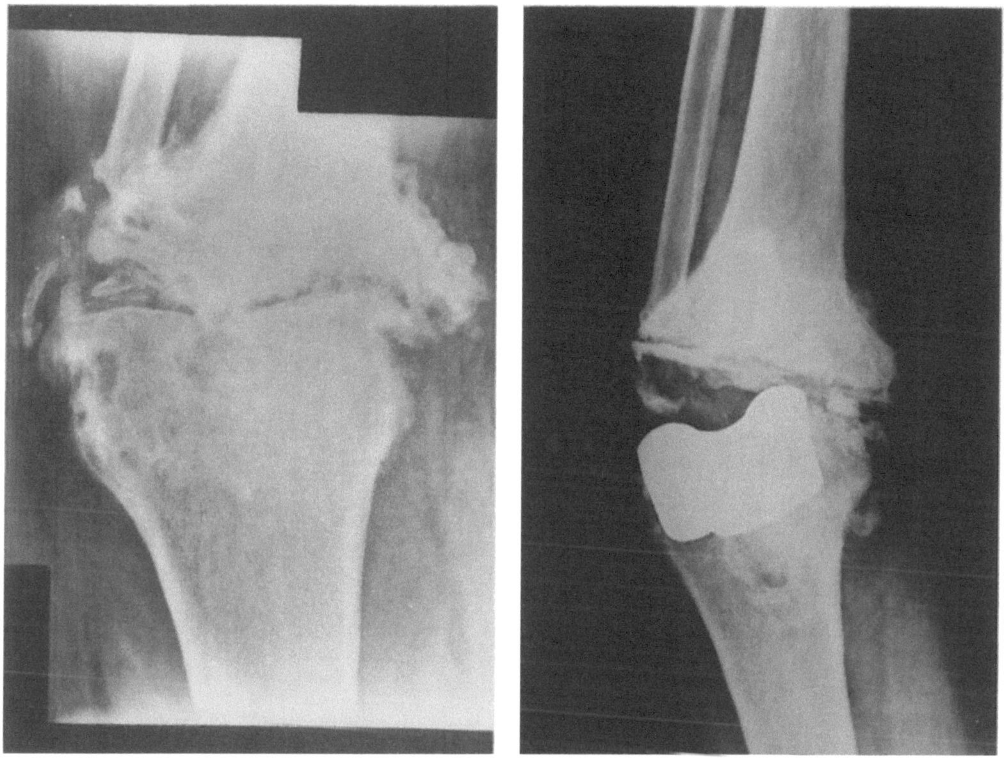

a b

Fig. 7.12

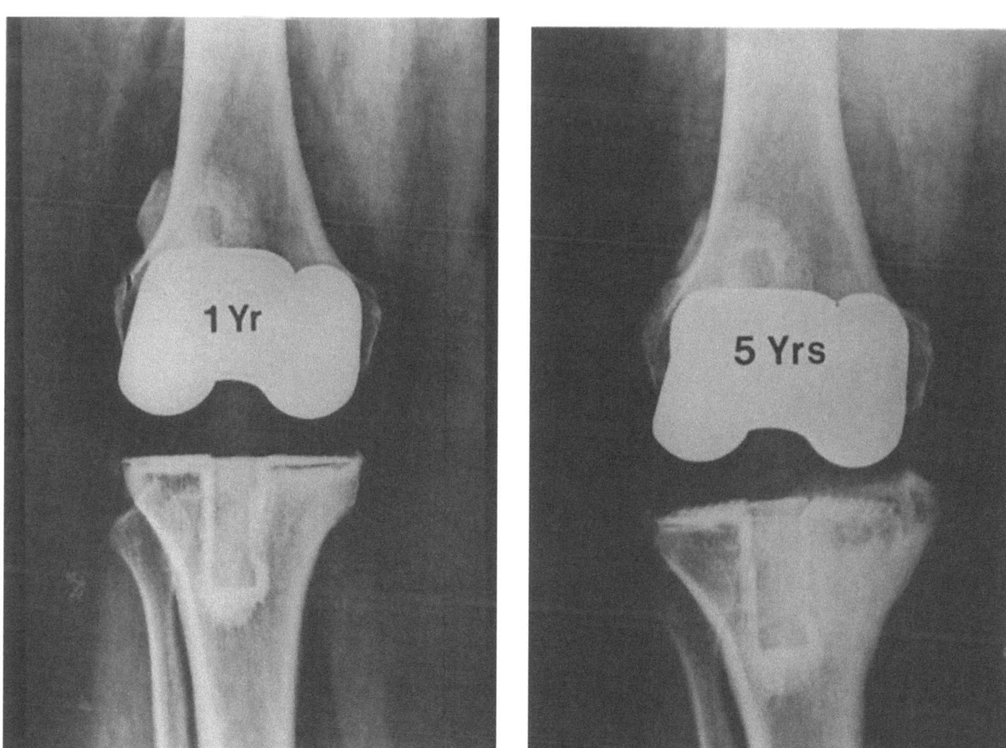

a b

Fig. 7.13

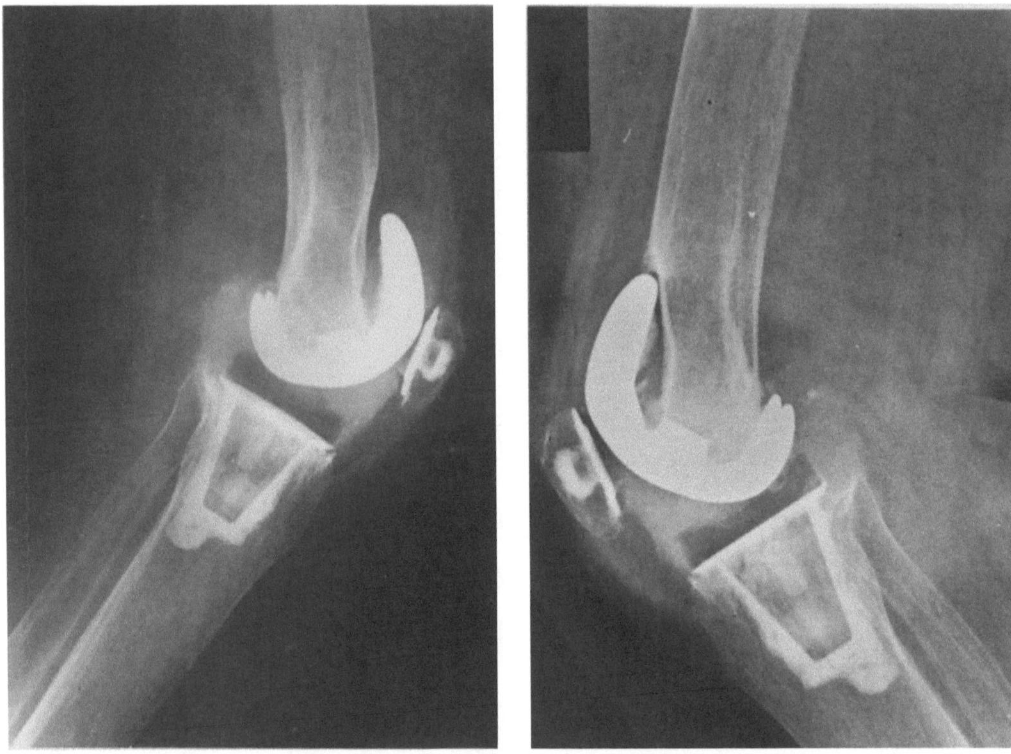

a b

Fig. 7.14.a Unusual resorption of anterior femoral bone 2 years post arthroplasty. At the time of surgery, intimate contact had been achieved between the bone, cement and the component. **b** Femoral component now grossly loose. Evaluation for infection yielded negative results. Allergy skin testing was positive for chrome combalt salts, raising the question of metal sensitivity with resultant osteolysis. A successful revision was performed with a custom-made titanium prosthesis.

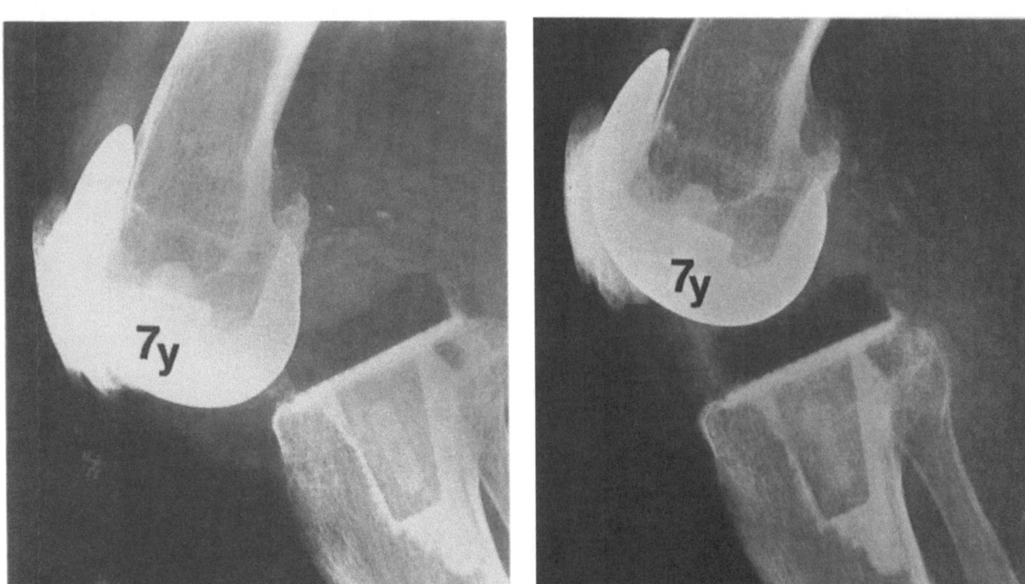

a b

Fig. 7.15. Posterior tibial dislocation. This patient was able to reduce the arthroplasty and preferred a brace over revision surgery.

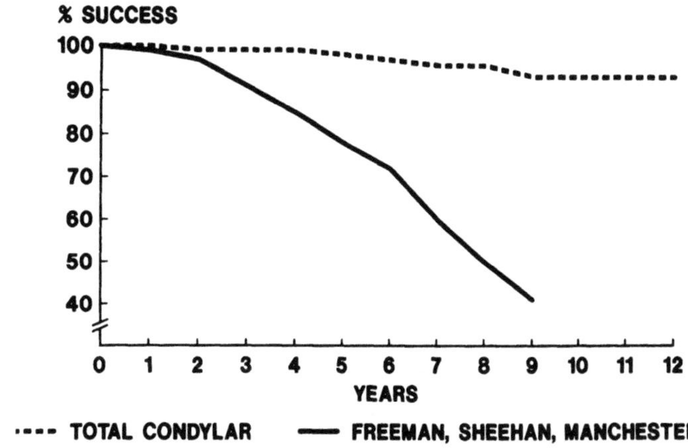

Fig. 7.16. A comparison of Total Condylar survivorship curves with a combined group of Freeman, Sheehan and Manchester arthroplasties.

from their experience with Total Condylar arthroplasties, and covers radiography, radionuclide scanning and arthrography. The complications of Total Condylar and some other knee arthroplasties have been characterized in detail.

Results from Independent Institutions

The first report on the Total Condylar prosthesis from an institution other than the Hospital for Special Surgery was published in 1981 by Laskin (1981). He described its use exclusively in patients with rheumatoid arthritis after a minimum 2 year follow-up. The paper focused on the successful application of soft tissue releases to correct varus and valgus deformities without compromising stability, in conjunction with the relatively conforming articular surface of the prosthesis. Results were not reported with HSS knee scores, but with a detailed analysis of function. Eighty-six per cent of patients were either completely pain free or suffered mild barometric discomfort at 2 years; 88% had markedly increased walking ability as a result of arthroplasty. Four patients (3.4%) required repeat surgery for: (a) progressive, painful varus-valgus instability at 8 months, (b) complete loosening of the patellar dome, (c) immediate postoperative varus-valgus instability and (d) necrosis of the patellar ligament requiring arthrodesis. No deep infections occurred (Laskin 1981).

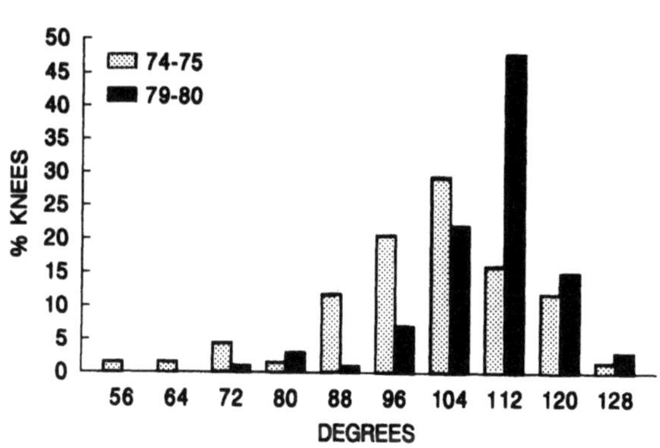

Fig. 7.17. Total Condylar flexion. Mean flexion of about 95° was achieved with the 1974 and 1975 cohort of Total Condylar prostheses. Total Condylar arthroplasties performed in 1979 and 1980, when the prosthetic device was available in a greater range of sizes and when surgical technique had been refined, had a mean flexion of 109°. The distribution of results suggests that 95° of flexion may not be an inherent limit to this prosthesis.

Further evaluation of this cohort by Laskin (1990) at a minimum 10 year follow-up demonstrated the problems of arthroplasty inherent in the rheumatoid patient. Chronic corticosteroid therapy had been used in 89% of the 117 Total Condylar replacements. Of 80 knees available for assessment, 19 had required further surgery during the intervening decade – 15 for tibial loosening (12.8%) and 4 (3.4%) for sepsis. One patient had a loose patellar component and four suffered patellar fragmentation; none required additional surgery. There was one supracondylar femur fracture related to a notch of the anterior femoral cortex. The presence of radiolucencies correlated with varus alignment and knees with varus alignment of the tibial component were also likely to have overall tibiofemoral varus. Knee scores declined with age because of general debility rather than decreased knee performance. Pain relief was enduring. The relatively high rate of tibial component loosening was related not only to alignment in these arthroplasties (done between 1975 and 1978), but doubtless also due to the extremely poor quality of bone in these patients on corticosteroids. This suggests that component loosening results from collapse of the underlying bone as has been observed by other surgeons (Rand and Coventry 1980).

In another publication, Laskin reviewed a group including patients with rheumatoid and osteoarthritis. He noted that radiolucencies were more common in arthroplasties with varus alignment and that three of 302 knees (0.99%) developed nonseptic loosening of implants by 6 years post surgery (Laskin 1984).

Borden and colleagues (1982) from the Cleveland Clinic reported their experience with 192 Total Condylar knees in 161 patients 45–75 months after surgery. They used the Total Condylar prosthesis for a wide variety of indications, including revision surgery, and described reliable pain relief (better with patellar resurfacing), generally improved function, and correction of deformity with preservation of stability. Patellar dislocation occurred in three cases (1.5%) and five knees (2.6%) had deep infections. While radiolucent lines were common, no surgery was required for component loosening. This early series reported seven knees with posterior tibial dislocation in flexion (3.6%). Three of these were revision procedures and no mention is made of how many had undergone patellectomy. While posterior tibial dislocation was the most common complication in the first 250 procedures the incidence was "markedly reduced" in the subsequent 300 Total Condylar prostheses implanted at the Cleveland Clinic. These surgeons identified correction of angular deformity as the most rewarding aspect of Total Condylar arthroplasty, but felt that greater flexion could be achieved with cruciate retaining designs (Borden et al. 1982).

The Cleveland Clinic later reported an 8.3–10.8 year follow-up for the first 129 consecutive Total Condylar arthroplasties. They had revised nine knees for infection, instability or loosening and were able to assess 64 of the original knees. They found 41% excellent, 36% good, 16% fair and 7% poor results. The average flexion for the group was 101°, and there was a 4% tibial component loosening rate that correlated with varus alignment (Schurman et al. 1987).

Aglietti, trained by Insall, returned to the Orthopedic Clinic of the University of Florence and began to use the Total Condylar in January 1975, soon after its introduction. He and Rinonapoli reported the results at 24–70 months in 48 knees with 62.5% excellent, 27% good, 8.5% fair and 2% poor results. Of two loose tibial components one had varus alignment. They found that maximum scores were achieved by the first year after surgery, and did not report any cases of posterior tibial instability or patellar problems in this first study (Aglietti and Rinonapoli 1981).

They later reported the 5 year results with 37 Total Condylar knees, finding 64% excellent, 21% good, 9% fair and 6% poor results by HSS knee scores; not appreciably different from their early report (Table 7.1). The two poor results were due to tibial component loosening in knees that had been implanted with a varus alignment. Instability occurred in two cases: due to intraoperative damage to the medial collateral ligament and the use of a tibial component that was too thin (Aglietti and Rinonapoli 1984).

Posterior tibial dislocation is usually associated with laxity of the flexion gap – either the knee is globally unstable because the polyethylene spacer is too thin or else the flexion gap is wider than the extension gap. In the latter situation, if the tibial component is chosen to fit the extension gap, the arthroplasty will be unstable in flexion. If the knee is stabilized in flexion, then the polyethylene spacer will be too large in extension and the patient will be unable to fully extend the knee. Another cause of posterior instability has been described by Bargren (1980), resulting from rotational malposition of a Total Condylar tibial component. The error of aligning a tibial component parallel to the posterior tibial cortex, instead of directing it towards the tibial tubercle contributes to posterior dislocation.

The longest duration follow-up of the Total Condylar prosthesis published by an institution other than the Hospital for Special Surgery, appears from Case Western Reserve in Cleveland (Goldberg et al. 1988). The study was directed by Goldberg who had been trained at the Hospital for Special Surgery prior to the introduction of the Total Condylar. These results

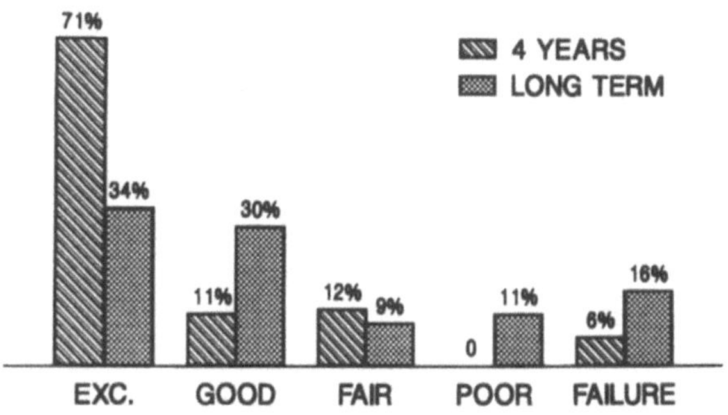

Fig. 7.18. Goldberg et al. (1988) noted a decline in knee scores from the interim 4 year follow-up to the final 9 to 11 year point. Patients continued to report excellent resolution of pain, but had a general deterioration in functional status over time.

had been presented in 1988 on the same program at the annual meeting of the American Academy of Orthopaedic Surgeons as the 10–12 year results from the Hospital for Special Surgery (Vince et al. 1987). The Total Condylar had been in use in Cleveland since May 1975 and arthroplasties performed from that time until the end of 1979 were included. There were 153 Total Condylar replacements in 113 patients, of whom 30 (42 knees) died and one (2 knees) was lost to follow-up. This left 109 arthroplasties in 82 patients for evaluation. These surgeons used nonmetal-backed tibial components exclusively, with standard soft tissue releases to correct deformity. Patella resurfacing was initially elected at the time of surgery in selected cases, but was eventually performed universally.

Arthroplasties were evaluated using the rating scale of the University Hospitals of Cleveland, which differs from the Hospital for Special Surgery knee scores. There had been a gradual decline of scores when the interim, 4 year results were compared with those at 7–11.5 years (Fig. 7.18). This reflects a general deterioration in function resulting from advancing age, with patients nonetheless describing consistent pain relief. Despite different scoring systems, the same observation was made in the Hospital for Special Surgery long term study (Vince et al. 1987, 1989). As others have consistently noted, superior results were recorded when the patella had been resurfaced.

A deficiency of the study by Goldberg and colleagues was the failure to describe the postoperative alignment in the arthroplasties, which complicates explanation of the failures. There were six loose tibial components, three posterior tibial dislocations (one of which was revised) and one infection. Three patients had supracondylar fractures, two of whom required revision arthroplasty (Goldberg et al. 1988). We do not know whether these complications are due to factors associated with the design of the prosthesis or to surgical technique.

Radiolucencies between methylmethacrylate cement and bone have long been a subject of interest and confusion in the literature on knee arthroplasty. Clearly, once a prosthesis has loosened, wide radiolucencies may be expected. However, it is difficult to position the knee and radiography equipment with sufficient accuracy and reproducibility to assess progression of lucencies. Ecker, Lotke and colleagues (1987) have addressed radiolucencies in detail with respect to the Total Condylar prosthesis. They reviewed 102 consecutive Total Condylar knee arthroplasties that had surgery between 1975 and 1978 (3–7 year follow-up) and noted a 4% clinical loosening rate. Using their own knee rating form, they found 44% excellent, 27% good, 22% fair and 7% poor results. A radiolucent line was present in 65% of knees. In 36% the line was defined as "thin" or less than 2 mm and located under *either* the medial or lateral tibial plateau. Thin lines under *both* plateaus were noted in 22% of knees. This distribution is similar to that reported in other studies. In 7% of knees, circumferential lines of 2 mm or more were present. These surgeons seem to have interpreted the significance of these lines constructively. The thick, circumferential lines occurred in one infected knee and in both knees that had subsided and were later revised in an obese male. Two patients with gelling, first step pain and mild symptoms not requiring revision also had wide radiolucencies as did two other knees that were asymptomatic. The knees with thick radiolucencies had generally poorer postoperative radiographic scores indicating poor positioning of components. There was, however, no correlation between the occurrence of *thin* radiolucent lines in any location and the eventual postoperative clinical score.

Furthermore, these investigators found in a cadaver study with the Total Condylar that if the prosthesis was rotated or flexed more that 5° that a 1 mm thick radiolucency could not be seen. This lucency was similarly obscured by angulation of the X-ray beam by more than 6° or displacement of the central beam more than 2.5 cm from the tibial plateau. Metal-backed prostheses made it even more difficult to see radiolucencies. We certainly shared this experience in the long term assessment of Total Condylar knees, trying to compare radiographs of a decade earlier with current studies. In general, conclusions based on the appearance or progression of radiolucencies alone should be evaluated cautiously.

Dorr and colleagues, working with the Total Condylar, provided some of the only clinical data on the importance of conservative resection of proximal tibial bone. They noted an increased incidence of radiolucencies and loosening when excessive amounts of bone were removed (Dorr et al. 1985).

Hvid and Nielsen (1984) published a 3 months to 2 year follow-up of the Insall-Burstein version of the Total Condylar prosthesis. A built-in posterior slope on the tibial component constituted the major departure from the original design. These Scandinavian surgeons concluded that progressive radiolucencies were most apparent in patients with rheumatoid arthritis whose knees had been aligned in varus. They experienced inconsistent success in achieving satisfactory postoperative alignment – 37% of knees were outside the desired 2–12° of valgus alignment. Each of the three prostheses that loosened in this short duration follow-up had been aligned in mechanical varus. No scores were provided.

In 1985, Nielsen, Hvid and Sneppen (1985) reviewed 238 Insall-Burstein Total Condylar prostheses including those in the aforementioned study, with a minimum 2 year follow-up. An unspecified number were performed as revision arthroplasties. Two knees required repeat surgery for infection or tibial component loosening. Three additional knees were considered to have tibial component loosening and one to have patellar component loosening. At the time they published their study, these knees had not had repeat surgery. The fair and poor results included patients with reflex sympathetic dystrophy and polyarticular disease that generally limited function. The failures were attributed to malalignment. No cases of posterior tibial subluxation or dislocation were noted when this Total Condylar prosthesis with a built-in posterior slope was used (Nielsen et al. 1985).

Doctors Hvid and Sneppen (Hvid et al. 1987) participated in a 1987 study that reviewed 95 knees in 65 patients with rheumatoid arthritis. They restricted the Insall-Burstein Total Condylar to varus or valgus deformities less that 35° and flexion deformities less than 30°. Like Laskin, they noted uniform pain relief at the 4-6 year follow-up. Function was generally improved, although scores were impaired by general debility. They had two knees with late deep infections that were treated with debridement and arthrodesis. Despite only moderate success in restoring alignment (22% in mechanical varus), no knees had been revised for aseptic loosening though two knees were "radiologically" loose.

The experience of this group with 103 osteoarthritic knees at 4–6 years was similarly good: 56% excellent, 33% good, 7% fair and 4% poor by HSS scores (Kjaersgaard-Andersen et al. 1989). Loosening of one Insall-Burstein Total Condylar occurred in an arthroplasty implanted in 4° of varus with 5° of anterior tilt on the tibial component. One patellar fracture in a psychiatric patient, persistent unexplained knee pain in a patient with porphyria and deep infection with *Staphylococcus albus* and *Escherichia coli* after skin necrosis accounted for the other three poor results.

An independent Danish group (Nafei et al. 1990) recently prepared the results from 4–8 years with the Total Condylar prosthesis in a combined group of rheumatoid and osteoarthritic patients. They noted generally successful results, but with superior scores amongst the patients with osteoarthritis, due to a higher level of general function.

Sneppen and colleagues (1985) published a study in 1985 that focused on patellofemoral function with the Total Condylar arthroplasty. Interestingly, in 100 primary arthroplasties they reported doing no lateral patellar retinacular releases. At a minimum 1 year follow-up they experienced no cases of patellar fracture or dislocation although moderate residual pain was present on walking in 12 knees. In six of these it was located anteriorly and attributed to the patellofemoral joint. These surgeons found no correlation between postoperative anterior knee pain and any preoperative variable (patellofemoral score, knee deformity) with the exception of fixed flexion deformity, which had a mild correlation. This correlation would of course be expected if the flexion contracture had been corrected by resection of additional distal femur, inevitably creating patella infera. After arthroplasty, patellar tilt had a slight but statistically insignificant effect. They concluded that patellar resurfacing with the Total Condylar usually produces stable and painless patellofemoral function.

In contrast to Sneppen's technique, Tauber and associates performed lateral patellar retinacular releases in a high percentage of Total Condylar arthroplasties, especially in knees with preoperative valgus deformity. Women, presumably because of increased Q-angles, received a release in more than 50% of their cases. Tauber and colleagues did not report any patellar fractures or dislocations (Tauber et al. 1986, 1987).

Again considering the patellofemoral joint, in a study of 111 patients who had Total Condylar arthroplasties from 1976 to 1980, Clayton and Thirupathi (1982) reported ten patellar complications: six fractures, two subluxations, one quadriceps tendon defect and one loosening of the patellar button. Five of the six fractures were treated surgically and the loose prosthesis was simply removed.

Schurman and colleagues (1985) from Stanford University published a short duration study of Total Condylar knee arthroplasties in 1985 concentrating on factors that influence range of motion. They reviewed 55 patients with 71 replacements after a minimum of 2 years and observed a definite regression toward the mean. Knees that had pre-operative flexion greater than 100° had lost motion at the time of follow-up while those with flexion less than 100° had gained. This association between pre- and postoperative flexion is consistent with Ritter's findings with the Total Condylar prosthesis (Ritter and Stringer 1979). The mean flexion for Schurman's entire group at 2 years was 106.8°, similar to Ranawat's experience (109°), (Ranawat and Hansraj 1989) and exceeding the 95° that has been generally associated with the Total Condylar.

Schurman's group found that "for the patients whose pre-operative flexion contracture was 10° or more, virtually all improvement in the contracture occurred at the time of surgery". Tibial femoral alignment had no measurable effect on flexion, although the more accurately aligned knees had less postoperative flexion contracture. This may reflect generally more adept surgical technique. Like others, Schurman and his colleagues hypothesized that posterior tilt of the tibial component would result in more flexion. However, close assessment of their results did not disclose any difference in flexion related to the position of the tibial component (Schurman et al. 1985).

There has been considerable interest in the Total Condylar arthroplasty and similar designs in Japan (Eto et al. 1988; Ueno et al. 1985), where there is a cultural requirement for full knee flexion to facilitate taking meals together while kneeling (Yoshino and Shoji 1987). As a result, knee arthroplasty was generally slow to gain acceptance in the Orient.

Eto and colleagues, from Nagoya, Japan implanted 367 Total Condylar arthroplasties in 250 patients between 1978 and 1985. They reported a 5–8 year follow-up of 75 arthroplasties in 55 patients. The average postoperative flexion was 88.5° in patients with rheumatoid arthritis and 93.9° in those with osteoarthritis (Eto et al. 1988). This is typically inadequate motion for much oriental custom.

Shoji developed a knee prosthesis with Yoshino that was based largely on the Total Condylar design. They believed strongly that the eventual limits of flexion depend more on the surface geometry of the arthroplasty and precise ligament tension in both flexion and extension than on the phenomenon of femoral rollback. Accordingly, they developed a meticulous technique using a tensor type of device that measures ligament tension in both flexion and extension (Shoji et al. 1987; Yoshino and Shoji 1987).

It is commonly argued by proponents of cruciate retention (Scott and Volatile 1986; Sledge and Walker 1984) – and often acknowledged by those who prefer to sacrifice the ligament – that the recreation of femoral rollback is important in gaining full flexion. Shoji and colleagues (1987) presented interesting evidence to the contrary. They published a series of lateral radiographs of a cadaver knee in positions of increased flexion. A second and third series were presented following sacrifice of the anterior and then the posterior cruciate ligament respectively. Each sequence demonstrated femoral rollback, which these investigators claim is the result of articular geometry and collateral ligament tension rather than cruciate ligament function.

The Yoshino-Shoji (Y/S) posthesis differs from the Total Condylar by a flattening of the posterior aspects of the tibial component. While the fear exists that this could allow excessive anterior tibial translation, the stabilizing effect of the hamstrings and posterior capsule is clearly prominent. These surgeons, using a surgical technique that quantifies ligament tension, did not experience any cases of instability. While their prosthesis includes a posterior cut-out on the tibia to accommodate surgeons who prefer to save the ligament, Shoji and colleagues sacrificed the ligament in each case. Interestingly, the patella was never resurfaced and they reported a mean postoperative flexion of 126.8° with a range of 95–165° – clearly superior to what is generally reported and accepted (Shoji et al. 1987).

Few aspects of the cruciate ligament controversy are known with certainty, except that the surgical exposure is facilitated when the ligament is removed, and some compensatory increase in prosthesis conformity will be needed (Freeman et al. 1977; Insall 1984; Thatcher et al. 1987). Much has been made of gait studies with respect to preservation or sacrifice of the cruciate ligament. It is generally acknowledged that even asymptomatic patients with excellent clinical results have some subtle abnormality of gait after knee arthroplasty. Some investigators have argued that patients with the less constrained cruciate retaining designs more frequently have gait patterns resembling normal, especially during stair climbing (Andriacchi and Galante 1982). By contrast, Colwell presented gait laboratory analysis that demonstrated near normal stair climbing ability by patients with Total Condylar replacements (Colwell et al. 1988). As detailed as these studies are, they are based on relatively small numbers, with variations in surgical technique such as alignment and ligament tension. The respective and lengthy arguments have been made in favor (Freeman et al. 1977; Freeman and Railton 1988) and against cruciate sacrifice (Andriacchi 1988; Scott and Volatile 1986; Sledge and Walker 1984). While it is clear that excellent results can be achieved with both classes of prosthesis, the issue itself is far from resolved.

Summary

The Total Condylar prosthesis has been in continuous clinical use for 16 years, invariably with methylmethacrylate cement fixation. It is best classified as a cruciate sacrificing design, with articular geometry that is more conforming to provide stability. This makes it a "semiconstrained" prosthesis. It was largely with this prosthesis that currently accepted techniques for correction of deformity with soft tissue releases were developed. The published clinical experience with this prosthesis has emphasized the importance of valgus tibial-femoral alignment to successful long term fixation. Patellar complications have been noted with relatively low frequency, and there is general agreement that patellar resurfacing with a polyethylene dome is preferable. A characteristic complication in the early experience with the prosthesis was posterior tibial dislocation resulting directly from failure to balance flexion and extension gaps and exacerbated by prior patellectomy and an anterior slope to the tibial articular surface.

While clinical performance as measured by knee scores declines after a decade, this is due to general deterioration in the functional status of an ageing population. There is virtually no change in pain relief at this point and the predicted survivorship at twelve years hovers around 90% in several studies.

The prosthesis and design principles it is based on are sound. It is unlikely to become obsolete until these clinical results are surpassed.

References

Aglietti P, Rinonapoli E (1981) Results of the total condylar knee prosthesis. Ital J Orthop Traumatol 7:17
Aglietti P, Rinonapoli E (1984) Total condylar knee arthroplasty: a five year follow-up study of 33 knees. Clin Orthop 186:104–111

Aglietti P, Insall J, Walker P, Trent P (1975) A new patellar prosthesis, its design and application. Clin Orthop 107:175
Andriacchi TP (1988) Retention of the posterior cruciate in total knee arthroplasty. J Arthroplasty S13–19
Andriacchi TP, Galante JO (1982) Influence of total knee replacement design on walking and stair climbing. J Bone Joint Surg (Am) 64:1328–1335
Armitage P (1971) Statistical methods in medical research. John Wiley and Sons, New York, pp 408–414
Bargren JH (1980) Total knee dislocation due to rotatory malalignment of tibial component: a case report. Clin Orthop 147:271–274
Behrens JC, Walker PS, Shoji I (1974) Variations in strength and structure of cancellous bone at the knee. J Biomech 7:201–207
Borden LS, Heyne T, Belhobek G et al. (1982) Total condylar prosthesis. Orthop Clin N Am 13:123–130
Burstein AH (1984) Biomechanics of the knee. In: Insall JN (ed) Surgery of the knee. Churchill Livingstone, New York, pp 21–40
Campbell WC (1931) Physiology of arthroplasty. J Bone Joint Surg (Br) 13:223
Campbell WC (1940) Interposition of vitallium plates in arthroplasties of the knee. Am J Surg 47:639
Clayton ML, Thirupathi R (1982) Patellar complications after total condylar arthroplasty. Clin Orthop 170:152–155
Colwell CW et al. (1988) Gait analysis of total condylar knee arthroplasty during stair ascent. Orthop Trans 12:591
Coventry MB (1979) Two-part total knee arthroplasty: evolution and present status. Clin Orthop 145:29–36
Dorr LD (1988) Technique of correction of varus deformity. Technique Orthop 3:77–86
Dorr LD, Boiardo RA (1986) Technical considerations in total knee arthroplasty. Clin Orthop 205:5–11
Dorr LD, Conaty JP, Schreiber R, Mehne DK, Hull D (1985) Technical factors that influence mechanical loosening of total knee arthroplasty. In: Dorr LD (ed) The knee, Papers of the first scientific meeting of the Knee Society. University Park Press, Baltimore, pp 121–135
Ducheyne P, Kagan A, Lacey JA (1978) Failure of total knee arthroplasty due to loosening and deformation of the tibial components. J Bone Joint Surg (Am) 60:384–391
Ecker ML, Lotke PA, Windsor RE, Cella JP (1987) Long term results after total condylar knee arthroplasty. Clin Orthop 216:151–158
Eto Y, Nagaya I, Saito S (1988) Value of the total condylar knee arthroplasty. In: Nina S, Paul JP, Yamamoto S (ed) Total knee replacement. Springer-Verlag, Tokyo, pp 63–70
Finerman GA, Coventry MB, Riley LH, Turner RH, Upshaw J (1979) Anametric total knee arthroplasty. Clin Orthop 145:85–90
Freeman MAR (1984) Surgical pathology of arthritis. In: Insall JN (ed) Surgery of the knee. Churchill Livingstone, New York, pp 505–526
Freeman MAR, Railton GT (1988) Should the posterior cruciate ligament be retained or resected in condylar nonmeniscal knee arthroplasty? The case for resection. J Arthroplasty S3–12
Freeman MAR, Swanson SA, Zahin A (1972) Total knee replacement of the knee using a metal-polyethylene two part prosthesis. Proc Soc Med 65:374
Freeman MAR, Insall JN, Besser W, Walker PS, Hallel T (1977) Excision of the cruciate ligaments in total knee replacement. Clin Orthop 126:209
Goldberg VM, Figgie MP, Figgie HE, Heiple KG, Sobel M (1988) Use of a total condylar knee prosthesis for treatment of osteoarthritis and rheumatoid arthritis. J Bone Joint Surg (Am) 70:802–811
Goodfellow JW, O'Connor J (1986) Clinical results of the Oxford knee: surface arthroplasty of the tibiofemoral joint with a meniscal bearing prosthesis. Clin Orthop 205:21–42
Gunston FH (1971) Polycentric knee arthroplasty: prosthetic simulation of normal knee movement. J Bone Joint Surg (Br) 53:272–277
Haberman ET (1986) Total joint replacement: an overview. Semin Roentgenol 21:7–19
Hamilton LR (1982) UCI total knee replacement. A follow-up study. J Bone Joint Surg (Am) 64:740–744
Hood RW, Vanni M, Insall JN (1981a) The correction of knee alignment in 225 consecutive total condylar knee replacements. Clin Orthop 160:94–105
Hood RW, Wright TM, Burstein AH, Insall JN (1981b) Retrieval analysis of seventy total condylar knee prostheses. Orthop Trans 5:319
Hood RW, Wright TM, Burstein AH, Insall JN (1981c) Retrieval analysis of twenty polyethylene patellar buttons. Orthop Trans 5(2):291–292
Hood RW, Wright TM, Burstein AH (1983) Retrieval analysis of total knee prosthesis: A method and its application to 48 total condylar prostheses. J Biomed Mater Res 17:829–842
Hsieh HH, Walker PS (1976) Stabilizing machanisms of the loaded and unloaded knee joint. J Bone Joint Surg (Am) 58:87–93
Hvid I, Nielson S (1984) Total condylar knee arthroplasty: Prosthetic component positioning and radiolucent lines. Acta Orthop Scand 55:160–165
Hvid I, Kjaersgaard-Andersen P, Wethelund JO, Sneppen O (1987) Knee arthroplasty in rheumatoid arthritis: Four to six year follow up study. J Arthroplasty 2:233–239
Inglis A, Lane L (1978) Total knee replacement using the duo-patella prosthesis. Orthop Trans 2:202
Insall JN (1984) Total knee replacement. In: Insall JN (ed) Surgery of the knee. Churchill Livingstone, New York, pp 587–696
Insall JN, Aglietti P (1980) A five to seven year follow-up of unicondylar arthroplasty. J Bone Joint Surg (Am) 62:1329–1337
Insall JN, Kelly M (1985) The total condylar prosthesis. Clin Orthop 205:43–48
Insall JN, Tria AJ (1979) The total condylar knee prosthesis type II. Presented at AAOS Meeting in San Francisco, California.
Insall JN, Ranawat CS, Aglietti P et al. (1976a) A comparison of four models of total knee replacement prostheses. J Bone Joint Surg (Am) 58:754–765
Insall JN, Ranawat CS, Scott WN, Walker P (1976b) Total condylar knee replacement. Preliminary report. Clin Orthop 120:149
Insall JN, Scott WN, Ranawat CS (1979a) The total condylar knee prosthesis. J Bone Joint Surg (Am) 61:173–180
Insall JN, Tria AJ, Scott WN (1979b) The total condylar knee prosthesis: The first 5 years. Clin Orthop 145:68–77
Insall JN, Hood RW, Flawn LB, Sullivan DJ (1983) The total condylar knee prosthesis in gonarthrosis. J Bone Joint Surg (Am) 65:619–628
Jones E, Insall JN, Inglis AE, Ranawat CS (1979) Guepar knee arthroplasty: Results and late complications. Clin Orthop 140:145–152
Jones R (1908) On the production of pseudoarthrosis of the hip without disarticulation of the head. Br Med J 494
Kjaersgaard-Anderson P, Hvid I, Wethelund JO, Sneppen O (1989) Total condylar knee arthroplasty in osteroarthritis: A 4 to 6 year follow-up evaluation of 103 cases. Clin Orthop 238:167–173
Laskin RS (1978) Unicompartmental tibiofemoral resurfacing arthroplasty. J Bone Joint Surg (Am) 60:182–185
Laskin RS (1981) Total condylar knee replacement in rheumatoid arthritis. J Bone Joint Surg (Am) 63:29–35

Laskin RS (1984) The total condylar and Richards maximum contact (RMC) knees: results. In: Laskin RS (ed) Replacement of the knee. Springer-Verlag, New York, pp 175–204
Laskin RS (1990) Total condylar knee replacement in rheumatoid arthritis. J Bone Joint Surg (Am) 72:529–535
Laskin RS, Matsen F (1987) The influence of joint line position during total knee replacement. Orthop Trans 11:535
Lewis JL, Michale JA, Donald PJ (1982) A comparative evaluation of tibial component designs of total knee prosthesis. J Bone Joint Surg (Am) 64:129–135
Lotke PA, Ecker ML (1977) Influence of positioning of prosthesis in total knee replacement. J Bone Joint Surg (Am): 59:77–79
MacIntosh DL (1958) Hemiarthroplasty of the knee using a space occupying prosthesis for painful varus and valgus deformities. J Bone Joint Surg (Br) 40:1431
MacIntosh DL (1966) Arthroplasty of the knee in rheumatoid arthritis. J Bone Joint Surg (Br) 48:179
Mallory TH (1982) Townley anatomic total knee arthroplasty using total tibial component with cruciate release. Clin Orthop 169:197–201
Markolf KL, Bargar WL, Shoemaker SK et al. (1981) The role of joint load in knee stability. J Bone Joint Surg (Am) 63:570–585
Marmor L (1985) Unicompartmental and total knee arthroplasty. Clin Orthop 192:75–81
McKeever D (1955) Patellar prosthesis. J Bone Joint Surg (Am) 37:1074
McKeever D (1960) Tibial plateau prosthesis. Clin Orthop 18:86–95
Merkel KD, Johnson EW (1986) Supracondylar fracture of the femur after total knee arthroplasty. J Bone Joint Surg (Am) 68:29–42
Miller A, Friedman B (1952) Fascial arthroplasty of the knee. J Bone Joint Surg (Am) 34:55
Moller JT, Boe S, Vang PS (1983) Total condylar prosthesis placement in knee arthroplasty. Biomechanic analysis of human knee preparation. Acta Orthop Scand 54:708–713
Nafei A, Steinke MS, Horlyck E (1990) Total condylar knee arthroplasty in the treatment of osteoarthritis and rheumatoid arthritis: A comparative study at 4–8 years follow-up. Am J Knee Surg 3:59–64
Nielsen S, Hvid I, Sneppen O (1985) Total condylar knee arthroplasty. Arch Orthop Trauma Surg 104:227–232
Ranawat CS (1985) Surgical technique of total condylar knee arthroplasty. Technique of bone cuts with conventional instruments. In: Ranawat CS (ed) Total condylar knee arthroplasty. techniques, results and complications. Springer-Verlag, New York, pp 54–68
Ranawat CS (1986) The patellofemoral joint in total condylar knee arthroplasty: Pros and cons based on five to ten year follow-up observations. Clin Orthop 205:93–99
Ranawat CS (1988) Total condylar knee arthroplasty for valgus and combined valgus-flexion deformity of the knee. Tech Orthop 3:67–75
Ranawat CS, Boachie-Adjei O (1988a) Survivorship analysis and results of total condylar knee arthroplasty. Eight to eleven year follow-up period. Clin Orthop 226:6–13
Ranawat CS, Boachie-Adjei O (1988b) Total condylar knee arthroplasty: 8–11 year follow-up. In: Nina S, Paul JP, Yamamoto S (ed) Total knee replacement. Springer-Verlag, Tokyo, pp 71–74
Ranawat CS, Dorr LD (1985) Surgical technique of total condylar knee arthroplasty: technique of total knee arthroplasty with precision cut instruments. In: Ranawat CS (ed) Total condylar knee arthroplasty, technique, results and complications. Springer-Verlag, New York, pp 69–83
Ranawat CS, Hansraj KK (1989) Effect of posterior cruciate sacrifice on durability of the cement bone interface: a nine year survivorship study of 100 total condylar knee arthroplasties. Orthop Clin N Am 20:63–70
Ranawat CS, Rose H (1985) Clinical and radiographic results of total condylar knee arthroplasty: a 3 to 8 year follow-up. In: Ranawat CS (ed) Total condylar knee arthroplasty, technique, results and complications. Springer-Verlag, New York
Ranawat CS, Sculco JP (1985) History of the development of total knee prosthesis at the Hospital for Special Surgery. In: Ranawat CS (ed) Total condylar knee arthroplasty, technique, results and complications. Springer-Verlag, New York, pp 3–6
Ranawat CS, Jordan L, Straub LR (1973) MacIntosh hemiarthroplasty in rheumatoid knee. Acta Orthop Belg 39:102–112
Ranawat CS, Insall JN, Shine J (1976) Duocondylar knee arthroplasty – the Hospital for Special Surgery design. Clin Orthop 120:76–82
Ranawat CS, Bryan WJ, Inglis AE (1983) Total knee arthroplasty in juvenile arthritis. Arthritis Rheum 26(9)1140–1144
Rand JA, Coventry MB (1980) Stress fractures after total knee arthroplasty. J Bone Joint Surg (Am) 62:226–233
Ritter MA, Stringer EA (1979) Predictive range of motion after total knee replacement. Clin Orthop 143:115–119
Rose HA, Hood RW, Otis SC et al. (1982) Peroneal nerve palsy following total knee arthroplasty. A review of the Hospital for Special Surgery experience. J Bone Joint Surg (Am) 64:347–351
Schneider R, Soudry M (1986) Radiographic and scintigraphic evaluation of total knee arthroplasty. Clin Orthop 205:108–120
Schneider R, Hood RW, Ranawat CS (1982) Radiologic evaluation of knee arthroplasty. Orthop Clin N Am 13:225–244
Schneider R, Abenavoli AM, Soudry M et al (1984) Failure of total condylar knee replacement. Radiology 152:309
Schurman DJ, Parker JN, Ornstein D (1985) Total condylar knee replacement: a study of factors influencing range of motion as late as two years after arthroplasty. J Bone Joint Surg (Am) 67:1006–1014
Schurman JR, Borden LS, Wilde AH (1987) Long term results of total condylar knee prosthesis. Orthop Trans 11:443
Scott RD, Santore RF (1981) Unicondylar unicompartmental replacement for osteoarthritis of the knee. J Bone Joint Surg (Am) 63:536–544
Scott RD, Volatile TB (1986) Twelve years' experience with posterior cruciate retaining total knee arthroplasty. Clin Orthop 205:100–107
Scott WN, Rozbruch JD, Otis JC et al. (1978) Clinical and biomechanical evaluation of patella replacement in total knee arthroplasty. Orthop Trans 2:203
Shoemaker SC, Markolf KL, Finerman GAM (1982) In vitro stability of the implanted total condylar prosthesis. J Bone Joint Surg (Am) 64:1201–1213
Shoji H, Yoshino S, Komagamine M (1987) Improved range of motion with the Y/S total knee arthroplasty system. Clin Orthop 218:150–163
Sledge CB, Walker PS (1984) Total knee replacement in rheumatoid arthritis. In: Insall JN (ed) Surgery of the knee. Churchill Livingstone, New York, pp 697–715
Smith-Petersen MN (1939) Arthroplasty of the hip. A new method. J Bone Joint Surg 21:269
Sneppen O, Gudmundsson GH, Bunger C (1985) Patellofemoral function in total condylar arthroplasty. Int Orthop 9:65–68
Soudry M, Iusim M, Mendes DG (1980) Total knee arthroplasty. Harefuah 98:488

Soudry M, Iusim M, Mendes DG (1981) Total condylar prosthesis. Orthop Rev 7:41
Soudry M, Mestriner LA, Binazzi R, Insall JN (1986a) Total knee arthroplasty without patellar resurfacing. Clin Orthop 205:166
Soudry M, Menachem A, Iusin M, Mendes DG (1986b) Experience with total condylar knee prostheses. Harefuah 110:172–4 (English abstract)
Speed JS, Trout PC (1949) Arthroplasty of the knee. A follow-up study. J Bone Joint Surg (Br) 31:53
Tauber C, Bar-On EB, Ganel A, Malkin C (1986) The total condylar knee prosthesis: a review of 71 operations. Arch Orthop Trauma Surg 104:352–356
Tauber C, Eichenblatt M, Noff M, Malkin C (1987) Lateral patellar release and bone grafting of the tibial plateau in total condylar knee arthroplasties. Arch Orthop Trauma Surg 106:257–259
Tew M, Waugh W (1982) Estimating the survival time of knee replacements. J Bone Joint Surg (Br) 64:579
Thatcher JC, Zhou XM, Walker PS (1987) Inherent laxity in total knee prostheses. J Arthroplasty 2:199–207
Townley CO (1985) The anatomic total knee resurfacing arthroplasty. Clin Orthop 192:82–96
Ueno T, Okumura H, Yamamuro (1985) Clinical experience with the total condylar type knee system. Jpn J Rheum Joint Surg 4:73
Venable CS, Stuck WB (1938) Electrolysis controlling factor in the use of metals in treating fractures. JAMA 111:1349
Vince K, Dorr LD (1987) Surgical technique of total knee arthroplasty: Principles and controversy. Tech Orthop 4:69–82
Vince K, Insall JN (1988) Long term results of cemented total knee arthroplasty. Orthop Clin N Am 19:575–580
Vince K, Insall JN, Kelly M, Silva M (1987) Total condylar knee prosthesis: Ten to twelve year follow-up and survivorship analysis. Orthop Trans 11:443
Vince K, Insall JN, Kelly M, Silva M (1988) Long term assessment of joint line position and motion in a cruciate sacrificing knee arthroplasty. Orthop Trans 12:710
Vince K, Insall JN, Kelly M, Silva M (1989) Total condylar knee prosthesis: ten to twelve year follow-up and survivorship analysis. J Bone Joint Surg (Br) 71:793–797
Walker P (1977) Historical development of artificial joints. In: Walker PS (ed) Human joints and their artificial replacements. Charles C Thomas, Illinois, pp 253–275
Walker P (1985) The total condylar and its evolution. In Ranawat CS (ed) Total condylar knee arthroplasty, technique, results and complications. Springer-Verlag, New York, pp 7–16
Walker P, Hajeck JV (1972) The load-bearing area in the knee joint. J Biomech 5:581
Walker PS, Hsieh HH (1977) Conformity in condylar replacement knee prostheses. J Bone Joint Surg (Br) 59:222–228
Walker PS, Ranawat C, Insall JN (1976) Fixation of the tibial components of condylar replacement knee prostheses. J Biomech 9:269–275
Wang CJ, Walker PS (1974) Rotatory laxity of the human knee joint. J Bone Joint Surg (Am) 56:161–170
Werner F, Foster D, Murray DG (1978) The influence of design on the transmission of torque across knee prostheses. J Bone Joint Surg (Am) 60:342–348
Wright TM Bartel DL (1986) The problem of surface damage in polyethylene total knee components. Clin Orthop 205:67–74
Wright TM, Rimnac CM, Faris PM, Bansal M (1988) Analysis of surface damage in retrieved carbon fiber-reinforced and plain polyethylene tibial components from posterior stabilized knee replacements. J Bone Joint Surg (Am) 70:1312–1319
Yoshino S, Shoji H (1987) Yoshino-Shoji total knee system: its features and postoperative results. In: Niwa S, Paul JP, Yamamoto S (eds) Total knee replacement. Springer-Verlag, Tokyo, pp 221–225

Chapter 8

The Posterior Stabilized Knee Prosthesis

Kelly G. Vince

Introduction

If the Total Condylar prosthesis proved to be so successful, why then was the Posterior Stabilized version designed and introduced into clinical practice? There are several reasons. It must be remembered that the Total Condylar, a cruciate sacrificing design, was conceived from the outset as part of a system of progressively more constrained devices (Insall et al. 1979b). Eventually, specific clinical limitations of the Total Condylar became apparent, such as the risk of the tibia dislocating posteriorly in the presence of a patellectomy (Vince et al. 1989). In addition, the initial experience with the Total Condylar suggested that more motion was desirable. Because it is generally held that the posterior cruciate ligament causes the femur to "roll back" on the tibia during flexion, and that the phenomenon of "femoral rollback" is necessary for full flexion, it was concluded that mechanical restitution of this phenomenon would increase flexion (Insall 1984). Clearly, general improvements in surgical technique that had been developed by the time the Posterior Stabilized prosthesis was introduced also contributed to superior flexion with this design. These are discussed in detail below.

The early, progressively more constrained prostheses that accompanied the Total Condylar (or Total Condylar I) device included the Total Condylar II and the Stabilo-Condylar (Insall et al. 1979b; Ranawat and Brigham 1977). The Total Condylar II, introduced in 1976, featured a central post on the tibia that was intended to prevent the tibia from dislocating posteriorly in situations where the size of the flexion gap exceeded the dimensions of the extension gap. It was intended to substitute for the posterior cruciate ligament in this capacity only. Neither the Total Condylar II, nor the Posterior Stabilized that followed it provided any stability to varus or valgus stresses. Early results with the Total Condylar II design proved unsatisfactory (Insall and Tria 1979), with an unexpectedly high rate of tibial component loosening. It seems that this was due to the tibial spine functioning as an extension block against the femoral component, that wrenched the tibial component loose. The design was modified and became what we recognize as the Posterior Stabilized arthroplasty in 1978.

The Total Condylar III, derived from the Stabilo-Condylar prosthesis, provided constraint to varus and valgus forces and prevented posterior tibial dislocation in the presence of a disparity between flexion and extension gaps. This mechanical stability results from a tall and wide tibial spine that conforms to the size and shape of a femoral housing (Donaldson et al. 1988). The design is intended for use in knees without functioning collateral ligaments and is virtually identical to the current "Constrained Condylar Prosthesis".

The Posterior Stabilized arthroplasty was introduced into clinical practice in 1978 on the Knee Service at the Hospital for Special Surgery

(HSS). It was originally reserved for correction of severe deformity and revision arthroplasty, but within a short time it became the prosthesis of choice for primary surgery. It continues to be used for all these indications.

Design

The Posterior Stabilized prosthesis resembled the Total Condylar prosthesis with a cam added

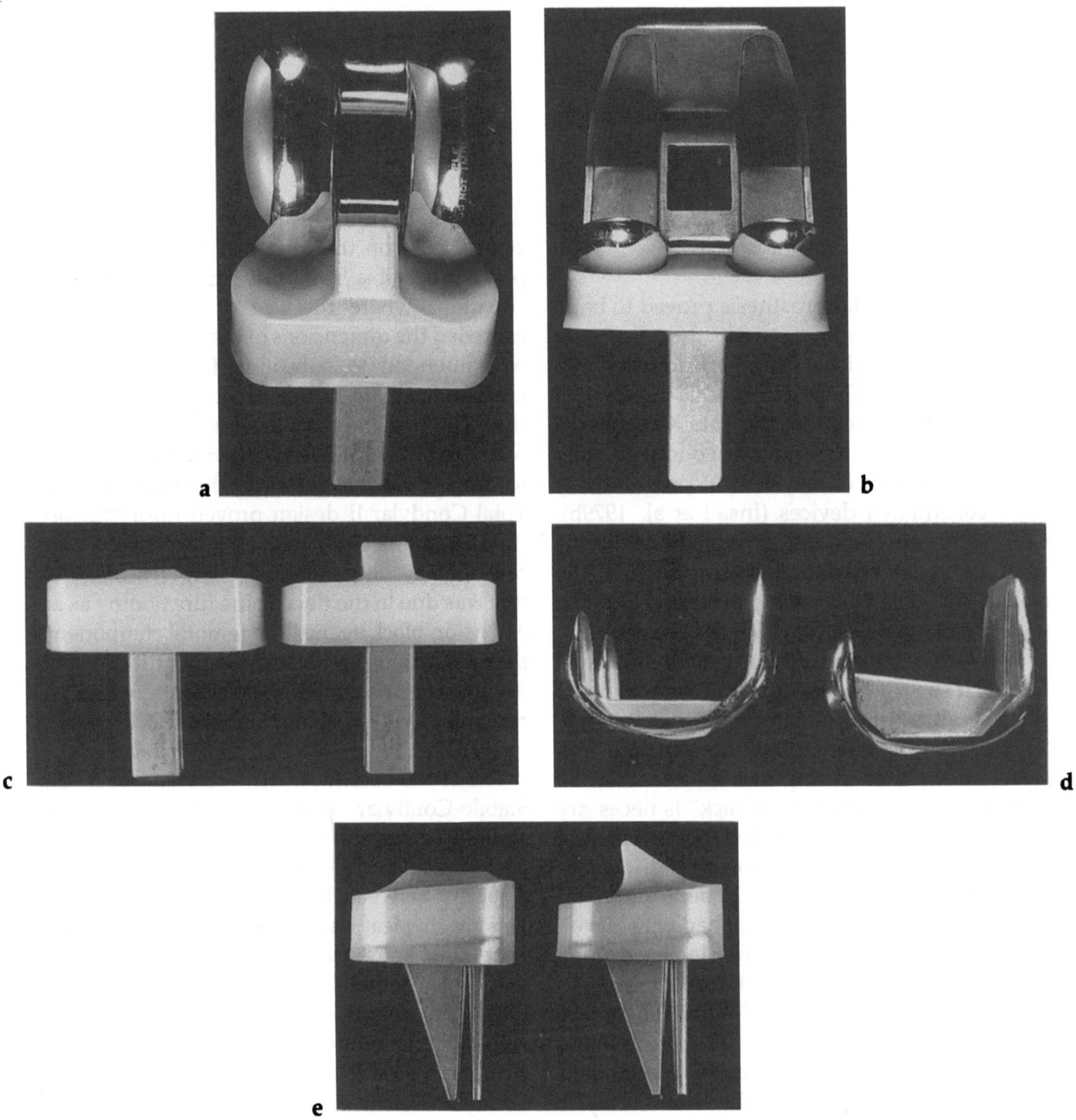

Fig.8.1. a Anterior view of a Posterior Stabilized (PS) knee prosthesis in flexion. The tibial spine has engaged the transverse cam on the femoral component. Other features resemble the Total Condylar (TC). **b** Posterior views. The tibial spine is hidden, in front of the femoral cam. **c** Anterior views of TC (left) and PS (right) prostheses. The PS tibia resembles the TC except for the addition of a prominent polyethylene spine. **d** Lateral views of TC (left) and PS (right) femoral components. The housing on the PS is prominent, and accommodates the tibial spine. **e** Lateral views of TC (left) and PS (right) tibial components, that are similar except for the spine on the PS. The built-in, posterior slope was not part of the original TC, but was introduced in the Insall-Burstein TC, and was retained for the PS. Posterior slope is believed to enhance flexion.

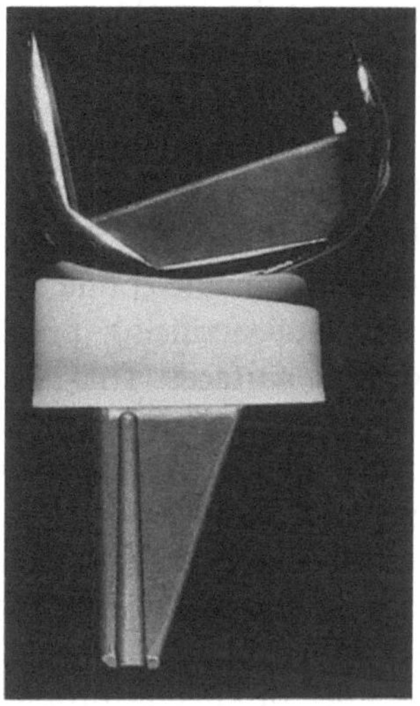

Fig.8.2. Lateral view of articulated Posterior Stabilized knee prosthesis. Slight hyperextension, though undesirable in the patient's knee, may be necessary to accomplish full extension depending on the relative positions of implanted components.

to the femoral component and a spine to the tibia (Fig. 8.1). Because of the general belief that posterior tibial tilt, resembling the anatomic angulation of the normal proximal tibia, enhances flexion and increases stability, this angle was built into the tibial component of the Posterior Stabilized. In this respect, it resembles the Insall-Burstein version of the Total Condylar prosthesis, allowing posterior tibial slope without impingement in extension. It differed most noticeably from the old Total Condylar II by the sloping anterior surface of the tibial spine. As the arthroplasty approaches full extension, this receding surface does not impinge on the femoral component until the prosthesis hyperextends about 15°. While hyperextension is undesirable in the reconstructed knee, the clinical situation sometimes arises that the femoral component has been implanted in a position of flexion relative to the long axis of the femur and the tibial component has several degrees of posterior tilt relative to the tibia. Accordingly, when the patient's knee is fully extended, the components themselves are relatively hyperextended (Fig. 8.2.). No impingement should result from these positions, within the limits of 10°–15° of hyperextension (Burstein and Insall 1981).

The articular geometry of the femoral and tibial condyles resembles the Total Condylar prosthesis; both devices function similarly in extension. The tibial component of the Posterior Stabilized has two wells which conform relatively to the femoral component (Fig. 8.3). The radius of curvature on the femoral component decreases posteriorly, such that the distal surface is flatter to enhance stability in extension. As the knee flexes, the contact area decreases and permits some rotation, that is limited by the spine and cam mechanism. The uphill stabilizing effect of the femoral condyles in the tibial wells is an integral part of both the Total Condylar and Posterior Stabilized designs. As the articular surfaces are sheared away from each other, the femoral component gradually rides up out of the tibial wells, tightening the collateral ligaments and preventing dislocation. The medial-lateral stabilizing effect of the central tibial eminence is increased by the tibial spine.

a 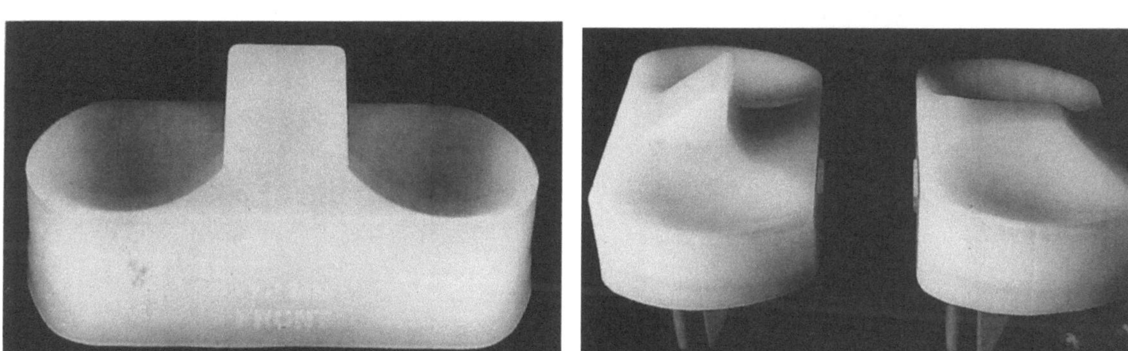 b

Fig.8.3. a Anterior view of Posterior Stabilized tibial articulation with conforming wells in each tibial condyle for the matching femoral condyle. The center of rotation of each femoral condyle during varus-valgus motion remains on the center of each tibial hemicondyle, avoiding edge loading. **b** Lateral views of Posterior Stabilized (left) and Total Condylar (right) components from above. The similarity of the conforming wells is apparent.

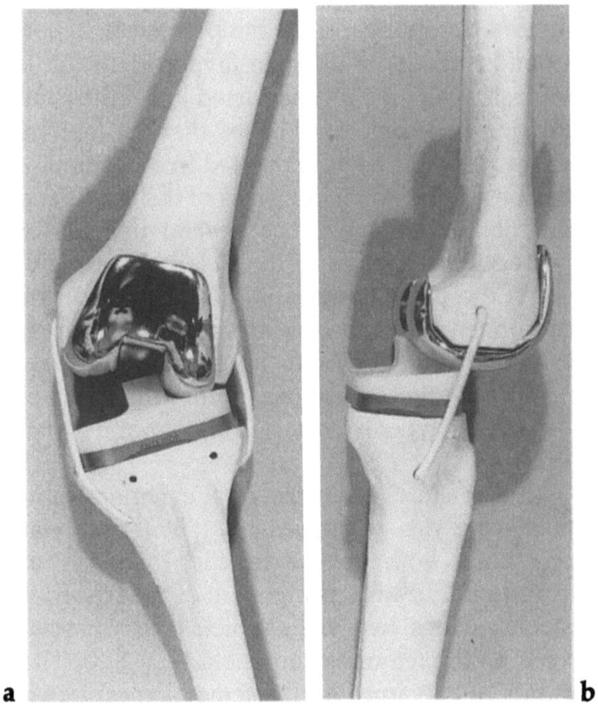

Fig. 8.4. a Anterior view of a Posterior Stabilized prosthesis installed on plastic model bones. There is no inherent mechanical stability to varus or valgus forces. In the absence of collateral ligaments, dislocation will occur. b The spine and cam cannot engage in extension and stability depends on soft tissues.

The similarity of the Total Condylar and Posterior Stabilized articular surfaces is the direct result of the fact that they are both cruciate-sacrificing designs that require inherent mechanical stability. In contrast to cruciate-conserving designs which require flatter tibial articular surfaces to avoid "kinematic conflict" (Insall 1984; Chap. 7), cruciate-sacrificing prostheses have more conforming surfaces. This results in better stress distribution, over a larger surface area, with a theoretically lower wear rate (Bartel et al. 1986; Wright and Bartel 1986). Wear has nonetheless been observed in both Total Condylar and Posterior Stabilized knee prostheses (Hood et al. 1983; Wright et al. 1988). Ewald (1991), with a vast experience of knee arthroplasty surgery, described his clinical impression that wear probably is greater with flatter, cruciate-retaining designs, but claims as well that the loosening rate of more conforming designs may be higher.

While the tibial spine and femoral cam mechanism increase constraint in this prosthesis, it is extremely important to understand precisely how and when this occurs. The Posterior Stabilized prosthesis provides absolutely no constraint to varus or valgus movements. The short-

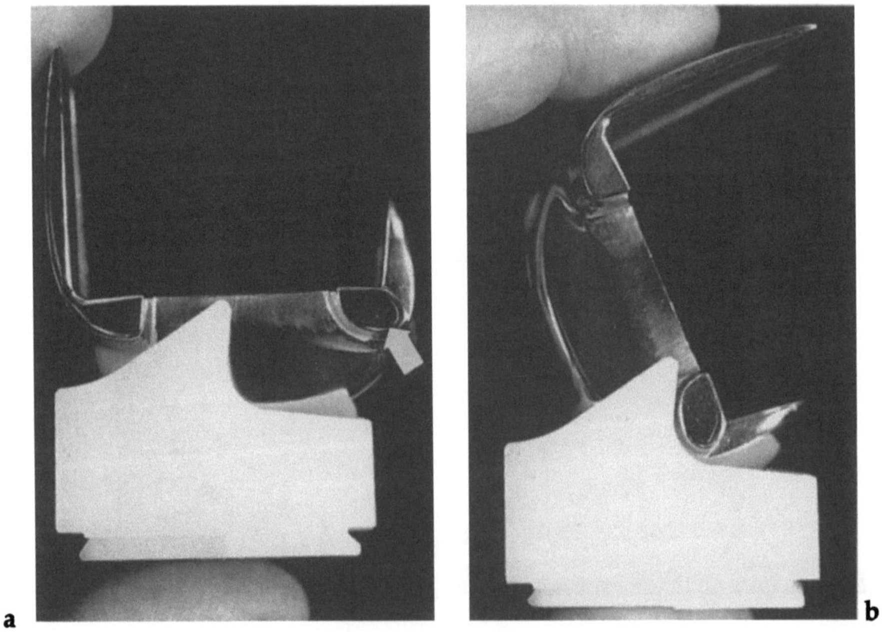

Fig.8.5 a,b. Cut-away cross-section of Posterior Stabilized prosthesis, anterior aspect facing to left side of photos. a The femoral cam (in cross-section and indicated by white arrow) does not make contact with the tibial spine until 50°–80° of flexion; b depending on the relative translation of the components in the anteroposterior plane.

ened tibial spine of the prosthesis will escape completely from the femoral housing in response to these stresses (Fig. 8.4a). Stability of the arthroplasty depends absolutely upon intact collateral ligaments. In addition, the tibial spine does not engage the femoral cam with the knee extended (Fig. 8.4b). The original design conceived that contact would occur somewhere between 40° and 50° of flexion (Burstein and Insall 1981). Peterson and Hillberry (1985) concluded, however, that the spine contacts the cam at between 80° and 86° of flexion depending on the loading situation, and that separation occurs during extension at about 79°. Clearly, if the concept of posterior stabilization is added to a prosthesis, the details of when contact occurs and precisely what type of constraint is imparted will have serious implications for function and fixation (Fig. 8.5).

Stability of the arthroplasty in extension, therefore, depends entirely upon precise soft tissue surgery and the conformity of the articular surfaces, just like the Total Condylar. It is in the position of flexion, where the hamstring muscles and iliotibial band contract in a direction favoring posterior dislocation of the tibia, that the cam and spine engage. The Posterior Stabilized prosthesis is particularly well suited to the reconstruction of knees that have undergone previous patellectomy. In these knees, the desirable anterior vector acting on the proximal tibia from the quadriceps has been severely compromised by the absence of a patella. The cam and spine mechanically prevent posterior dislocation in this situation and also provide a fulcrum around which the tibial component can rotate. In the absence of such a fulcrum, the effect of the hamstring muscles is to translate the proximal tibia posteriorly (Fig. 8.6).

The cam and spine reproduce femoral rollback. This means that as the knee flexes, the contact point of the femoral component with the tibial condyle moves further posteriorly (Fig. 8.7). This permits increased flexion without interference between the posterior surfaces of the femur and the tibial component. Restoration of femoral rollback is the usual explanation for the increased flexion that is seen with the Posterior Stabilized prosthesis.

The forces that result between the femoral and tibial components are affected by the spine and cam mechanism. The vector of the force that the femur applies to the tibial spine as the knee flexes is directed anteriorly. One would expect such a force acting in isolation to generate compression between the tibial component and bone anteriorly and tension posteriorly, effectively rocking or rotating the component. Fortunately, this is not an isolated effect because as the femur rolls posteriorly on the tibia the resultant joint reaction force has the converse effect of compression posteriorly and tension anteriorly. The net resulting vector is more uniformly compressive and directed closer to the middle of the component (Fig. 8.8).

One aspect of knee arthroplasty kinematics and surgical technique that receives little attention is the effect of relative ligament tension in flexion and extension. It may, however, be a significant factor in the increased flexion reported with the Posterior Stabilized. Japanese surgeons (Shoji et al. 1987), for whose patients it is culturally important to kneel for social functions, developed a surgical instrument resembling a tensor to measure accurately ligament tension in both flexion and extension. They believe that it is desirable to construct a flexion gap with slightly less tension, such that the arthroplasty is relatively tighter and more stable in extension. Many patients are able to flex further with their knees less tight. Yoshino and Shoji (1987) developed a prosthesis, similar to the Total Condylar, that they implanted with sacrifice of the cruciate ligaments, but with which they reported, however, a mean flexion exceeding 125°.

The priority that surgeons implanting the Total Condylar prosthesis have recognized is the absolute necessity of adequate stability in flexion to reduce the risk of posterior tibial dislocation. With the Posterior Stabilized prosthesis, however, the knee can be implanted with *slightly* less tension in the flexed position, yet giving the surgeon confidence that dislocation will not occur because of the presence of the tibial spine. While this may contribute to enhanced flexion with the Posterior Stabilized prosthesis, no data are available to confirm this hypothesis. While the device was designed to accommodate about 120° of flexion, a well-motivated, thin patient with excellent pre-operative motion may achieve more (Fig. 8.9).

It must be remembered that despite the spine and cam mechanism, the Posterior Stabilized

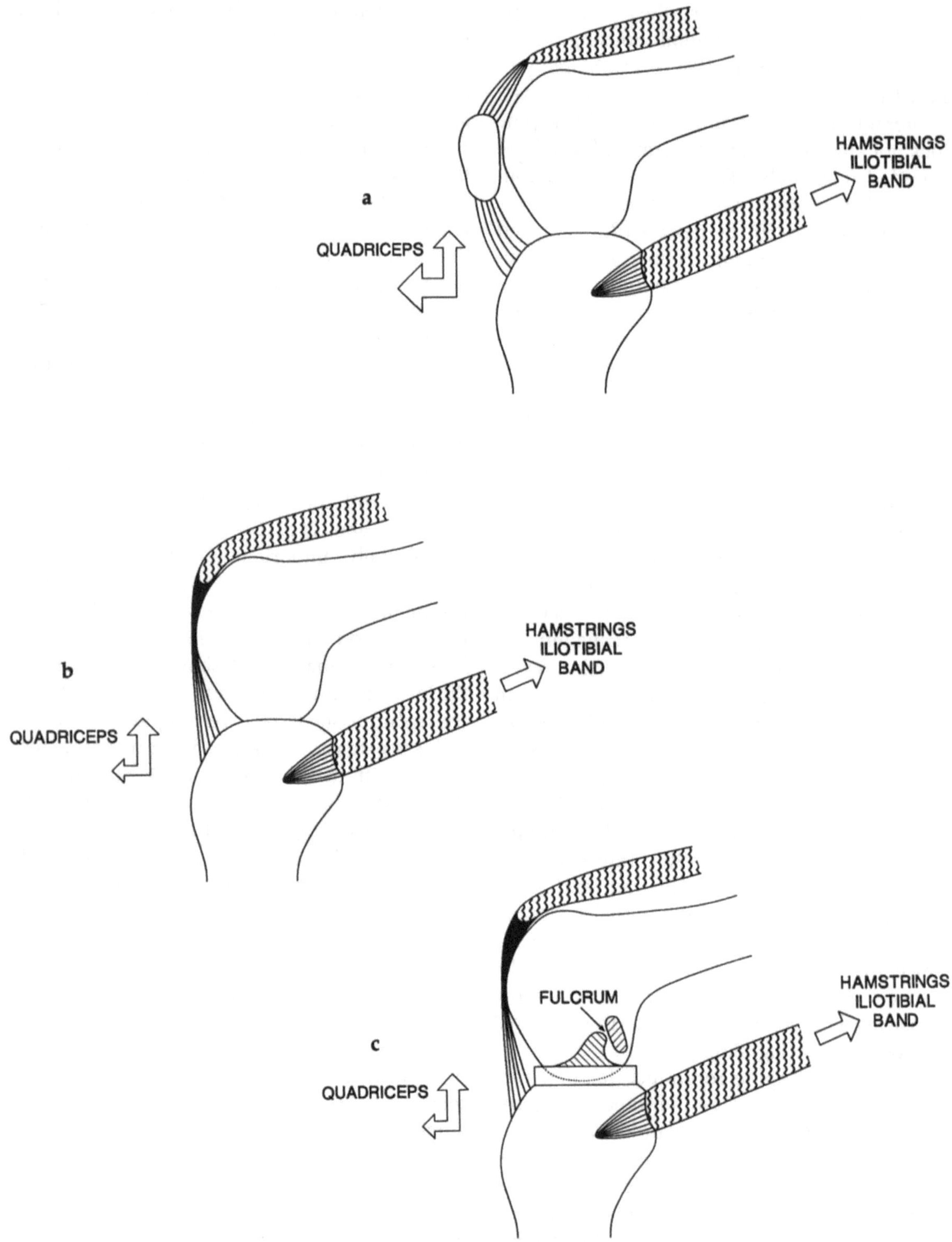

Fig.8.6. a Schematic diagram of normal knee from lateral side. The anteriorly directed vector of the extensor mechanism is enhanced by the patella. The hamstrings and iliotibial band normally function as knee flexors, but also tend to pull the tibia posteriorly. This is opposed by the extensor mechanism and resisted by collateral and cruciate ligaments. **b** In the absence of a patella, the anteriorly directed vector of the extensor mechanism is compromised. Any arthroplasty placed in the absence of a patella will depend heavily on functional posterior cruciate and collateral ligaments to avoid posterior tibial dislocation. **c** The spine and cam mechanism of the Posterior Stabilized furnishes a fulcrum for the flexing knee, such that the hamstrings and iliotibial band will flex, rather than dislocate the knee. This effect becomes more important in the absence of the patella.

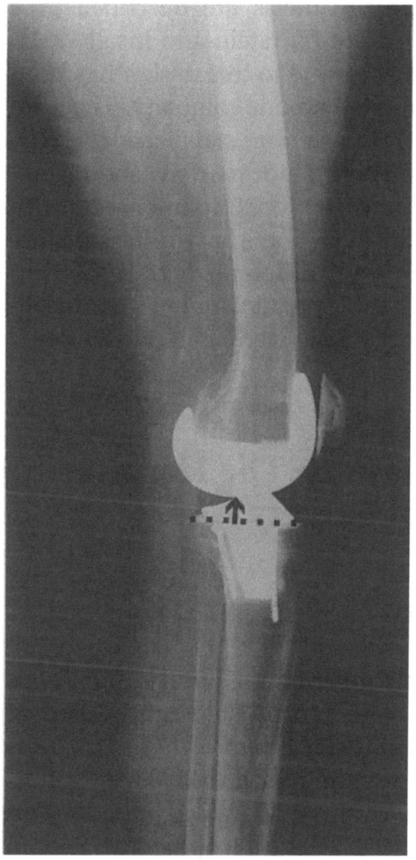

a

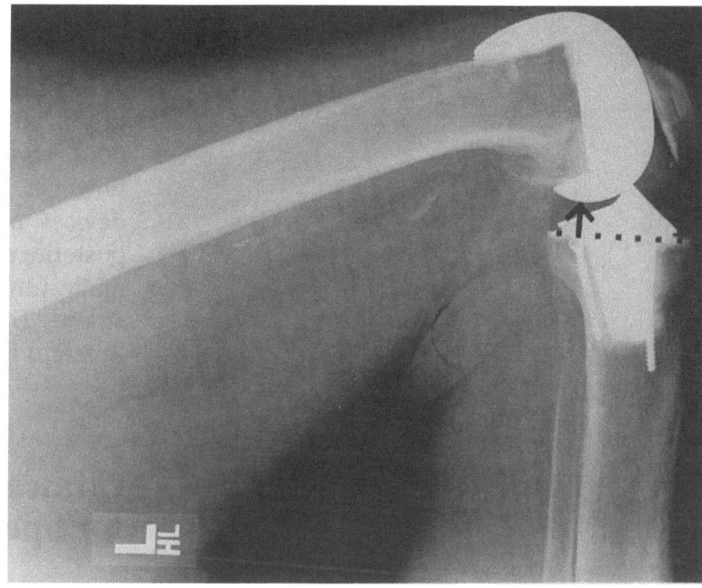

b

Fig.8.7 a,b. Lateral radiographs of a Posterior Stabilized arthroplasty. **a** In extension, the tibial-femoral contact point is just posterior to center. **b** With flexion, the femur moves posteriorly on the tibia. This is "femoral rollback", believed to increase flexion in the arthroplasty.

arthroplasty may still dislocate, and two such cases out of a series of 832 Posterior Stabilized (0.24%) replacements have been reported by Galinat et al. (1988) of Jefferson Medical College. Interestingly, both patients had valgus knees pre-operatively, requiring extensive release of lateral structures. A rotational mechanism of dislocation was postulated that presumably

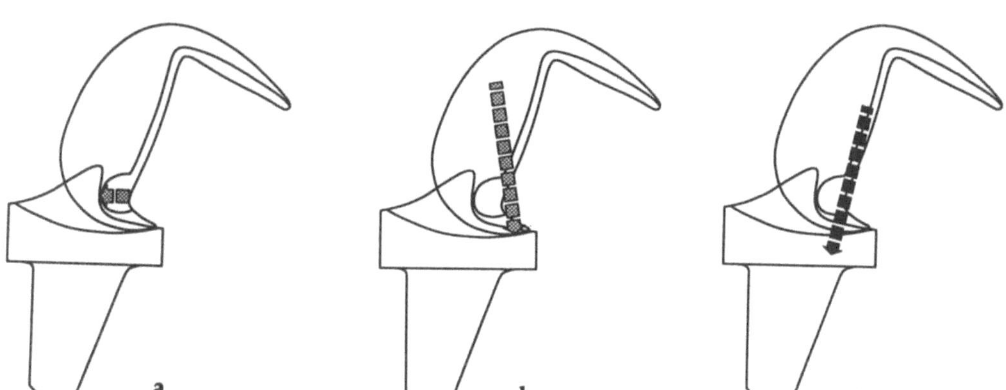

Fig.8.8. **a** Schematic lateral view of Posterior Stabilized prosthesis showing force vector resulting from the action of the spine and cam mechanism. The femoral cam imparts a force directed anteriorly, tending to compress the tibia anteriorly and lift the component posteriorly. **b** Femoral rollback moves the contact point of the femur with the tibia posteriorly so that the joint reaction force tends to compress the posterior tibia and lift the component anteriorly, the converse of that shown in **a**. **c** The resultant vector of **a** and **b** is thus almost all compression, balanced over the keel. (Adapted from Insall et al. (1982) with permission.)

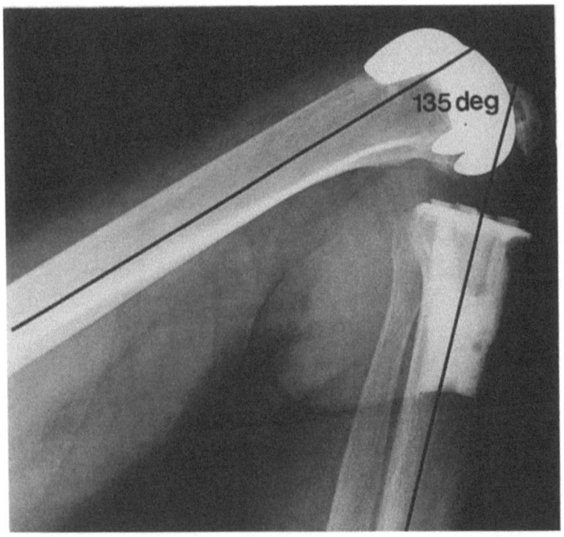

Fig.8.9. Lateral radiograph of a Posterior Stabilized arthroplasty. Flexion to 135°.

began at about 20° of flexion. Both dislocations were easily reduced without requiring sedation, and neither recurred within 18 months. The danger of posterior dislocation of the tibia also increases with maximum flexion if the femoral cam actually rides up and over the tibial spine (Fig. 8.10).

Characteristics of the Insall-Burstein Posterior Stabilized knee prosthesis are described in a United States patent (Burstein and Insall 1981). A prosthetic device true to this design has been produced by more than one company. The term (and concept) "posterior stabilization" has, however, been applied more widely, and several devices now offer optional components with posterior stabilization. Some have different kinematic function with different degrees of constraint. This chapter pertains only to the Insall-Burstein Posterior Stabilized knee prosthesis.

Clinical Results: The Hospital for Special Surgery

Early Reports

The first report describing clinical results with the Posterior Stabilized prosthesis appeared in 1981 (Hood et al. 1981). The prosthesis had been introduced in 1978 and by early 1980, 221 primary and revision arthroplasties had been done on the Knee Service at the Hospital for Special Surgery with this device. The title of the paper,

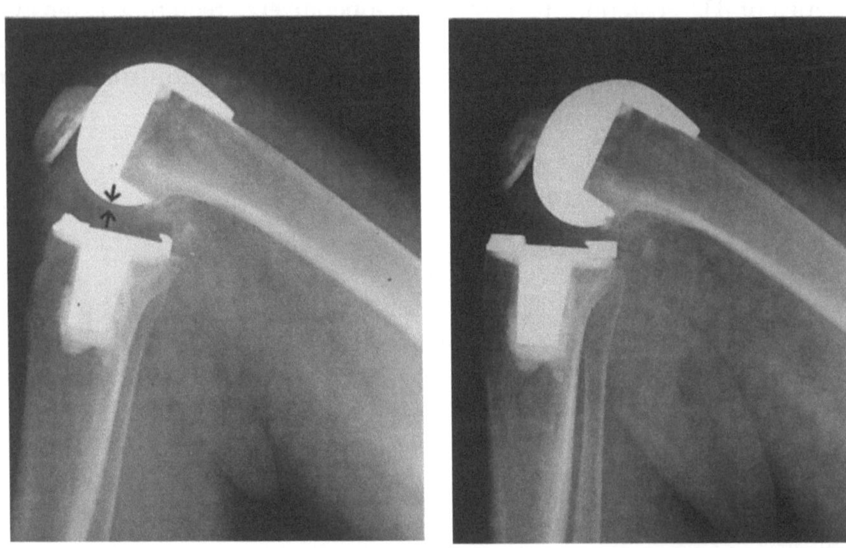

a b

Fig.8.10. **a** Lateral radiograph of a Posterior Stabilized arthroplasty where the tibia has dislocated posteriorly. The radiographic appearance is subtle, with separation between the femoral condyle and tibial polyethylene (arrows) and no femoral rollback. The clinical presentation is not subtle as the knee is locked painfully in this position. This patient dislocated while vigorously flexing her arthroplasty beyond 130° wearing ankle weights. Laxity of the flexion gap will contribute to tibial dislocation. **b** The arthroplasty is easily reduced without anesthesia by applying longitudinal traction to the flexed limb and performing an anterior drawer test maneuver or by hyperflexing the dislocated knee.

"The Correction of Knee Alignment in 225 Consecutive Total Condylar Knee Replacements", is somewhat misleading. As stated in the materials and methods section of the manuscript, the Insall-Burstein Posterior Stabilized Condylar prosthesis was used, not the Total Condylar. The title refers to the Posterior Stabilized generically as a "total condylar type"replacement. This distinction was emphasized in later publications.

The thrust of the 1981 paper was the successful application of soft tissue releases to the correction of deformity and restoration of stability using a prosthesis that offered no inherent varus-valgus constraint. Notable in this group of severely deformed knees was that no arthroplasty was complicated by posterior tibial dislocation, one of the problems experienced with the Total Condylar. In this short duration follow-up no data were offered regarding complete HSS Knee Scores or knee motion. Three failures were reported, due to sepsis in one knee and component loosening in two obese patients, one of whom had undergone Posterior Stabilized arthroplasty as a revision procedure.

In 1982, the first formal review of Posterior Stabilized arthroplasties appeared with a 2–4 year follow-up of 118 primary procedures (Insall et al. 1982). Ninety-seven per cent good to excellent results were reported by HSS Knee Rating Scores. The study concluded that mean flexion with this device was 115° as compared with 95° in the original Total Condylar studies (Insall et al. 1979a). As the mean pre-operative flexion was 95° in both the Total Condylar and Posterior Stabilized cohorts, this was not a confounding variable. The true gain due to the Posterior Stabilized design alone may not, however, have been a full 25°. A later study of Total Condylar arthroplasties done with uniform surgical technique and full availability of component sizes reported a mean flexion of 109° (Ranawat and Hansraj 1989). Comparing an early study of the Total Condylar, function was better with the Posterior Stabilized (Insall et al. 1982) as three times as many patients (76%) could ascend stairs and rise from a chair than could patients with Total Condylar replacements (22%) (Insall et al. 1979a).

Patellar complications were reported in thirteen Posterior Stabilized arthroplasties (11%). Two (1.7%) of these were lateral subluxations and ten (8.4%) were stress fractures. These data have at times been misquoted (Scuderi and Insall 1989; Sneppen et al. 1985; Wetzner et al. 1985) with all 13 patellar complications attributed to fracture. While most fractures were comminuted and displaced, eight of ten patients achieved excellent knee scores without quadriceps weakness or extensor lag after conservative therapy. The average range of motion in the knees with a patellar fracture had been 119° prior to fracture; and remained so after healing. The incidence of fracture was double when the 38 mm patellar resurfacing dome was used as compared with the 35 mm patellar prosthesis. Whether this relates to the size of the component or the size and weight of the patient is unknown, but no fractures were encountered in patients with 32 mm patellar replacements. One patient without a fracture had pain that resolved when a fibrotic peripatellar nodule was removed. Complete arthroplasty failure occurred in three (2.5%) patients due to tibial component loosening, femoral component loosening and deep sepsis.

Comparing the Posterior Stabilized at 5–7 Years with the Total Condylar at 10–12 Years

When we reviewed the original 128 Posterior Stabilized prostheses at 5–8 years post surgery (Vince et al. 1988c) the clinical performance compared favorably with the long term results of the Total Condylar (Vince et al. 1989), without any increased number of failures due to aseptic loosening. The two groups were similar though not identical prior to surgery (Table 8.1).

The Posterior Stabilized arthroplasties in the 5–8 year review had been implanted into 74 women and 28 men with 26 bilateral arthroplasties. Age, weight and diagnoses are tabulated (Table 8.1). Thirteen patients weighed more than 100 kg, and 87% exceeded their ideal body weight. Obesity alone was not regarded as an absolute contra-indication to surgery, although patients were warned of the increased risk of loosening. The pre-operative diagnosis was predominantly osteoarthritis or osteonecrosis. Four

Table 8.1. Comparison of Total Condylar and Posterior Stabilized pre-operative variables
(a) Original Cohort

	Total Condylar	Posterior Stabilized
Implantation:	1/74–12/75 (24 months)	1/78–12/79 (24 months)
Knees	130	128
Patients	104	102
Male	22	28
Female	82	74
Age (range)	67 (39–87)	65 (36–87)
Weight (range)	76 kg (43–113)	77 kg (46–139)
OA/ON	100	108
RA	30	12
Traumatic	0	8

(b) Available at follow-up

	Total Condylar I	Posterior Stabilized
Duration of follow-up	10–12 years	5–8 years
Original number of knees	130	128
Knees available (%)	74 (57)	96 (75)
Dead or lost or invalids	56	32
% Dead or lost	43	25
Mean pre-op score	45	49

patients (6 knees) died within months of surgery and without any postoperative evaluation of the arthroplasty. Except for one myocardial infarction, these deaths were unrelated to knee surgery. An additional three patients with unilateral replacements were lost before the first annual follow-up. None of these seven patients (9 knees) could be included in the study, leaving 95 patients (119 knees) for inclusion in a survivorship analysis.

The Total Condylar group had undergone surgery on average 4–5 years earlier and were correspondingly older at follow-up evaluation. Their mean age at surgery was also slightly older at 67 years (Table 8.1). The average weight was comparable at 76 kg, but with fewer very heavy patients in the Total Condylar group. The distribution by gender and diagnosis was similar, although only the Posterior Stabilized group included posttraumatic arthritis.

Alignment was corrected in all cases with conventional soft tissue releases described previously (Hood et al. 1981), although these had been refined by 1978 when the Posterior Stabilized was introduced. As confidence in these techniques grew, more severely deformed knees were reconstructed and so the Posterior Stabilized group included, on average, more knees with significant deformity (Fig. 8.11).

Survivorship Analysis and Failures

Using the method described by Armitage, survivorship tables were constructed for both groups (Table 8.2) and survivorship curves were plotted from these (Fig. 8.12). According to this method each arthroplasty is entered into the study once, as either a success or failure, at the time of last assessment. Failure was defined as revision arthroplasty having been recommended or performed. The seven failures in the Total Condylar group have been described (Vince et al. 1989). There were four amongst the Posterior Stabilized group, three of which occurred within 3 years after surgery.

One Posterior Stabilized failed due to sepsis occurring 15 months postoperatively with non-Group A hemolytic streptococcus. The infection was treated with removal of the prosthesis,

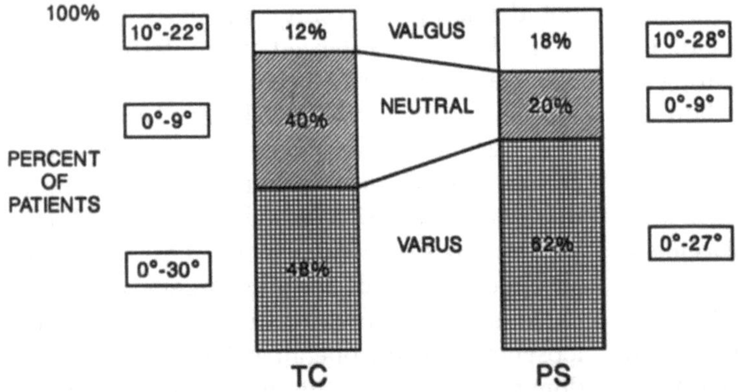

Fig.8.11. Comparison of pre-operative deformity in a group of HSS patients who had Total Condylar arthroplasties with patients who had Posterior Stabilized replacements. With increased confidence in the soft tissue techniques for correction of deformity, more severely deformed knees were reconstructed by the time the PS was available.

Table 8.2. Survivorship lifetables
(a) Total Condylar

Interval since operation, years x to x+1	Last reported during this interval: Failed (dx)	Intact (wx)	Living at start of interval (nx)	Adjusted number at risk (n'/x)	Estimated probability of death (qx)	Estimated probability of survival (px)	Percentage of survivors after x years (1x)
0–1	0	5	124	121.5	0.0000	1.0000	100.0
1–2	1	14	119	112.0	0.0089	0.9911	99.1
2–3	0	5	104	101.5	0.0000	1.0000	99.1
3–4	0	0	99	99.0	0.0000	1.0000	99.1
4–5	1	19	99	89.5	0.0112	0.9888	98.0
5–6	1	4	79	77.0	0.0130	0.9870	96.7
6–7	1	0	74	74.0	0.0135	0.9865	95.4
7–8	0	2	73	72.0	0.0000	1.0000	95.4
8–9	2	2	71	70.0	0.0286	0.9714	92.7
9–10	0	31	67	51.5	0.0000	1.0000	92.7
10–11	0	36	36	18.0	0.0000	1.0000	92.7
11–12	0	6	0				
Total	6	124					

(b) Posterior Stabilized

Interval since operation, years x to x+1	Last reported during this interval: Failed (dx)	Intact (wx)	Living at start of interval (nx)	Adjusted number at risk (n'/x)	Estimated probability of death (qx)	Estimated probability of survival (px)	Percentage of survivors after x years (1x)
0–1	0	4	119	117.0	0.0000	1.0000	100.0000
1–2	2	15	115	107.5	0.0186	0.9814	98.1395
2–3	1	1	98	97.5	0.0103	0.9897	97.1330
3–4	0	3	96	94.5	0.0000	1.0000	97.1330
4–5	0	30	93	78.0	0.0000	1.0000	97.1330
5–6	1	21	63	52.5	0.0190	0.9810	95.2828
6–7	0	39	41	21.5	0.0000	1.0000	95.2828
7–8	0	2	2	1.0	0.0000	1.0000	95.2828
Total	4	115					

debridement and 6 weeks of intravenous antibiotics followed by a successful re-implantation that was rated "good" 5 years later.

Two failures, one of a femoral component and the other of a tibial component, resulted from aseptic loosening. Both patients weighed more than 100 kg. In the knee with tibial component loosening, a medial tibial defect had been filled with methylmethacrylate cement. When this extruded, the arthroplasty collapsed in varus.

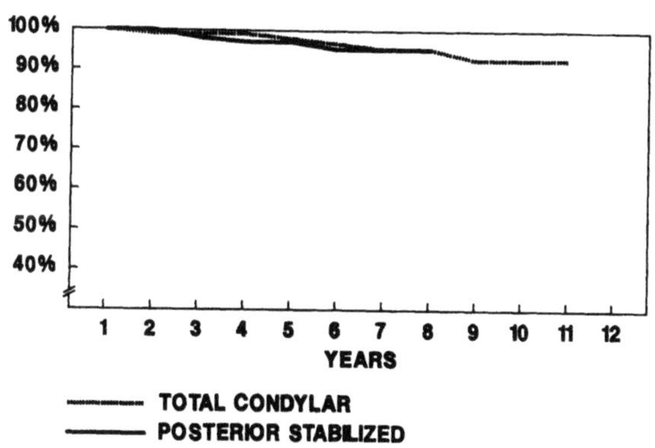

a

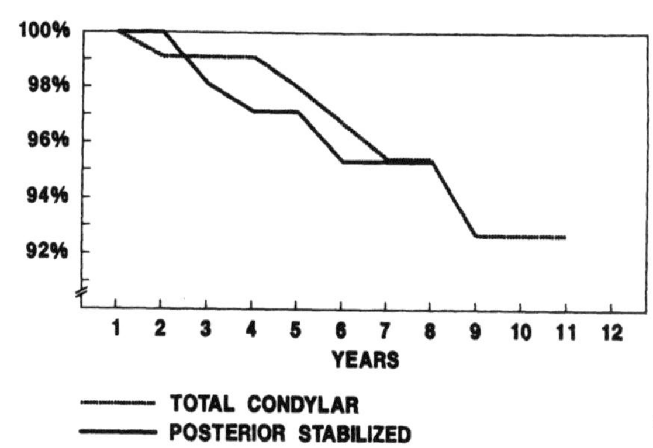

b

Fig. 8.12. a Survivorship curves of Total Condylar and Posterior Stabilized arthroplasties showing no difference by 8 years, with the Total Condylar data extending to 11 years. **b** Magnified view of same curves confirms their similarity.

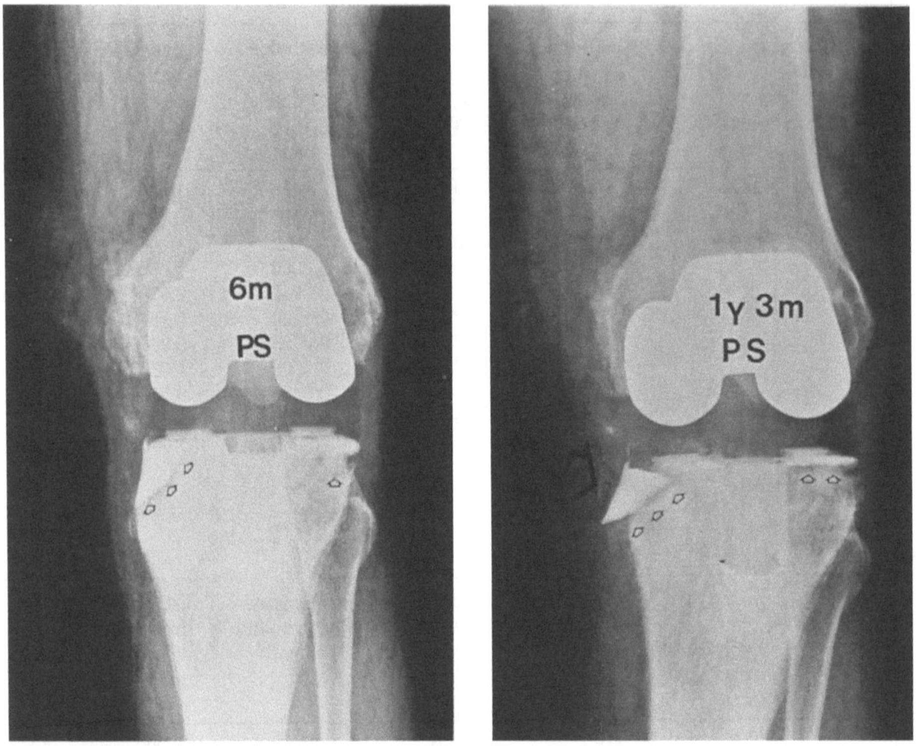

a b

Fig.8.13. **a** Posterior Stabilized arthroplasty at 6 months performed on an obese patient with a severe varus deformity and medial tibial plateau defect. All polyethylene component sits on an uncontained cement wedge in the defect. **b** This technique has been abandoned in favor of bone graft or metal wedge reconstruction, because of the failure of cement block, seen here extruded from the joint (three small arrows) with lifting of the lateral tibial component (two small arrows).

Revision with a custom component including a tibial wedge was rated as excellent 3 years later (Fig. 8.13).

The patient with a loose femoral component was revised with a Total Condylar III prosthesis that loosened within 18 months. A second revision, this time with custom components, was performed and was rated as "good" 2 years later.

The fourth failure occurred 66 months post arthroplasty due to femoral component loosening in a 65-year-old male weighing 84 kg. No organisms were isolated from multiple specimens taken at the time of revision surgery. In retrospect, this patient's past history of pneumocystis carinii pneumonia and contralateral lower limb Kaposi sarcoma indicated probable involvement with the Acquired Immune Deficiency Syndrome (AIDS). Unusual, difficult to isolate opportunistic organisms may have contributed to loosening. Successful revision surgery was performed, but the patient died of diseases related to AIDS within 18 months (Fig. 8.14).

The predicted survivorship for the Posterior Stabilized was therefore 95.2% at 8 years and for the Total Condylar was 92.7% at 12 years (Table 8.2).

Clinical Rating

Only those Posterior Stabilized arthroplasties with a 5–8 year follow-up, and the Total Condylar arthroplasties with a 10–12 year follow-up were included in the clinical assessment. All failures had been included in both the survivorship analyses and clinical evaluations.

Ninety-six Posterior Stabilized prostheses had an average pre-operative HSS knee score of 49 points and were followed for a minimum of 5 years at which time 76 (79%) were rated excellent, 16 (17%) were good, none were fair and four (4%) were rated poor (Fig. 8.15).

Seventy-four Total Condylar knees were evaluated at 10–12 years postoperatively: there were 38 excellent (51%), 27 good (37%), 3 fair

a
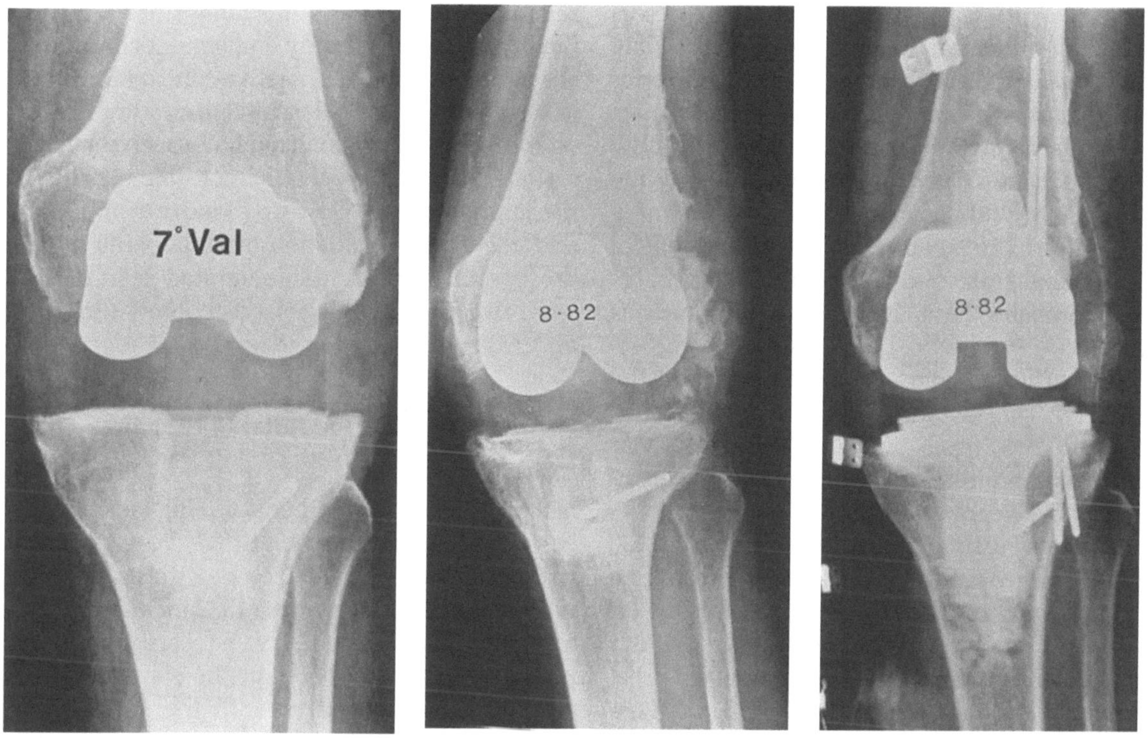

b,c

Fig.8.14. a Patient with well aligned, well fixed Posterior Stabilized arthroplasty who later (b) suffered painful loosening inexplicably. Diagnosis of AIDS was made later. While all intra-operative cultures were negative for infection, it is possible that sepsis from difficult to isolate organisms may have occurred. c Successful revision to custom Posterior Stabilized components was performed, but the patient succumbed to AIDS within 18 months.

(4%) and 6 poor (8%) results (Fig. 8.15). Because of the longer duration of follow-up in this latter group, the patients were about 5 years older on average than those in the Posterior Stabilized group. Scores decline with age due to general debility unrelated to function of the arthroplasty (Goldberg et al. 1988; Vince et al. 1989).

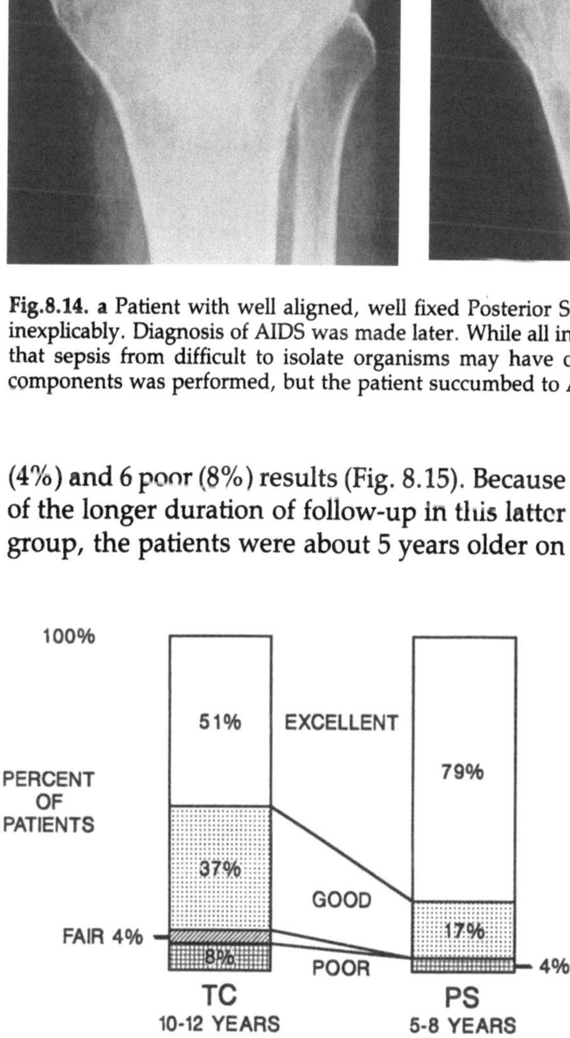

Fig.8.15. Comparison of Total Condylar HSS knee scores at 10–12 years with Posterior Stabilized scores at 5–8 years. The higher percentage of good and excellent scores amongst the Posterior Stabilized patients reflects modest increases in flexion and generally better function. The lower Total Condylar scores result from the advanced age of patients in that cohort.

The great concern with the introduction of the Posterior Stabilized prosthesis was whether the modest increase in constraint (mostly rotational) would result in an increased rate of prosthetic loosening. The survival curves, however, with failure defined as prosthetic removal having either been performed or recommended, were not significantly different. If one considers failure due to aseptic component loosening alone, the differences between the two groups are even less.

In the Total Condylar cohort, the greatest single factor associated with failure was malalignment. As has been reported countless times, varus alignment leads to tibial component loosening. The Posterior Stabilized prostheses were implanted on average a few years after the Total Condylar prostheses. This was a critical era in the development of surgical techniques for the correction of deformity and maintenance of stability. While malalignment was a rare occurrence in the Posterior Stabilized group, generally heavier patients were treated with the Posterior Stabilized prosthesis and at the time, techniques for reconstructing tibial defects were not fully developed. This has been demonstrated by the arthroplasty with cement reconstruction of a tibial defect. The advent of superior methods of using bone graft and augmented prostheses would probably have averted a failure such as this.

We concluded from our comparison that the improved clinical function of the Posterior Stabilized prosthesis over the Total Condylar was not compromised by a higher rate of loosening after 5–8 years of use.

A recent survivorship analysis of 1430 cemented knee arthroplasties performed over a 15 year period on the HSS Knee Service evaluated 224 Total Condylar prostheses with a polyethylene tibia, 289 Posterior Stabilized prostheses with a polyethylene tibia and 917 Posterior Stabilized prostheses with a metal-backed tibial component. Over the 15 year study period, there were 12 failures amongst the Total Condylars with an annual failure rate of 0.65% and a success rate of 90.56%. The Posterior Stabilized components with polyethylene tibial components had an annual failure rate of 0.27% and a 10 year success rate of 97.34%. The metal-backed tibial components had 0.19% failures annually and a 7 year success rate of 98.75%. No metal-backed tibial components needed revision during the seven years of the study (Scuderi et al. 1989).

The use of the Posterior Stabilized arthroplasty has been evaluated in several special situations. Ambulatory patients with arthritis and concomitant Parkinson's disease functioned well, after conventional surgical techniques were used to correct flexion deformities (Vince et al. 1988b). Posttraumatic arthritis poses specific problems, with surgical results that are often inferior to those after primary arthroplasty for arthritis (Zelicoff et al. 1988). Patients with psoriasis have generally good functional results, but are subject to inordinately high (17%) infection rates (Stern and Insall 1989), presumably from chronic bacterial skin colonization. The Posterior Stabilized prosthesis offers the advantage of increased posterior stability for revision knee arthroplasty (Insall and Dethmers 1982) and reimplantation after infection (Insall 1986). Neuropathic arthropathy and similar conditions are often regarded as a relative contra-indication to knee arthroplasty. Reasonable surgical results with the Posterior Stabilized have been reported for a small series of Charcot joints with a medium duration follow-up (Soudry et al. 1986a) and a 2–9 year evaluation of 70 patients under the age of 55 years demonstrated results that were superior to high tibial osteotomy (Stern et al. 1990).

Clinical Results: Hospitals other than HSS

Norman Scott of the Lennox Hill Hospital in New York has reported an extensive experience with the Posterior Stabilized prosthesis since its inception. His first report in 1982 included primary arthroplasties done for osteoarthritis in 34 patients, rheumatoid arthritis in 5, and revision surgery in 4. Consistent with the series from HSS, the average age of patients at Lennox Hill was 65 years (range 25–84), with a predominance of women. The Lennox Hill group included some profound deformities: 45° of varus, 35° of valgus and 80° of flexion contracture.

Results by HSS knee scores were poorest for the revisions and best for patients with osteoarthritis. Using manipulation under general anesthesia in 14 patients (24%), the average motion for the entire group was 112° with 120° for patients with osteoarthritis, 104° for rheumatoid arthritis and 88° for posttraumatic arthritis. The complications in this early series included two deaths, two infections, one transient peroneal nerve palsy and two cases of myositis ossificans. No mention was made of patellar fractures (Scott and Schosheim 1982).

Scott and Rubinstein (1986) published an interim report of 56 knees with follow-up of 3–6 years. This series was distinguished by an unusually even division by gender with 20 women and 18 men. All but one arthroplasty received a patellar dome. The average age of 67.7 years (range 27–84) and weight of 165 pounds (102–235) were comparable to other series. The majority of patients had osteoarthritis or osteonecrosis (82%) with rheumatoid arthritis (14%) and old tibial plateau fractures (4%) comprising the balance.

With an average pre-operative knee score of 46.9 points, the clinical results at follow-up were 87% excellent, 7% good, 2% fair and 4% poor (Fig. 8.16). Data regarding knee motion were not included. The notable finding in this study, however, was the occurrence of patellar fractures in three knees (5.3%). All of these were sustained by patients who had received the 41 mm polyethylene button, which is thicker as well as having a larger diameter. It is difficult to ascribe fractures to the size of the component alone as larger sized patella prostheses are used in larger, heavier patients who tend to be male. This interim follow-up did not report any cases of tibial component loosening.

Scott and associates (1988) later published a 2–8 year follow-up of 119 primary arthroplasties. This group of patients resembled the HSS cohorts with respect to age, weight and diagnosis. Three arthroplasties radiographically showed subsidence of the tibial component including one patient with bilateral replacements who declined revision. The third case was revised. Infection complicated two other surgeries and was treated by resection arthroplasty in one patient and staged re-implantation in another. In this review, by HSS knee scores, 83% of the arthroplasties were rated excellent, 15% good, none fair and 2% as poor (Fig. 8.16).

Patellar fractures occurred in six knees (5%), all within the first year after arthroplasty. Five patients healed spontaneously without additional surgery and eventually enjoyed excellent results. One was treated with a patellectomy. Each patient with a fracture had received a lateral patellar retinacular release with transection of the lateral geniculate arteries. Dr. Scott and his associates attributed patellar fracture in large part to avascularity (W.N. Scott et al. 1988) and later pursued elegant studies of patellar bone scans after lateral retinacular release that are discussed below (Scuderi et al. 1987).

Recognizing that pre-operative motion is a major factor in determining post arthroplasty flexion, Scott and associates noted that the 49 arthroplasties that gained less than 100° of flexion had an average pre-operative flexion of 77°. By excluding these 49 knees, they found an overall arc of flexion of 114° in the remaining 70. This, however, is not consistent with how motion has been reported in the past and is not easily compared with the results of other series.

Lombardi et al. (1988) reviewing 47 Posterior Stabilized knee arthroplasties done by or under the supervision of Dr Thomas Mallory in Columbus, Ohio, reported an 85% survival rate at 6 years. This resulted from four failures in three patients (one infection, two aseptic loosenings, and one painful and stiff). The presence of radiolucent lines, although nonprogressive in the five knees where they occurred, correlated with malalignment. This report did not comment on the problem of patellar fractures.

Aglietti, who had published his results with the Total Condylar (Aglietti and Rinonapoli 1984), collaborated with Mazzotti for his first report in English of a series of Posterior Stabilized arthroplasties. Twenty-two cases were evaluated between 6–21 months. No failures were noted at this early stage and 91% of patients enjoyed good or excellent results. Most of the manuscript was devoted to a detailed description of the prosthesis and surgical technique (Aglietti and Mazzotti 1981). A second report had an average 3½ year follow-up with a familiar patient group that averaged 65 years of age (range 22–77) and had 73% women. The distribution of diagnoses were osteoarthritis or osteonecrosis in 72%, and rheumatoid arthritis in 28%. Pre-operative deformities were similar to other reports, but included a relatively high percentage (17.5%) of patients who had significant flexion contractures, with a mean of 37° (range 20°–80°). Data were presented for 70 knees (85% of entire cohort). The results were excellent in 72%, good in 22%, fair in 4% and poor in 2% (Aglietti et al. 1986) (Fig. 8.16).

Three fair results were related to varus instability after lateral collateral release, subsidence of a tibial component into varus and a severe patellar click, that improved after surgical resection of a peripatellar fibrotic nodule. Two poor results were due to infection and loosening of both components in obese patients. Suppression with antibiotics (though not the preferred treatment in ideal circumstances) was elected for the first patient, and arthrodesis was performed for the second (Aglietti et al. 1986).

Aglietti and Buzzi (1988) published a 3–8 year follow-up of Posterior Stabilized arthroplasties in 1988. They reviewed 85 knees out of 95 that had received this prosthesis. There was a predominance of women (87%) with other variables similar to previous studies. Excellent results

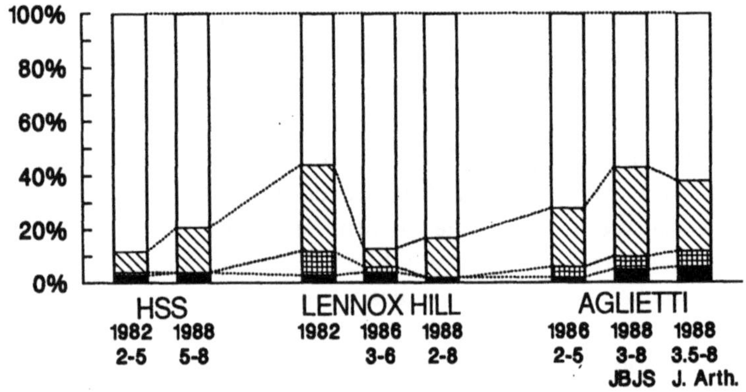

EXC	88	79	56	87	83	72	57	62
GOOD	8	17	32	7	15	22	33	26
FAIR	1	0	9	2	0	4	5	6
POOR	3	4	3	4	2	2	5	6

Fig.8.16. Comparison of HSS knee scores amongst several studies of the Posterior Stabilized prosthesis: HSS (left), Lennox Hill (center) and Aglietti (right). The 1982 Lennox Hill scores were compromised by inclusion of patients with posttraumatic arthritis, and revision arthroplasties. The patient cohorts differ in each study although good and excellent results dominate.

were noted in 57%, good in 33%, fair in 5% and poor in 5% (Fig. 8.16). "Probable" radiographic loosening was diagnosed in 2 of 33 all polyethylene tibial components and 3 of 50 metal-backed devices. The incidence (6%) is identical in both groups. Only one of these cases was confirmed by revision surgery, and the others continued to function without revision at the time of publication.

They did not experience any patellar stress fractures in their series despite having performed lateral retinacular releases in 48% of knees, without preserving the geniculate arteries. These surgeons felt that the modest average flexion of 98° (70°–130°) in their series (being less than the HSS patients) may have protected the patella.

Aglietti and Buzzi (1988) were, however, disturbed by a 20% incidence of patellofemoral impingement (Table 8.3), which they attributed to proximal soft tissues rubbing against the anterior edge of the femoral component. They observed a reduction in the frequency of this problem after the anterior femoral flange was redesigned with a smoother contour in 1982. A low position of the patella relative to the joint line (patella baja) was identified as the major associated factor in their patients with patellofemoral problems (Aglietti et al. 1988).

Laskin and associates (1988), having an extensive experience with cruciate sacrificing, cruciate sparing and posterior stabilized designs, reviewed a large group of arthroplasties that had been performed in arthritic knees with severe

Table 8.3. Patellofemoral problems

	Prosthesis[a]	Fracture (%)	Subluxation (%)	Impingement (%)
Insall et al. (1982)	PS	8.4	1.7	2.5
Scott W.N. and Rubinstein (1986)	PS		5.3	
Scott W.N. and Schosheim (1982)	PS		5.0	
Aglietti and Buzzi (1988)	PS		0.0	20
Scott R.D. (1982)	Duopatella	RA:0.7 OA:3.5		
Ranawat et al. (1984)	TC	0.0		
Ritter and Campbell (1987)	Not specified	Release No release	1.5 3.6	

[a]PS, Posterior Stabilized; TC, Total Condylar

fixed deformities. Each knee had > 15° of fixed varus and all but five had a concomitantly severe flexion contracture.

These arthroplasties were divided into three groups: (1) Severe deformities reconstructed with a variety of posterior cruciate retaining prostheses. (2) Severe deformities reconstructed with the Insall-Burstein Posterior Stabilized prosthesis. (3) A control group with neither fixed varus nor valgus deformities, and with flexion contractures of < 5°, where a posterior cruciate retaining device was used. The three groups were comparable for all other pertinent variables, with pre-operative HSS knee scores of 59, 57 and 59 points for groups 1 to 3 respectively and postoperative scores of 80, 88 and 86 respectively. While the differences in scores were not statistically significant, the ability to eliminate flexion contractures (Fig. 8.17a) and restore desired valgus alignment (Fig. 8.17b) was better with the Posterior Stabilized prosthesis. The results with the Posterior Stabilized prosthesis in the deformed knees were similar to those with cruciate retaining devices in the undeformed knees. In addition, the mean flexion for group 1 was 83° and for group 2 was 113°, implying that it is more difficult to restore flexion and retain a functional posterior cruciate ligament in the deformed knee than it is mechanically to substitute for the function of the PCL (Fig. 8.17c). This paper is one of the few recent studies to critically compare subtle aspects of different designs and indicate specific situations where one design may be preferable to another (Laskin et al. 1988).

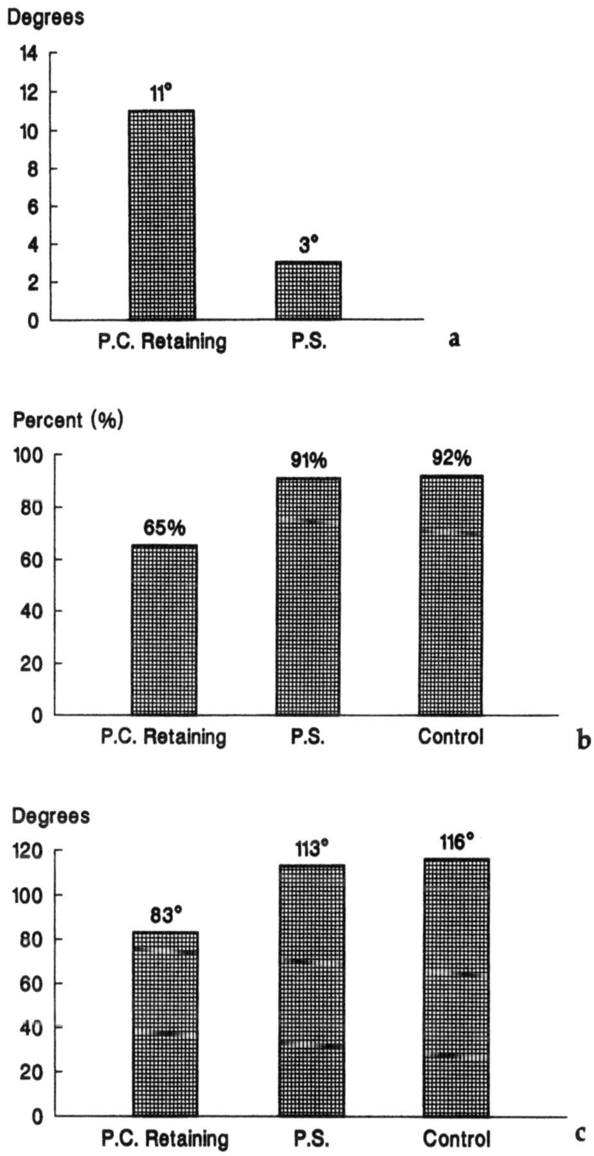

Fig. 8.17. a–c. Comparing the Posterior Stabilized (P.S.) total knee prosthesis in knees with severe fixed deformity with a similarly deformed group and a nondeformed control group using posterior cruciate (P.C.) retaining devices. **a** Mean residual flexion contracture postarthroplasty. **b** Percentage of patients with desired 7° (±2°) valgus alignment, implying that correction of deformity may be more easily achieved after resection of the cruciate ligament. **c** Mean flexion in each group demonstrating mean of 113° in severely deformed knees treated with the Posterior Stabilized prosthesis that is superior to mean of 83° with posterior cruciate retaining devices in deformed knees and comparable to results with posterior cruciate retaining devices in nondeformed knees. (from Laskin et al. (1988) with permission.)

Patellofemoral Complications

The patellofemoral joint is one of the most problematic aspects of knee arthroplasty. Insall et al. (1985) have described it as the major residual complication in an otherwise successful surgical procedure. The topic merits detailed attention in a discussion of the Posterior Stabilized arthroplasty, as patellar fracture and "patellar catch syndrome" have been identified specifically in patients with this prothesis.

The decision to resurface the patella emerged from some basic trade-offs. If the patella is left unresurfaced, about 30% of patients will suffer persistent pain and compromised function of the extensor mechanism (R.D. Scott 1979; R.D. Scott et al. 1982; W.N. Scott et al. 1978). While universal resurfacing has been favored, (Levai et al. 1983; Ranawat et al. 1984) the topic continues to receive attention (Shoji et al. 1989; Soudry et al. 1986b), largely because of complications that have resulted from resurfacing.

Fracture: Incidence and Etiology

While much has been written about patellar fractures, it is apparent that little is conclusive (Table 8.4). The complication is neither new to resurfaced patellae nor unique to the Posterior Stabilized prosthesis. Patellar complications occurred in offset hinge prostheses such as the Guepar and unconstrained devices such as the Geomedic, Townley, ICLH (Freeman and Hammer 1978) and the Duopatella, both with and without patellar resurfacing. Mochizuki and Schurman (1979) reviewed 32 unresurfaced patellae in offset hinges and described patellar subluxation in 37%, dislocation in 10%, generalized wear of the patellar cartilage and bone in 4% and localized wear in 6%. The complications were fewer with unconstrained devices (without patellar resurfacing) where 3% and 6% had subluxation and generalized wear respectively. Persistent pain, thought to originate in the patellofemoral joint, was common in their study, but no fractures of the patella were noted. Perhaps pain protected the patella by diminishing the patients' activities. Roffman et al. (1980) described an unusual case where a Total Condylar patellar dome was used with a Guepar arthroplasty and a patellar fracture resulted.

Table 8.4. Factors contributing to fatigue fracture of resurfaced patella

(a) Demand
1. Weight (Thompson et al. 1981; Dupont and Baker 1982)
2. General activity (Insall et al. 1982)
3. Flexion (Insall et al. 1982; Aglietti et al. 1988. Contrary: Simison et al. 1986)

(b) Patellofemoral component design
5. Increased thickness (W.N. Scott and Schosheim. 1982)
6. Lug length (R.D. Scott et al. 1982)

(c) Weak bone
7. Osteopenia (R.D. Scott et al. 1982)
8. Steroid therapy (Dupont and Baker 1982)
9. Thermal necrosis due to PMMA (Berman et al. 1984; Clayton and Thirupathi 1982)

(d) Surgery
10. Patellar cut
    - (i) Removal of excess bone to weaken patella (R.D. Scott et al. 1982; Levai et al. 1983)
    - (ii) Removal of inadequate bone to increase forces (Bryan 1988)
    - (iii) Removal of peripheral bone (R.D. Scott et al. 1982; Thompson et al. 1981)
    - (iv) Removal of lateral facet subchondral bone (Ranawat et al. 1984)
11. Avascular necrosis due to lateral release (R.D. Scott et al. 1982; Clayton and Thirupathi 1982. Contrary: Aglietti et al. 1988)
12. Lateral shear of patella (Ritter and Campbell 1987; Thompson et al. 1981)
13. Increased tension in extensor mechanism due to: Anterior tibial displacement and increased distance from tibial tubercle to origin of extensors (Ranawat et al. 1984; Roffman et al. 1980; Simison et al. 1986)
14. General malalignment of any of the arthroplasty components (Figgie et al. 1989)

(e) Fixation failure
15. Loosening of patellar component (Thompson et al. 1981)

The Duopatellar prosthesis was one of the first knee arthroplasties to provide patellar resurfacing. Richard Scott and colleagues described their experience in 1982 with Duopatellar arthroplasties implanted between 1975 and 1980. This prosthesis, along with the Total Condylar, evolved directly from clinical experience with the Duocondylar (R.D. Scott 1982; Chap. 7). During that period, Richard Scott and associates resurfaced all patellae in patients who had rheumatoid arthritis to eliminate the antigenic stimulus of residual articular cartilage and so minimize the chance of recurrent effusions. They were, however, selective about resurfacing patellae in the presence of osteoarthritis, citing a stronger quadriceps moment by Cybex testing without a patellar prosthesis and a 3.5% incidence of stress fracture through the fixation lug when the dome was used (R.D. Scott and Reilly 1980). In their patients without patellar resurfacing, there was one fracture in 588 rheumatoid knees (0.2%) and no fractures among 253 osteoarthritic knees. These surgeons identified avascular, necrotic bone at the time of repeat surgery on some of the knees with patellar fractures and concluded that the lateral patellar retinacular release, including transection of the geniculate arteries, was largely responsible for the fractures. In addition, they noted fewer fractures after reducing the size of the lug such that a more shallow hole was drilled in the patella (R.D. Scott et al. 1982).

The Attenborough knee replacement evolved similarly; no provision was made for patellar resurfacing initially, but the high incidence of patellofemoral pain (56%) led to the introduction of patellar resurfacing. While the pain was remedied by patellar resurfacing, patellar fracture complicated 17.5% of these knees. The fragmentation differed in extent, from small fractures of the pole to general comminution. The fractures occurred spontaneously (except for one patient who fell), were identified incidentally on routine radiographs and happened within 12 months of surgery in the majority of patients. The extent of flexion was modest in this study group, with 61% achieving 90° or less motion and only 3% achieving more than 110°. The Attenborough prosthesis is mechanically stabilized by a bar that links the tibial and femoral components, and the patellar prosthesis features a relatively large central lug (Simison et al. 1986). A similarly high frequency of fractures was observed by Cameron and Fedorkow (1982) with the ICLH prosthesis when the drill hole intentionally broached the anterior cortex.

The Total Condylar arthroplasty, introduced in 1974, was initially implanted with selective patellar resurfacing at the Hospital for Special Surgery. However, the results with a patellar dome proved superior in terms of pain relief and function with fewer cases requiring additional surgery for patellofemoral problems (W.N. Scott et al. 1978). Insall, Scott and Ranawat, in an early review of Total Condylar arthroplasties, reported one fracture of a resurfaced patella in 422 cases (0.2%) (Insall et al. 1979a). Roffman et al. (1980) reported a resurfaced Total Condylar patella complicated by fracture in 1980 and Clayton and Thirupathi (1982) reported ten patellar complications in 111 Total Condylar arthroplasties (9%), of which six (5%) were fractures. The average onset of these complications was early, at 1.4 years. Dupont and Baker (1982) reported six patellar fractures in 921 (0.65%) arthroplasties that included Total Condylar and Duopatellar prostheses. They identified obesity, rheumatoid arthritis and steroid therapy in the affected patients.

In a more comprehensive review of patellar fractures complicating Total Condylar knee arthroplasties at the Hospital for Special Surgery, Thompson, Hood and Insall identified 18 cases in 1030 (1.75%) knees from 1974–1980. The group with fractures was predominantly female (83%) and with an average age of 66 years (comparable to the cohort as a whole). All had osteoarthritis, with a mean weight of 188 lb and height of 5′2″. This mean weight exceeded that of the entire group by about 30 lb. The fractures were heralded by the appearance of a cement peg radiolucency in ten patients (55%) which some attribute to avascular necrosis. These fractures were diagnosed on average 15 months after arthroplasty (range 2–60 months). Fractures not associated with antecedent radiolucencies occurred earlier, at 7 months on average. All but three fractures were regarded as the result of fatigue failure rather than trauma. Conservative treatment yielded the best results when it was feasible (Thompson et al. 1981).

Grace and Sim (1986, 1988) reported 12 patellar fractures (0.15%) at the Mayo Clinic during a period when 8249 total knee arthroplasties had been performed. This likely represents underreporting as no mention is made of duration of follow-up or how many patients were lost. The different orientation of fractures suggested different etiologies to these surgeons: horizontally displaced fractures related to excessive lateral loading from incorrect tracking, and vertically displaced fractures were the result of weakness secondary to resection of the articular surface, the lug hole and perhaps avascularity.

The first formal review of the Posterior Stabilized prosthesis (Insall et al. 1982), as noted above, found that patients climbed stairs better and enjoyed more flexion than had been the experience with the Total Condylar. This was accompanied by an 8.4% incidence of patellar fractures, that was attributed to the larger polyethylene buttons, increased flexion and greater activity level in patients who had fractures. Because the spine and cam mechanism and the anterior displacement of the tibal tubercle that it produces actually increases the moment arm of the extensor mechanism, a lower quadriceps force would be expected for identical motion without the mechanism (Insall et al. 1982). Some have suggested, however, that anterior displacement of the tibia may also increase the distance from the origin to the insertion of the extensor mechanism. As flexion increases, so too does the tension in the patella (Ranawat et al. 1984). When combined with a thicker button, this tension may exceed the yield point of patellar bone.

In our review of a similar but not identical cohort of the early HSS Posterior Stabilized arthroplasties from 5 to 8 years, the incidence of patellar fracture had not increased from the first report (Vince et al. 1988c). All patellar fractures occurred within the first 3 years after surgery, a 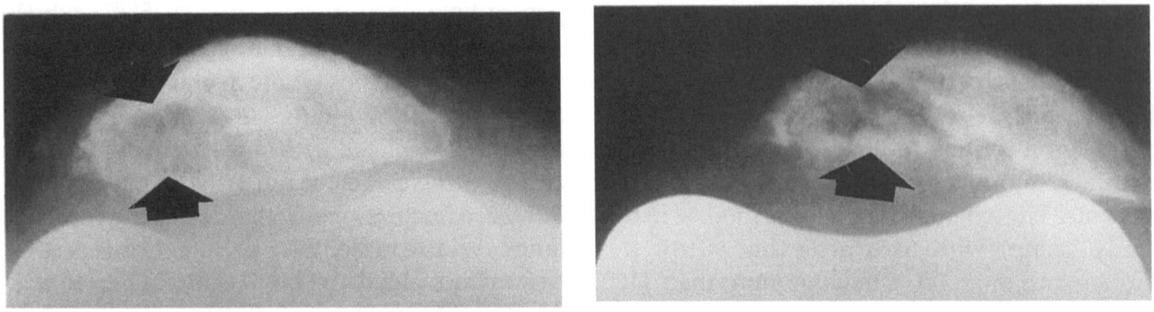 b

Fig. 8.18. a,b. Merchant patellofemoral radiographic views. Radiolucency that may represent avascular necrosis in an otherwise well fixed, centrally tracking patella (**a**) proved to herald loosening of the polyethylene dome and fracture of the patella (**b**).

and most within 2 years. This tendency has been observed in other reports of patellar stress fractures after knee arthroplasty (Clayton and Thirupathi 1982; Goldberg et al. 1988; Roffman et al. 1980; R.D. Scott et al. 1982; Simison et al. 1986), implying that a mechanical situation has been established by the knee arthroplasty that predisposes to fracture. If the cause of fractures were simply fatigue failure, then as more time passed the incidence of fractures would increase.

Richard Scott and associates, in comparing motion and incidence of fracture in the Duopatellar and Total Condylar arthroplasties, concluded that the greater flexion possible in cruciate retaining designs explained their higher frequency of patellar disruption (R.D. Scott et al. 1982). While excellent restoration of flexion, high activity level and heavy patient weight undoubtedly increase the forces on the patella, it would seem that increased stress is not sufficient cause for fracture. One series reporting mean flexion greater than 125°, with the Yoshino-Shoji knee reported no patellar fractures (Shoji et al. 1987). Increased flexion in conjunction with factors that weaken the patella, such as osteopenia (R.D. Scott et al. 1982), deep lug holes (R.D. Scott et al. 1982), removal of large amounts of bone in preparation for resurfacing and thermal necrosis of bone by methylmethacrylate (Clayton and Thirupathi 1982), may be responsible.

The implication of avascular necrosis of patellar bone secondary to a lateral patellar retinacular release has received considerable attention. Ranawat et al. (1984) published radiographs of a progressive lucency in a resurfaced patella that they attributed to osteonecrosis. While this case (in a Total Condylar knee arthroplasty) did not result in a patellar fracture, it undoubtedly weakened the patella and supports the observation of Thompson et al. (1981) that radiolucencies herald a fracture. I have observed a similar sequence of progressive radiolucency around the patellar component in a Posterior Stabilized arthroplasty, that culminated in a fracture (Fig. 8.18).

Several surgeons have investigated the relationship between lateral patellar retinacular release, avascular necrosis of the patella and patellar fracture. Release of the patella is, of course, essential in some cases to ensure smooth, central tracking of the extensor mechanism. Valgus alignment of the arthroplasty, trauma, malrotation of tibial or femoral components and failure to perform a release when necessary have all been identified as factors leading to dislocation of the patella. The type of prosthesis is not generally regarded as a factor in dislocation (Merkow et al. 1988). While the release is frequently performed in clinical practice, there is concern that interruption of the superior geniculate artery, especially in conjunction with resection of the patellar fat pad that carries the inferior geniculate artery will render the patella avascular (Scapinelli 1967; Clayton and Thirupathi 1982). There is also evidence, in a rabbit model, that polymethylmethacrylate cement can cause thermal necrosis of bone (Berman et al. 1984).

Wetzner et al. (1985) studied 41 knee arthroplasties of unspecified design with ^{99m}Tc-MDP bone scan before and 6–17 days after arthroplasty to assess patellar vasculature. Believing that avascular bone places an arthroplasty patient at greater risk of patellar fracture, these surgeons restricted the activities of patients with cold bone scans and performed a follow-up examination 2–3 months postoperatively. Four patients had less uptake on the postoperative than pre-operative scan; three of them had been treated with lateral retinacular releases. Follow-up bone scans in these patients demonstrated progressively increased uptake of radionuclide. Of the other 36 arthroplasties with the expected postoperative increase in scan activity, ten had received lateral retinacular releases. No fractures occurred, and the effect of restricted activity is difficult to assess.

In a similar study, Scuderi et al. (1987) examined the relationship of lateral releases to patellar viability in 36 Insall-Burstein Posterior Stabilized knee arthroplasties, performed by or under the direction of Norman Scott at the Lennox Hill Hospital. A variety of prosthetic patellar button sizes had been used and the scans were performed at varying intervals after surgery (24 hours to 7 days). Scans showed that 56.3% of patellae with a lateral release and 15% of those without a release sustained an avascular insult, but neither group had radiographic abnormalities. Sequential scans of the 12 cold patellae taken 3–10 months after surgery showed a progressive increase in the patellar radionuclide uptake, indicating revascularization. The only patellar fracture occurred in one knee of a patient who had undergone bilateral arthroplasties, with both patellae appearing cold on scan. The fracture occurred 8 months after arthroplasty and was treated successfully without surgery (Fig. 8.19). Late revascularization of the patella may come from the prepatellar vessels as indicated by Kayler and Lyttle (1988).

The association between lateral patellar retinacular releases and at least temporary avascularity if not necrosis has been established. Necrotic bone, which may be a causal, resultant or independent factor has been identified histologically in some fractured patellae (R.D. Scott et al. 1982). However, the hypothesized causal link between lateral releases and fracture has not been confirmed. Ritter and Campbell (1987) sought, but did not find, a relationship between performing the lateral retinacular release and the occurrence of patellar fracture. By contrast, they found 17 patellar fractures amongst 471 arthroplasties (3.6%) where no release had been performed and a single fracture amongst 84 arthroplasties (1.5%) when a release had been performed. They concluded that increased lateral pull on an unreleased patella was in fact largely responsible for increased tensile force and fracture.

Figgie et al. (1989) applied their concept of a "neutral range" of component position (Figgie et al. 1986) to the evaluation of 36 condylar type arthroplasties with patellar fractures. They found that none of these patients had components aligned in the neutral range and the greater the malalignment, the more severe the fracture. Unlike other surgeons who have focused on local factors, Figgie et al. cite overall arthroplasty alignment as a major source of problems.

Treatment of Patellar Fracture

Fractures of a resurfaced patella may often be treated without surgery. Certainly, the reduced mass of bone, especially if avascular, is rarely amenable to open reduction and internal fixation. Goldberg, as the first author of a collaborative study on patellar fracture type and prognosis in condylar total knee arthroplasties classified these complications in 36 cases (Table 8.5). No data were offered regarding the type of prosthesis involved although radiographs of several Posterior Stabilized devices were

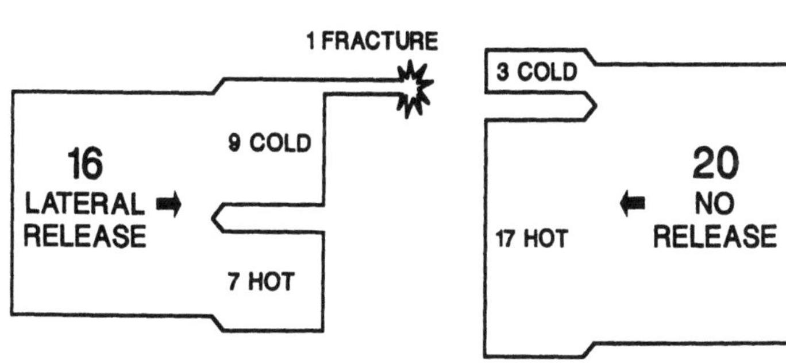

Fig.8.19. Flow chart indicating the occurrence of cold and hot bone scans after lateral patellar retinacular release. Despite small numbers, it seems that this release, by violating the geniculate vessels, is more likely to cause a vascular insult to the patella. To what extent this results in patellar fractures is unknown (Scuderi et al. 1987).

Table 8.5. Goldberg classification of patellar fractures in total knee replacement

I. Not involving the implant/cement composite or quadriceps mechanisms
II. Involving the implant/cement composite and/or quadriceps mechanisms
III. a. Inferior pole fractures *with* patellar ligament rupture
 b. Inferior pole fractures *without* patellar ligament rupture
IV. Fracture dislocations

included. They concluded that fractures not associated with loosening of the patellar component, disruption of the extensor mechanism (Type I or III B) or major implant malalignment may be treated nonoperatively. All 15 knees with these types of fractures received an excellent or good rating, without surgical intervention. They observed mixed results after surgery on all patellae with a fracture dislocation, with fractures disrupting the bone/implant/cement composite (Type II) and fractures with extensor mechanism disruption (Goldberg et al. 1986).

In general, loosening of the patellar dome is a compelling indication for surgery. This may be apparent on plain radiographs or, as with some all polyethylene designs, will be best demonstrated with an arthrogram (Fig. 8.20). It is frequently useful to temporize if the extensor mechanism is intact even if the dome is loose, to allow some consolidation of fracture fragments to occur. This will maximize the prospect of resurfacing the patella at surgery. When resurfacing is not feasible, it is preferable to shape the remaining bone rather than perform a patellectomy.

Patellar Tracking and Impingement

Problems with tracking are largely avoidable by correct component positioning in conjunction with a lateral patellar retinacular release (Merkow et al. 1988; Leblanc 1989). Other soft tissue problems of the resurfaced patellofemoral joint remain problematic and at times puzzling. Insall, Lachiewicz and Burstein (1982) described a painful Posterior Stabilized knee arthroplasty that was improved by removal of a peripatellar fibrotic nodule. They also noted painless grating and clicking during extension of the knee that was suggestive of a similar lesion in two other patients. The source of symptoms and pain seemed to be soft tissue impingement against the anterior margin of the intercondylar box of the femoral component in the original Posterior Stabilized design. Accordingly, this contour was smoothed and the femoral flange was extended further posteriorly in an early modification of the design. The Insall-Burstein II Posterior Stabilized prosthesis, released in 1989 includes further changes to smooth the patellofemoral articulation (Insall et al. 1982). The catch may still occur, however.

The appearance of peripatellar fibrotic nodules as a cause of pain was later corroborated in a case report by Pettine and Bryan (1986), but with a prosthesis other than the Posterior Stabilized. They were unable fully to explain this occurrence except as an aberration of healing. In another article, Bryan (1988) described the problems of patella infera and fat pad hypertrophy after total knee arthroplasty that result in persistent pain and compromised flexion. While these are two distinct problems, one relating to patellar height and the other to fibrotic nodules about the patella, they appear to be related.

Figgie et al. (1986) at the Case Western Reserve examined 116 consecutive Posterior Stabilized arthroplasties from 2½ to 5 years after surgery. They focused on patellofemoral symptoms including pain, clicking, catching and locking. They concluded that these problems were related to mechanical variables and surgical technique: anterior-posterior positioning of the tibial implant, height of the patella above the joint line, and change in the position of the joint line above the prosthesis. A *neutral range* of component position was determined as that which resulted in: (1) The center of the tibial component being situated at the same position or posterior to the center line of the tibia. (2) A change in the location of the joint line of 8 mm or less. (3) A patellar height of 10–30 mm above the joint line. Only 35% of the cohort fell into this neutral range (Table 8.6), but these knees had uniformly superior results by scores, motion and pain relief.

Patella infera is probably the worst outcome of the three variables studied. Each patient in whom the inferior pole of the patella lay distal to the surface of the joint had pain or diminished function. Figgie and associates explained that

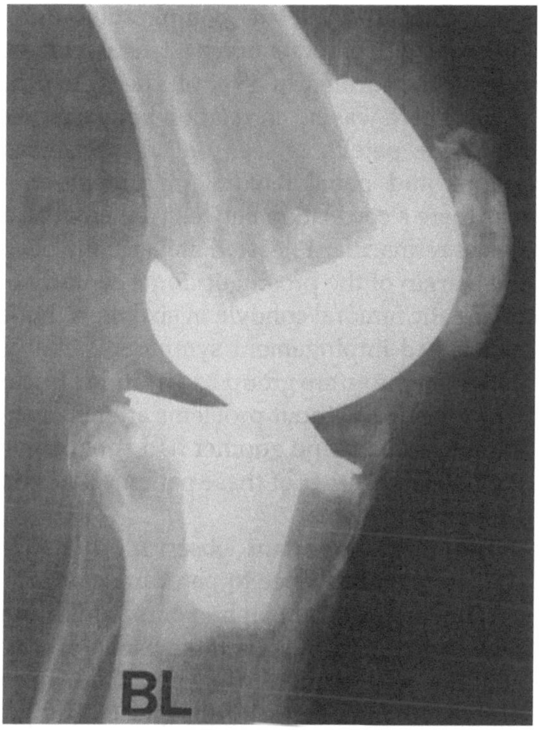

a

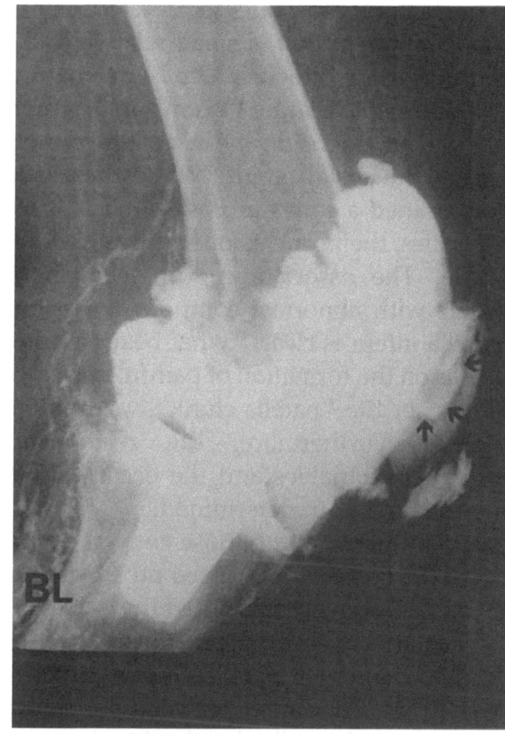

b

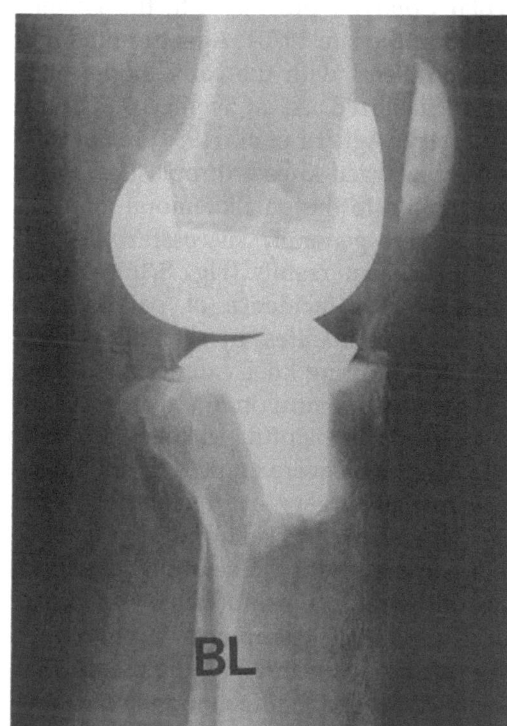

c

Fig. 8.20. **a** Lateral radiograph of a Posterior Stabilized arthroplasty that was painful. Despite the presence of a fragment superiorly, loosening of the dome was not apparent. **b** Lateral arthrogram with dye completely surrounding polyethylene dome, confirming the need for revision surgery. **c** Revised patella feasible because of adequate residual patellar bone.

Table 8.6. The influence of tibial-patellofemoral location on function in patients with the Posterior Stabilized condylar knee prosthesis (Figgie et al. 1986)

	In neutral range	Out of neutral range
% of entire group	35% 41/116	65% 75/116
Mean score	96±2.5 points	84.9±11.5 points
Excellent	39	36
Good	2	25
Fair	Nil	4
Poor	Nil	10
Mean ROM	110±13	96±22
Patellofemoral symptoms		
Pain	Nil	23
Mechanical	Nil	22
Vague ache	Nil	22
Manipulation	Nil	9
Reoperation	Nil	8

patella infera occurs most commonly in patients whose patellae were relatively low with respect to the joint line pre-operatively. We found this to be a common factor compromising the results of total knee replacement after high tibial osteotomy, presumably due to contracture of the patellar tendon itself (Windsor et al. 1988). Two other factors identified by Figgie and associates that lead to patella infera are: anterior positioning of the femoral component and selection of a femoral component that is small relative to the anterior-posterior dimension of the natural femur. Both lead to a larger flexion gap that must be balanced in extension by resection of more bone from the distal femur. While these surgeons examined a series of Posterior Stabilized arthroplasties, their conclusions are more widely applicable. The association of patellofemoral symptoms with abnormal component position and patella infera is clear – what bearing a low patella has on the formation of painful peripatellar nodules or the "patella clunk" syndrome is unspecified. Furthermore, the relationship between these variables and the occurrence of patellar fractures is undetermined.

Aglietti and associates (whose general experience with the Posterior Stabilized prosthesis has been reviewed above) contributed the only work on the Posterior Stabilized prosthesis that has specifically examined patellofemoral function and drawn an association between soft tissue impingement and patellar height. Moving from the Total Condylar prosthesis to the Posterior Stabilized in the late 1970s, Aglietti noted more patellar problems with the early model of the Posterior Stabilized. At an average of 5.5 years after surgery, Aglietti et al. (1988) reviewed 73 Posterior Stabilized knee arthroplasties, paying close attention to the patellofemoral joint. The surgeries were generally successful with 93% good or excellent results (Fig. 8.16), but this included a 21% incidence of patellofemoral impingement as manifest by catching (11%) or locking (10%) during knee extension. Catching was somewhat painful in 6 cases (8%) and locking was mildly painful in 4 knees (5%). Pain from locking was severe enough in one knee to indicate further surgery, at which time a peripatellar proliferative synovial frond, that had been catching on the anterior edge of the intercondylar box of the femoral component, was excised. While the patient's symptoms improved, the overall result remained fair. Aglietti and colleagues found that the gliding motion of the patella was completely smooth in only 41 knees (56%).

The 1982 modification to the anterior box of the femoral component reduced the incidence of all impingement symptoms amongst Aglietti's patients from 25% to 15%. The more severe form of these problems, locking, was almost eliminated by the modification, having been reduced from 15% to 3%. This complication did not correlate with whether or not a lateral retinacular release (performed in 48% of knees) had been done. There was no correlation between medial tilt of the patella as seen on or sunrise radiographs and patellofemoral impingement, nor was there a correlation between a medial tilt and lateral retinacular release. Patellar bone beyond the margin of the prosthetic dome contacted the prosthetic femoral condyle in six knees, none of which had impingement symptoms. Only one patient in the entire group had a fatigue fracture, which healed without problems after 6 weeks of immobilization, and another had subluxation of the patella. Neither of these patients had impingement symptoms.

The most important observation made by Aglietti with reference to patellar impingement pertained to patellar height. For reasons of surgical technique, the height of the patella above the joint line was frequently lowered, from an average of 16 mm before arthroplasty (range 3–37 mm) to only 4 mm after surgery ($P < 0.001$), representing a mean lowering of 12 mm (range 0–28). The average height of the patella was 1.8 mm in patients with impingement problems, 2.2 mm in those with palpable crepitus, and 5.5 mm in knees with a normal gliding movement (difference between first and third variables $P < 0.005$). Patients with the original design of the femoral component were more susceptible to impingement in the presence of patella infera; with a patellar height less than 5 mm the incidence of impingement symptoms was 33%, but it was zero when patellar height exceeded 5 mm.

Aglietti found, consistent with several previous studies (Ritter and Stringer 1979; Vince et al. 1988a), that postoperative flexion correlated better with pre-operative flexion than with the height of the patella. Unlike Figgie and associates, Aglietti did not detect a difference in outcome based on sagittal positioning of the femoral or tibial components. Neither the diameter of the patellar implant (either 32 mm or 35 mm), nor the postoperative tibiofemoral angle, correlated with impingement.

Hozack, working with other surgeons in Philadelphia, specifically reported the "Patellar Clunk Syndrome" in Posterior Stabilized knee arthroplasties (Hozack et al. 1988). Vernace et al.

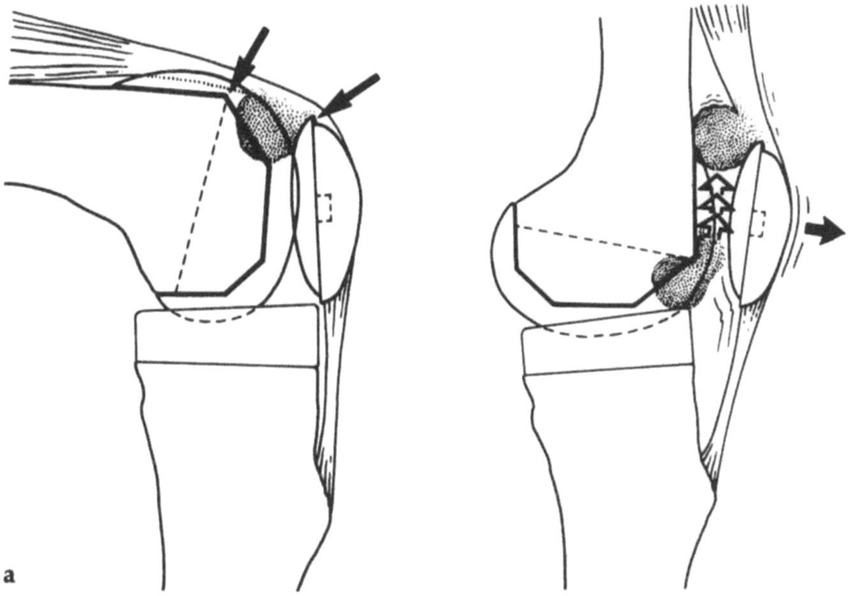

Fig. 8.21. **a** Patellar clunk syndrome resulting from impingement of fibrous tissue between patellar dome and anterior femoral condyle. **b** This usually causes pain during extension as the tissue is dragged over the condyle. Although this has been identified in some cases of Posterior Stabilized arthroplasty, it has also occurred with other prostheses. The offending fibrous tissue may be resected arthroscopically. (From Vernace et al. (1989) with permission.)

(1989), from the same group as Hozack, diagrammed the location of fibrous tissue that catches on the anterior femoral flange to produce the clunk, and described a method for its removal with arthroscopic techniques (Fig. 8.21). The success of this procedure assumes that the impinging fibrous tissue occurs idiosyncratically and is not the *result* of patella infera, otherwise it might be expected to recur.

The Posterior Stabilized implant, like many modern designs, gives reproducibly good surgical results with a satisfactory range of flexion and low incidence of complications. The problem of patellar fracture is largely unresolved, is not unique to this design and is relatively infrequent. The problem of the patellar impingement syndrome is more disturbing. Aglietti's work is extremely important, establishing the relationship with patella infera, and integrating several pertinent observations made by others. It seems that the incidence of symptomatic patellar impingement was lower after the 1982 femoral modification, *but* that serious impingement problems are definitely related to patella infera. These are difficult to correct, especially if the patient has a pre-existing contracture of the patellar tendon.

Surgical Technique

Insall-Burstein I

The Posterior Stabilized arthroplasty was originally implanted using a technique borrowed directly from the Total Condylar and based firmly on several principles of knee arthroplasty developed in the preceding decade (Vince and Dorr 1987). The primacy of soft tissue releases to the restoration of alignment and stability were integral to the procedure. These releases were based in turn on ideas about the pathology of the arthritic knee described by Freeman (1984) and Insall (1984). Minimal proximal tibia was resected to preserve the stronger subchondral bone and flexion and extension gaps were balanced formally using the tensor device. Norman Scott reduced the description of the original technique to a cogent sequence of five steps, which are paraphrased below. These are the "instrument steps" done after soft tissue releases have been completed (W.N. Scott et al. 1988).

Step 1. The anterior femur is cut flush with and parallel to the anterior femoral cortex.

Step 2. The posterior prominences of the femoral condyles are resected using the cutting block that corresponds to the prosthesis that will best approximate this dimension.

Of the five sizes of components in the original system, one (55 mm) was reserved for extremely small patients such as those with juvenile rheumatoid arthritis. The other four represented only two choices of anteroposterior (AP) dimension. The smaller two (58 mm and 65 mm) had the same anteroposterior dimension (44 mm) but differed in medial-lateral width. The same is true of the two larger sizes (66 mm and 72 mm) that shared an identical AP size (48 mm confirm). Consequently, the ability to reproduce the AP dimension was limited to two choices plus one for the extremely small patient.

Step 3. The proximal tibia is resected perpendicular to the axis of the bone using an extramedullary guide. A minimum of bone is removed from the proximal tibia.

Step 4. The level and angle of distal femoral resection is determined by either distracting the extended knee manually or with the use of a tensor device. The alignment, corresponding in large part to the angle of the distal femoral cut, must be valgus, but is determined to a great extent by ligament balance achieved earlier with soft tissue releases. The level of resection is determined by how much distal femur must be resected to create a space in extension that equals the space between the femur and tibia with the knee flexed at 90°.

Step 5. The finishing steps create chamfers and an intercondylar notch on the distal femur and the keel hole in the proximal tibia. The articular surface of the patella is resected and a central lug hole made to accept the prosthetic dome. The arthroplasty is evaluated with trial components before cementing the actual device in place.

Insall-Burstein II

The Insall-Burstein Posterior Stabilized II prosthesis was introduced in 1989 with modifications to the components and instruments reflecting changes in the concepts behind the operation. The contour of the femoral trochlea and the anterior edge of the intercondylar box were further smoothed to diminish patellar impingement. Each one of the five sizes of femoral component was given a discrete anteroposterior dimension, to improve the prospect of reproducing that anatomic dimension.

How a surgeon selects the anteroposterior size of the femoral component affects stability of the arthroplasty, motion of the knee and the height of the patella above the joint line. An oversized femoral component will tend to increase soft tissue tension of the flexion gap, and as a result, may decrease flexion. *Slightly* increased laxity in flexion is feasible with the Posterior Stabilized, because the spine and cam mechanism prevents posterior tibial dislocation within a narrow excursion, as compared with the Total Condylar. The published work of two experienced surgeons, W. N. Scott et al. (1988) and Figgie (1986), has important bearing on this concept. Norman Scott, describing his technique in 1988 explained, "the posterior prominences of the femoral condyles are resected and the widest possible trial femoral component is used, to minimize the amount of bone that is removed". The stated priority is to preserve bone, and maintain stability in flexion. Accordingly there would be a tendency, if the anatomic dimension is "between sizes", to increase the normal dimension and correspondingly increase tension in flexion. While this enhances stability, it may do so at the expense of flexion.

Figgie et al. (1986) as noted above, explained that reducing the AP dimension of the femoral component inevitably requires that more distal femur be resected in order to create equal flexion and extension gaps. Resecting distal femur moves the joint line proximally and creates patella infera.

The current recommendation with the Insall-Burstein II prosthesis is to opt for the smaller sized femur if the actual dimension falls between sizes. This has become safe only because of the larger number of femoral component sizes (AP dimensions) that are available. The associated limitations must be borne in mind – selecting a smaller component leads to patellar infera and a larger one to a tight flexion gap.

The greatest change in the Insall-Burstein II instrument system was the elimination of the tensor device, and introduction of an intramedullary femoral cutting guide. This decision seemed to ignore the principles of establishing equal flexion and extension gaps and the importance of soft tissue releases that had been empha-

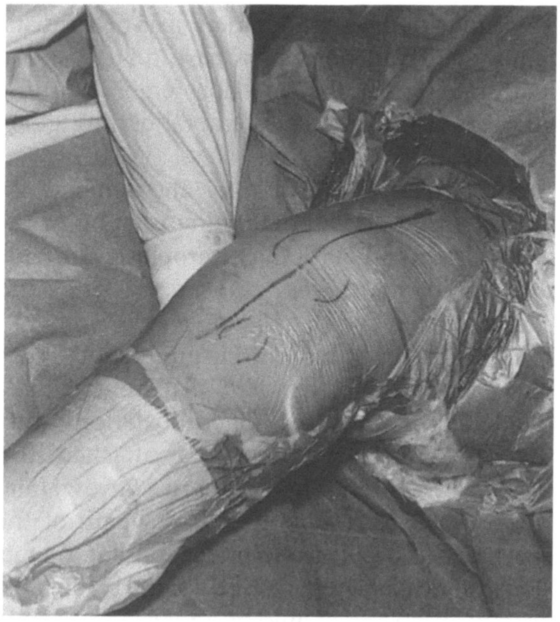

Fig.8.22. Standard anterior longitudinal skin incision, avoiding the bony prominence of the tibial tubercle on its medial side.

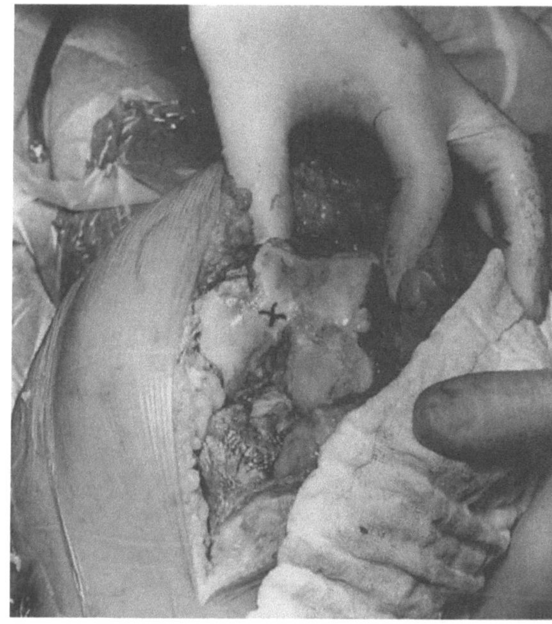

Fig.8.23. Entry point for the femoral intramedullary (IM) guide indicated by a "+", slightly medial to the center of the notch and corresponding with the center of the intramedullary canal.

sized in the original technique. To the contrary, however, these principles have neither been forgotten nor subverted and remain critically important to all arthroplasties. In some ways, too much was expected of the tensor device. It was used in one step to confirm the adequacy of ligament releases and determine the angle as well as the level of the distal femoral bone cut. All of this effectively hinged on how much torque the surgeon applied to the medial and lateral distracting screws of the tensor.

Additional principles have been adopted:

1. The angle of the distal femoral cut must be perpendicular to the mechanical axis of the limb irrespective of other variables. As such it bears a constant relationship to the long axis of the femur in a given individual (Moreland et al. 1987) and a single step in the surgical procedure is now devoted to establishing this angle.

2. Once the distal femoral angle that will restore mechanical alignment has been measured from full-length pre-operative radiographs, it can be most accurately cut using an intramedullary guide (Laskin and Turtel 1989).

3. The level of the joint line should be conserved within certain narrow limits, but neither at the expense of removing excessive proximal tibial bone nor of using articular polyethylene of inadequate thickness because of concern over polyethylene wear (Wright and Bartel 1986; Wright et al. 1988).

The standard anterior longitudinal skin incision that passes medial to the base of the tibial tubercle provides full exposure of the knee (Fig. 8.22). With the patella fully everted to the lateral side, and without risking avulsion of the patellar tendon from the tibial tubercle (arrow) a hole is drilled in the distal femur to admit the femoral intramedullary (IM) alignment guide. Note that the center of the medullary canal corresponds to a point that is slightly medial to the top of the intercondylar notch. (indicated by a "+") (Fig. 8.23).

The drill should not be inserted very far into the femur because of the danger of perforating the cortex, and the distal hole should be enlarged to allow egress of medullary contents (Fahmy et al. 1990). Plunging a long, thick rod into the canal threatens to drive marrow fat into the circulation where it will inevitably enter the pulmonary vasculature (Fig. 8.24).

The femoral IM alignment guide is available with a standard 9 in. long intramedullary rod

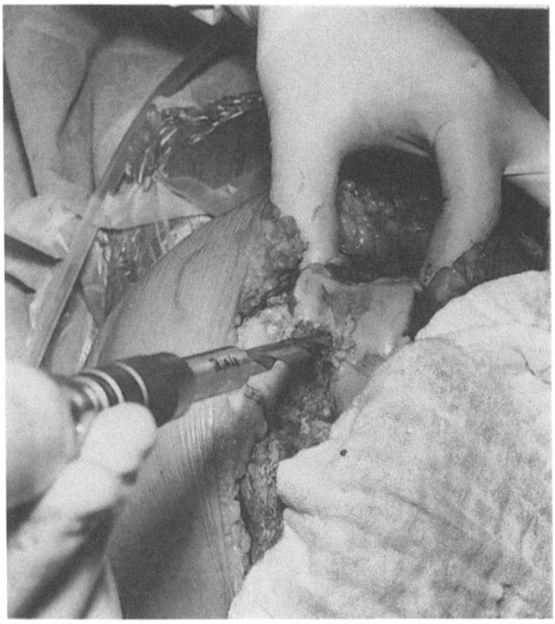

Fig.8.24. Enlarging the hole for the IM guide allows egress of marrow contents and reduces risk of driving fat into venous and eventually pulmonary circulation.

and a 4 in. version for special circumstances. This guide defines the anatomic axis of the distal femur, and functions as a base for two other instruments: (1) the anterior femoral cutting guide, and (2) the distal femoral cutting guide (Fig. 8.25).

The rotational position of the femoral IM alignment guide will determine rotation of the femoral component of the arthroplasty. Internal rotation compromises patellar tracking and should be avoided (Fig. 8.26).

The anterior femoral cutting guide slides into a track (arrow) on the femoral IM alignment guide (Fig. 8.27a), and is positioned posteriorly until the point of a curved metal bar attached to it contacts the anterior femoral cortex (arrow) (Fig. 8.27b). This corresponds with the path of the saw blade as it exits from the cutting slot. As this slot admits only a thin saw blade, the blade must be very sharp and should be advanced slowly to prevent it from bending during the cut (Fig. 8.27c). When the correct amount of external rotation has been selected, more bone will be

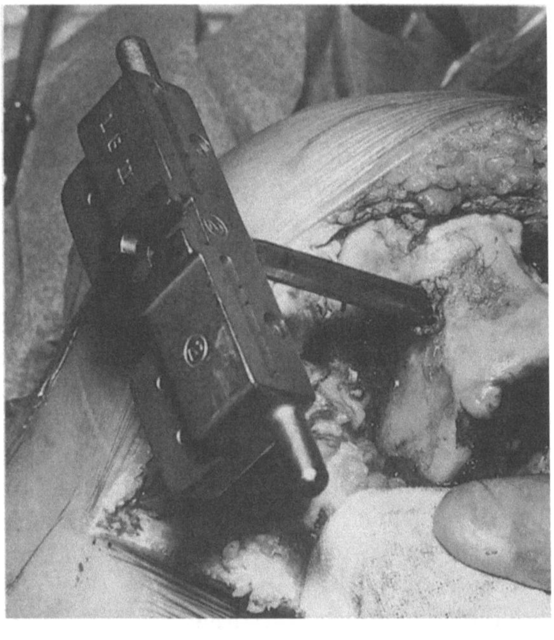

Fig.8.25. The femoral IM guide defines the anatomic axis of the femur and is the base to which the anterior femoral cutting guide and the distal femoral cutting guide are attached in sequence.

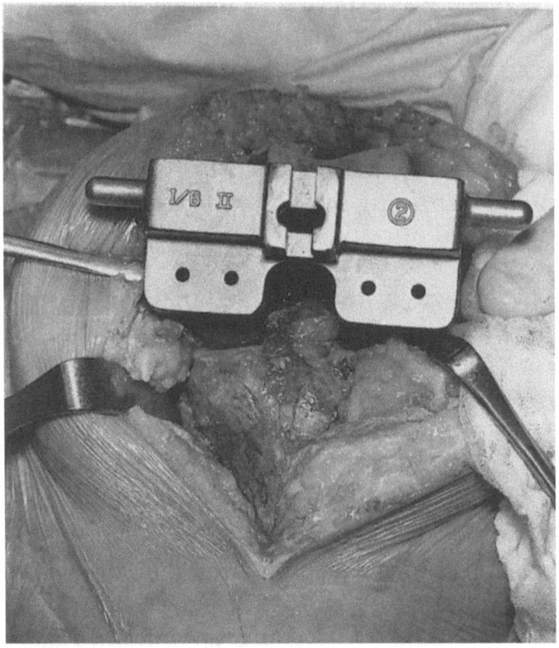

Fig.8.26. The rotational position of the femoral IM guide will determine the rotation of the femoral component. Avoid internal rotation.

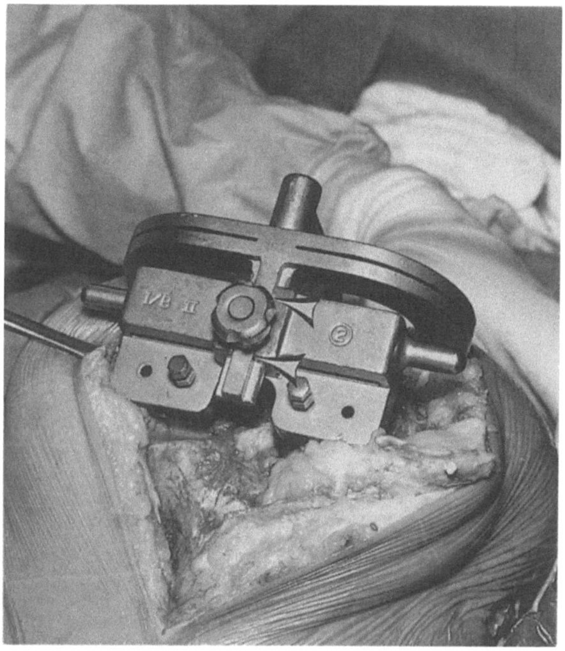

a

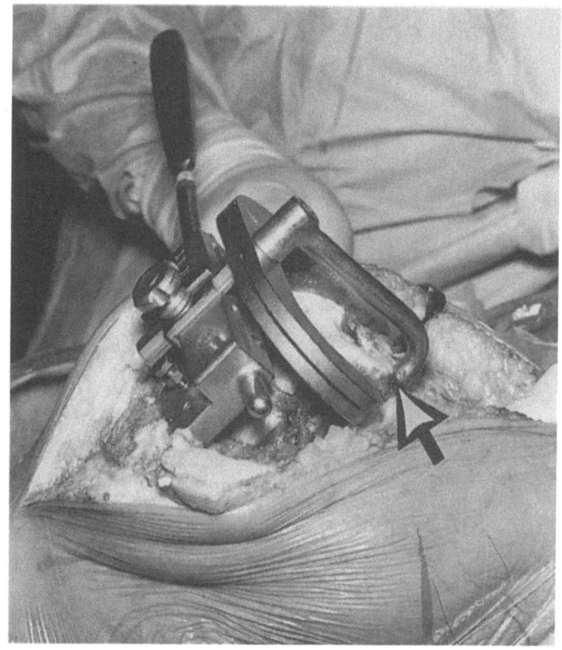

b

Fig.8.27. a The anterior femoral cutting guide slides into a track on the femoral IM alignment guide (arrows). b The tip of a curved metal bar, attached to the anterior femoral cutting guide corresponds with the path of the saw blade and should be placed against the anterior femoral cortex (arrow). c The thin saw blade required for the guide should be advanced slowly to avoid bending up during the cut.

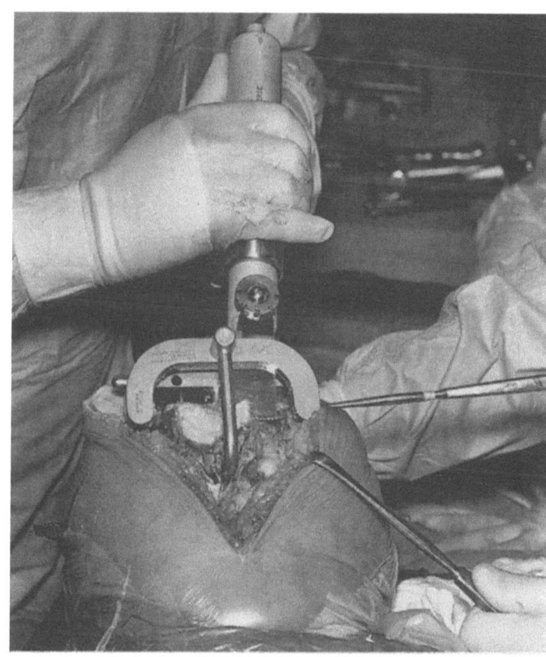

c

removed from the lateral trochlea than the medial, but no notch under the femoral cortex should result. The newly cut anterior femur provides an even surface for the next jig, and will later be revised to a slightly more flexed angle, that corresponds to the inner size and shape of the component.

The anterior femoral cutting guide may be removed and replaced by the distal femoral cutting guide. It has a peg which inserts into a designated hole on the femoral IM guide. The appropriate side of the distal femoral cutting guide (labeled "right or left") faces up, and the opposite side rests against the newly cut surface of the anterior femur. The correct angular orientation of the distal femoral cut will have been determined by measurements made on preoperative radiographs. This angle, between the distal cutting slot and the intramedullary rod is reproduced by inserting a pin into the hole on the instrument designated by that angle (Fig. 8.28) (arrow).

Two saw slots are available on the distal cutting guide. The standard, more distally located slot, resects an amount of distal femur equal in thickness to the femoral component. The more proximal slot is reserved for knees with fixed flexion contractures. The prudent choice is always the more distal slot as additional bone can be removed later with the distal femoral recutting guide if necessary.

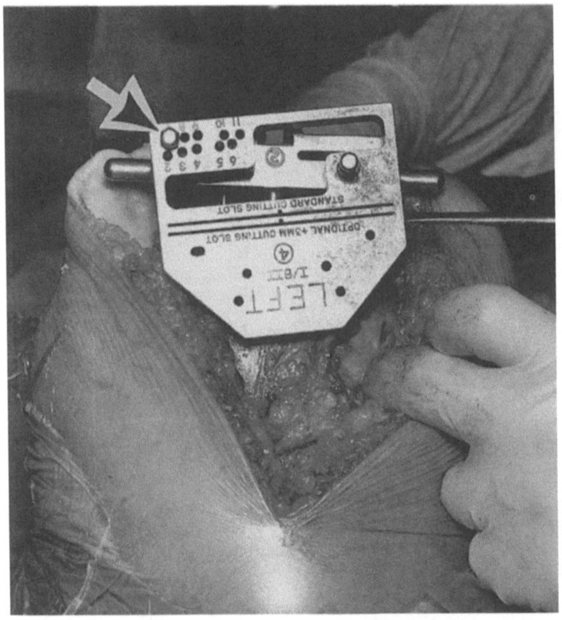

Fig.8.28. The angle between the anatomic axis of the femur and the distal femoral cut that will re-establish the mechanical axis of the lower extremity must be determined from full-length radiographs at the time of preoperative planning. This angle is selected by placing a pin in the appropriate hole on the distal femoral guide (arrow). The surgeon will view the guide upside down, as shown in this figure, while standing above the knee and looking down on the anterior thigh in surgery.

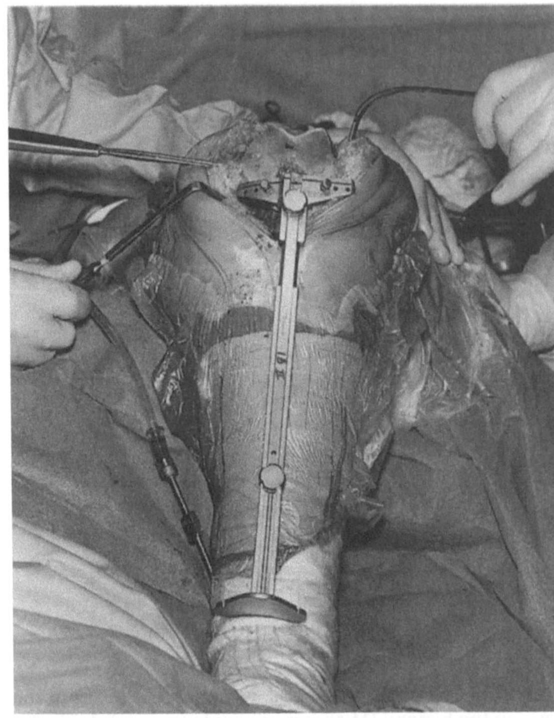

Fig.8.29. An extramedullary cutting guide is used for the tibia. Posterior slope is built into the component.

The extramedullary tibial cutting guide is positioned to cut the tibia at right angles to the long axis of this bone in two planes. A slight posterior slope to the proximal tibial cut is acceptable, remembering that a posterior slope is already "built into" the tibial component. Anterior sloping is unacceptable as it may compromise flexion by making the knee tighter the further it flexes (Fig. 8.29).

With the knee flexed to 90°, and after the proximal tibia has been removed, the posterior cruciate ligament should be severed from the posterior femur and its bulk excised, being careful not to damage structures in the popliteal fossa. Blood vessels in the remaining stump should be cauterized (Fig. 8.30).

The anteroposterior (AP) dimension of the distal femur, from resected anterior femur to the posterior femoral condyles, is measured with the femoral AP measuring guide. If the bone is between sizes, then the smaller component is usually selected, remembering that patella

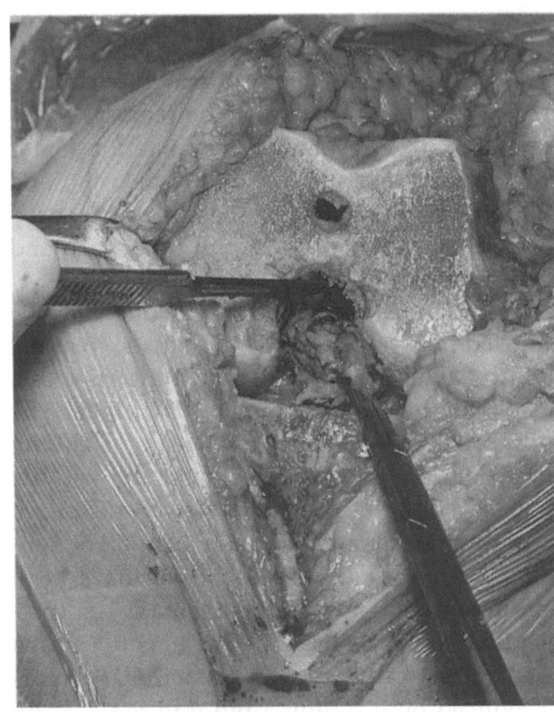

Fig.8.30. With the knee flexed to 90°, the posterior cruciate ligament is removed from its femoral attachment.

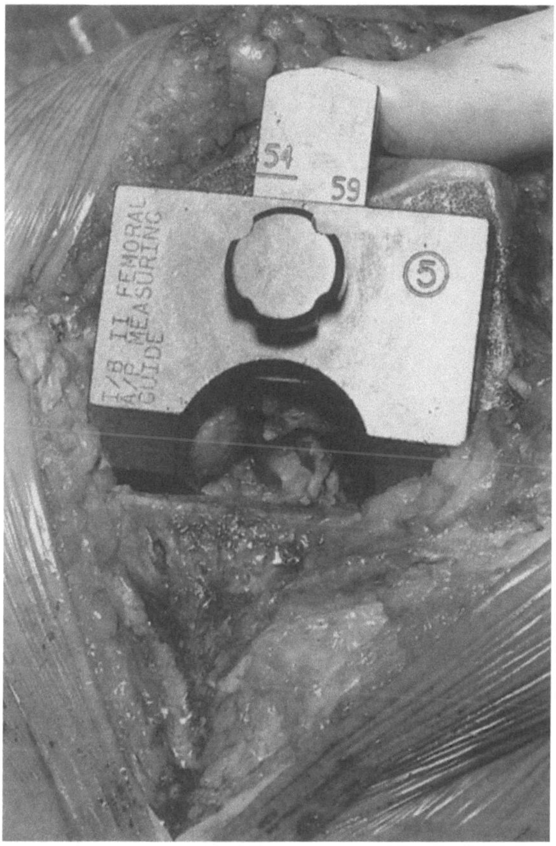

a

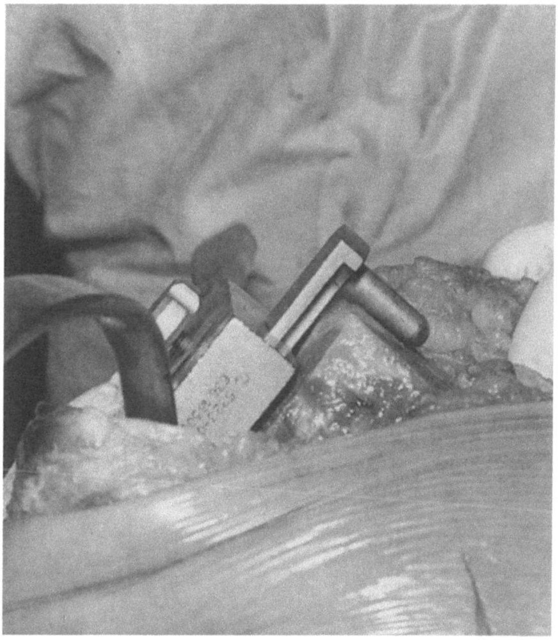

b

Fig.8.31. a,b. The anteroposterior (AP) dimension of the distal femur, from the resected anterior femur to the posterior femoral condyles is measured with the femoral AP measuring guide seen anteriorly (**a**) and laterally (**b**).

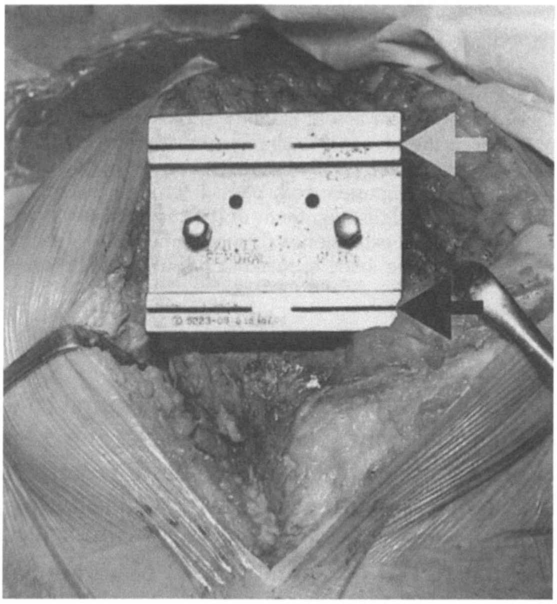

Fig.8.32. A femoral AP cutting block is available that corresponds to the size of each femoral component. There are two cutting slots: 1, to revise the preliminary anterior femoral cut (white arrow); 2, to resect the posterior femoral condyles (black arrow).

infera, instability and excess bone loss may result from selecting a component that is *too* small (Fig. 8.31a, b).

There is a specific femoral AP cutting guide for each size of femoral component. The guide has a flange that rests on the preliminary cut of the anterior femur; the bulk of the block should rest flat against the distal femur. The anterior slot on the guide will recut the anterior femur at a slightly flexed angle and the posterior cut will remove the posterior femoral condyles (Fig. 8.32).

Two laminar spreaders are opened inside the knee, one medially and one laterally to assess stability and symmetry of ligament balance in flexion (Fig. 8.33a). By this point, soft tissue releases will largely have been completed and the posterior cruciate ligament will have been excised. This means that all bone cuts and soft tissue releases that determine the flexion and extension gaps have been made. Access to the joint is excellent, and residual meniscal cartilage is easily removed. The size of the flexion gap and

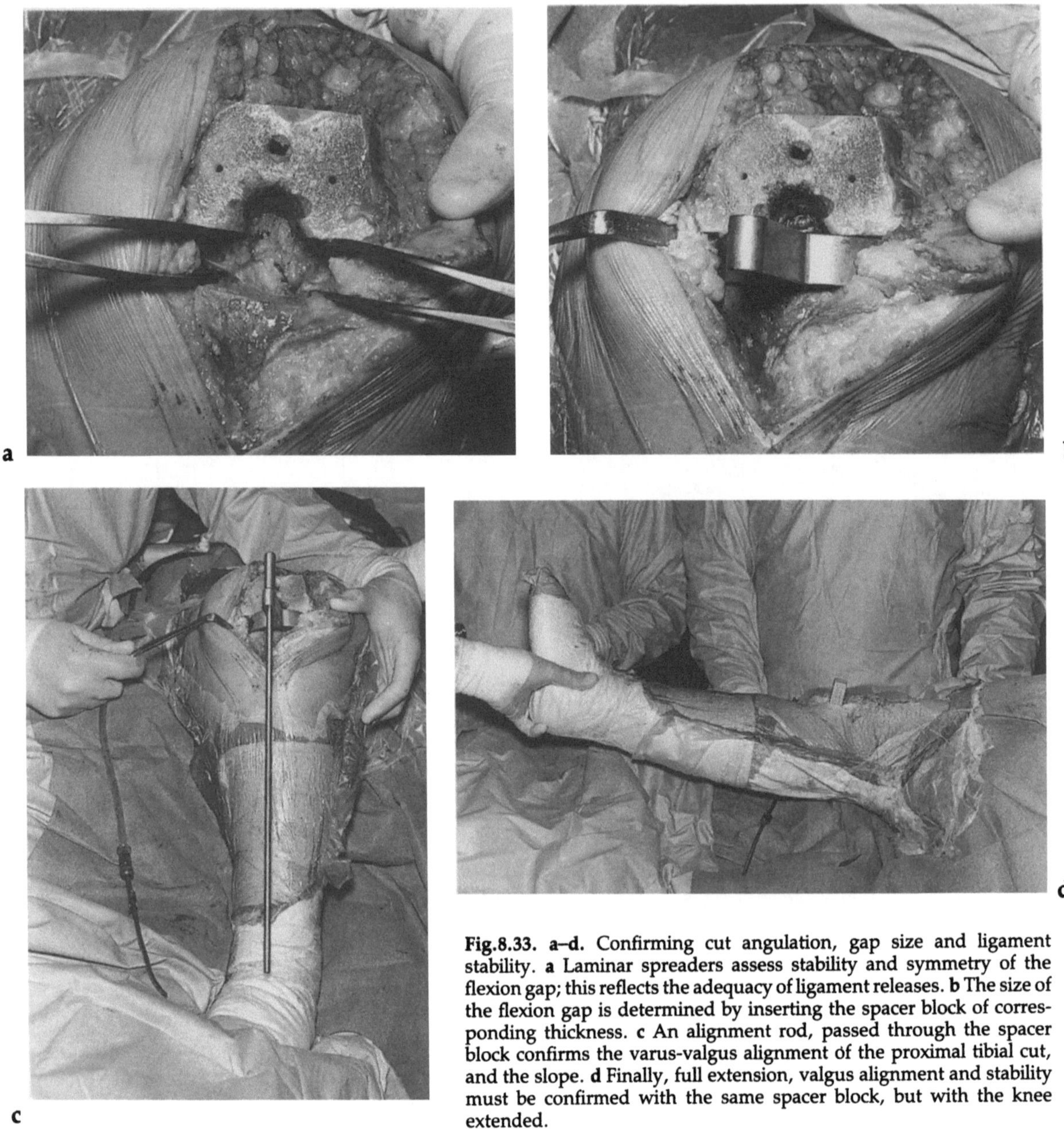

Fig.8.33. a–d. Confirming cut angulation, gap size and ligament stability. **a** Laminar spreaders assess stability and symmetry of the flexion gap; this reflects the adequacy of ligament releases. **b** The size of the flexion gap is determined by inserting the spacer block of corresponding thickness. **c** An alignment rod, passed through the spacer block confirms the varus-valgus alignment of the proximal tibial cut, and the slope. **d** Finally, full extension, valgus alignment and stability must be confirmed with the same spacer block, but with the knee extended.

the accuracy of the proximal tibial cut are confirmed with a spacer block and short alignment rod (Fig. 8.33b, c). The same spacer block should fit comfortably between the tibia and femur with the knee in extension. Three criteria must be satisfied at this point: (1) full extension of the knee, (2) stability to varus and valgus forces, (3) valgus alignment (Fig. 8.33).

If the spacer block fits comfortably between the tibia and femur in flexion, but the knee is too tight in extension, it may be necessary to elevate posterior capsule from behind the femoral condyles, release the posterior capsule or resect additional small amounts of distal femur. A distal femoral recutting guide is available for this optional step. Pins are slipped into the holes designated 2, 3 or 5 mm (arrow) of additional resection on the recutting block, which is positioned on the now final slope of the anterior femur. The pins rest against the distal femoral surface. The wedge shape of this cutting block, different from the initial distal femoral cutting

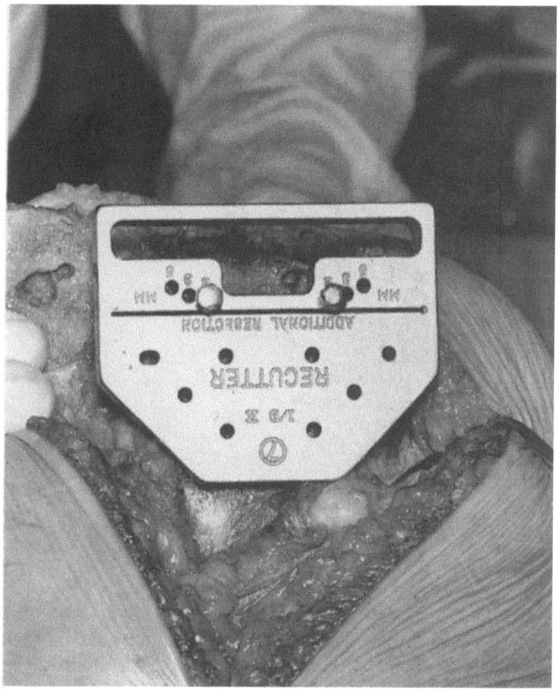

a

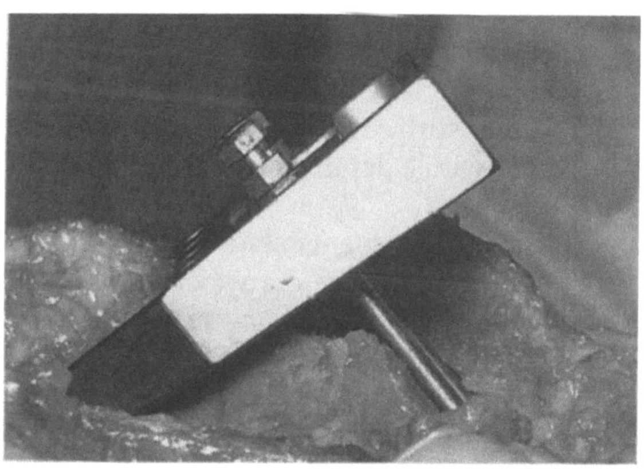

b

Fig.8.34. **a** If the extension gap is too tight, after checking with spacer blocks, a flexion contracture will result. A femoral recutter is available to guide resection of additional distal femur. The surgeon again will view the device "upside down" as shown, when looking at the distal femur from above the anterior thigh. **b** Recutting block seen from the side, with the distal femur at the right of the figure. The recutter is wedge shaped to compensate for the revised anterior femoral cut. This is an optional step to correct minor flexion contracture when present.

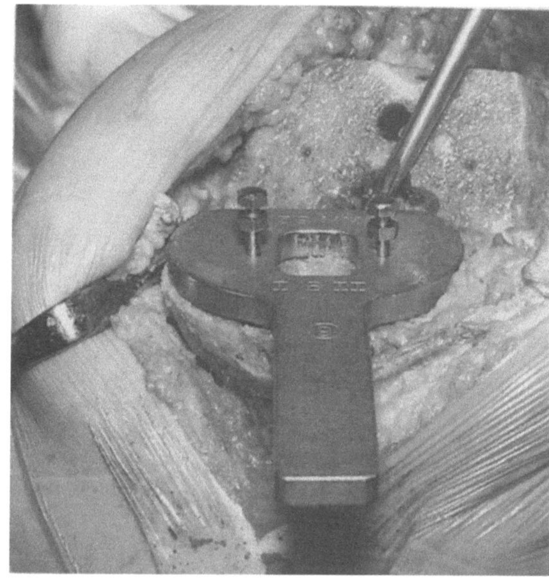

Flig.8.35. The tibial template determines the position of the tibial component. The keel hole is cut with an osteotome and shaped with the keel punch.

block, conserves the angle between the anterior and distal surfaces (Fig. 8.34a–b).

The tibial template positions and shapes the keel hole. It should be placed as far posteriorly as possible (Figgie et al. 1986), with rotation selected by the relative positions of the tibial tubercle, malleoli, and first metatarsal. The template should *not* simply be aligned parallel to the posterior tibial cortex (Fig. 8.35).

The femoral notch-chamfer cutting guide is positioned slightly lateral of mid-position to reduce overhang of the anteromedial flange of the femoral component. The chamfers are cut with a saw using the slotted guides (arrows).

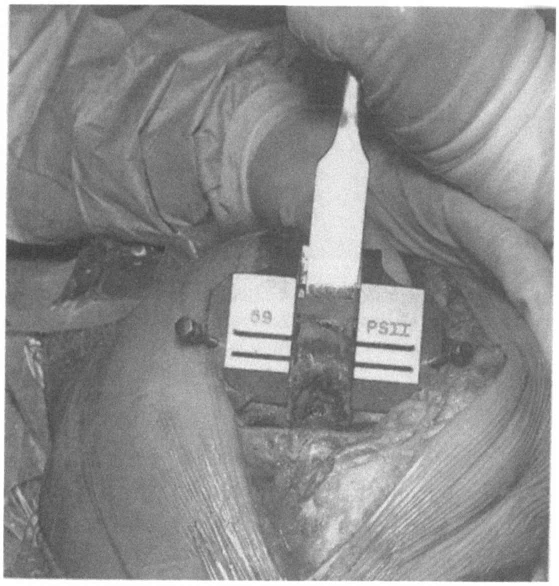

Fig.8.36. The femoral notch-chamfer cutting guide allows accurate creation of the chamfers and intercondylar notch.

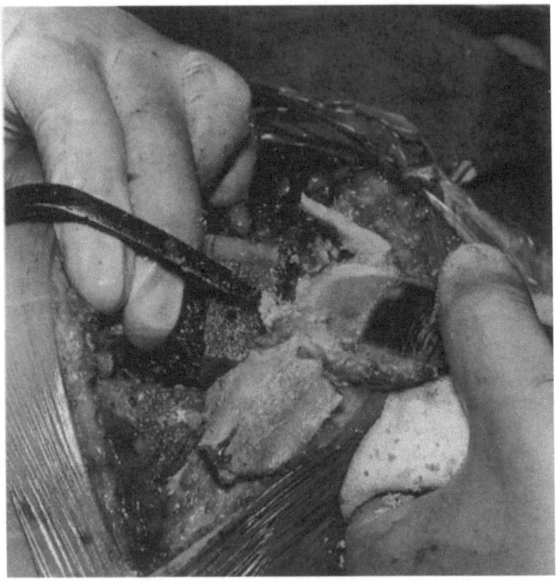

a

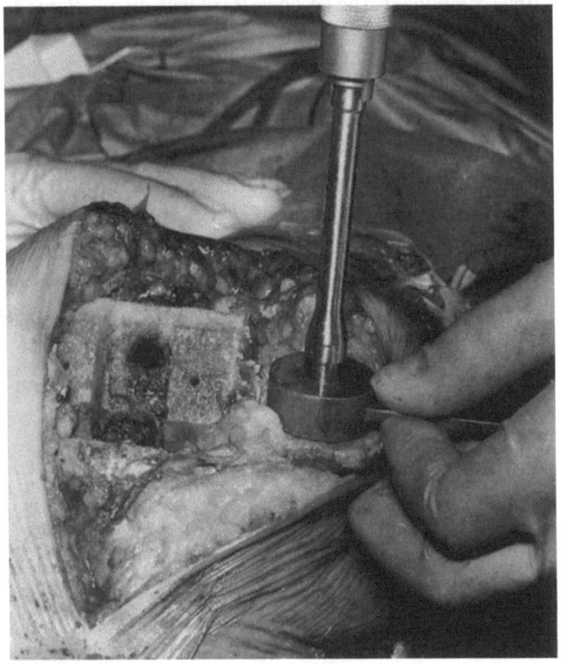

b

Fig.8,37. a The patella may be held by hand, with clamps or with specially designed clamps. A sharp saw blade is needed. **b** The central lug hole is drilled with a depth stop drill.

Once both medial and lateral sides of the notch are cut with a saw, the block of bone is removed from the intercondylar notch with an osteotome (Fig. 8.36).

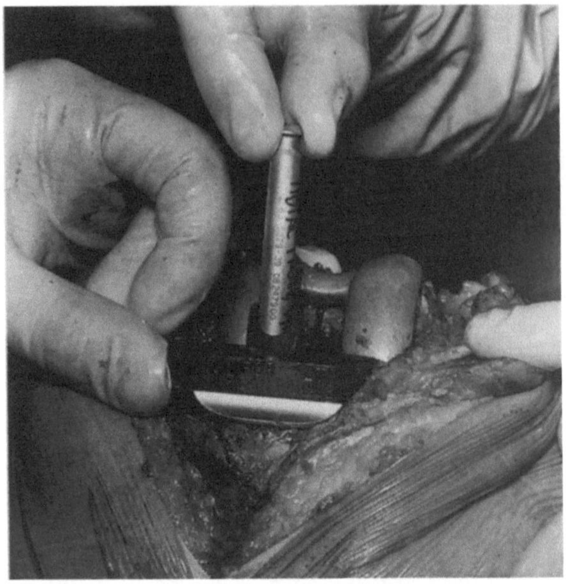

Fig.8.38. Trial components are impacted. Reduction may be tested with tibial inserts of different thickness, each of which slides into the trial tray and is then secured temporarily with a peg.

The patella may be held with clamps, by hand or with a specially designed instrument, while its articular surface is resected. The central hole is created with a depth stop drill and guide (Fig. 8.37a, b).

The trial components are inserted. The polyethylene tibial surface corresponding in thickness to the spacer block that was used to confirm the flexion and extension gaps slides into the tibial tray and is held during trial reduction with a peg (Fig. 8.38). Four criteria *must* be satisfied at this point: (1) full extension of the knee, (2) valgus alignment of the limb, (3) stability to varus and valgus forces, (4) central tracking of the patella.

All components are cemented into place (Fig. 8.39a, b). It is sometimes easier to cement the tibial tray first so that the femoral component does not interfere with rotational positioning. This sequence was not feasible with the original Insall-Burstein Posterior Stabilized prosthesis because of the single piece tibial component which made it difficult to insert the femoral component over the tibial spine. The tibial polyethylene articular surface is retained with a clip that is introduced from the front.

a

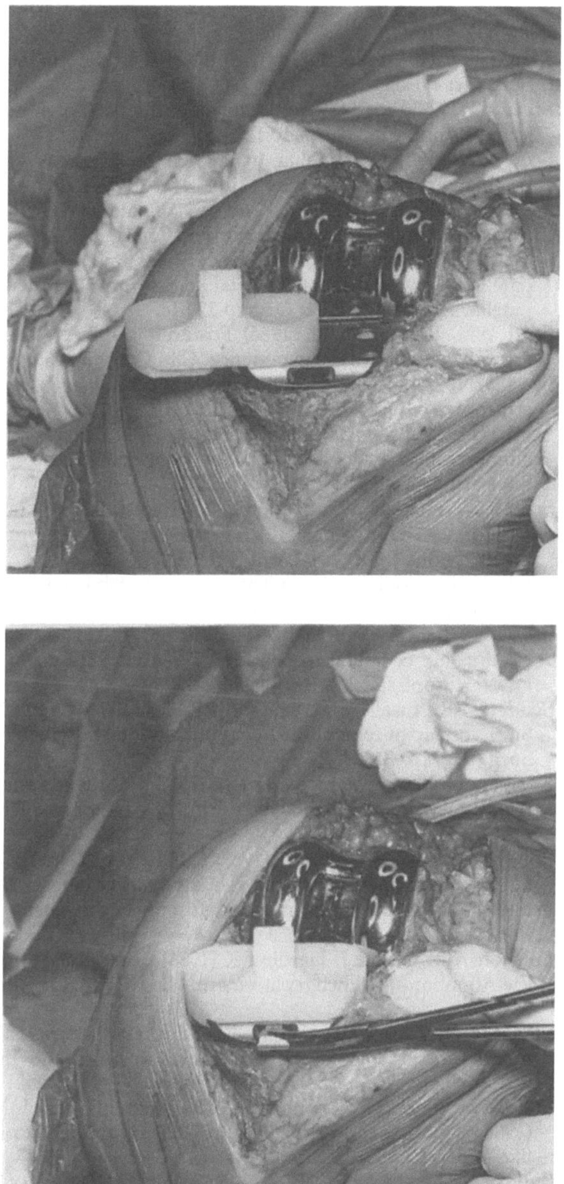

b

Fig.8.39. a After all components are cemented in place the articular polyethylene is slid into the tibial tray and, b secured with a two pronged retaining clip (that can be removed with a tonsil clamp).

References

Aglietti P, Buzzi R (1988) Posteriorly stabilized total condylar knee replacement. Three to eight years' follow-up of 85 knees. J Bone Joint Surg (Br)70:211

Aglietti P, Mazzotti GN (1981) Total knee prosthesis: evolution of the principles and technique and initial results obtained with the total condylar knee prosthesis "with Posterior stability". Ital J Orthop Trauma 7:181–194

Aglietti P, Rinonapoli E (1984) Total condylar knee replacement: A 5 year follow-up study of 33 knees. Clin Orthop 186:104

Aglietti P, Buzzi R, Pisaneschi A (1986) Total condylar knee prosthesis with posterior stability. A mid-term follow-up of 74 cases with severe deformity. Ital J Orthop Trauma 12:275

Aglietti P, Buzzi R, Gaudenzi A (1988) Patellofemoral functional results and complications with the posterior stabilized total condylar knee prosthesis. J Arthroplasty 3(1):17

Bartel DL, Bicknell MS, Wright TM (1986) The effect of conformity, thickness and material on stresses in ultrahigh molecular weight components for total joint replacement. J Bone Joint Surg (Am) 68:1042

Berman AT, Reid JS, Yanicko DR, Sih GC, Zimmerman MR (1984) Thermally induced bone necrosis in rabbits: relation to implant failure in humans. Clin Orthop 186:284

Bryan RS (1988) Patella infra and fat-pad hypertrophy after total knee arthroplasty. Tech Orthop 3:29–33

Burstein AH, Insall JN (1981) Posteriorly stabilized total knee joint prosthesis. United States Patent No. 4,298,992

Cameron HU, Fedorkow DM (1982) The patella in total knee arthroplasty. Clin Orthop 165:197

Clayton ML, Thirupathi R (1982) Patellar complications after total knee condylar arthroplasty. Clin Orthop 170:152

Donaldson WF III, Sculco TP, Insall JN et al. (1988) Total condylar III knee prosthesis. Long term follow-up study. Clin Orthop 226:21–28

Dupont JA, Baker SA (1982) Complications of patellofemoral resurfacing in total knee arthroplasty. Orthop Trans 6:369

Ewald FC (1991) Presidential address to the Knee Society: the second decade. Clin Orthop (in press)

Fahmy NR, Chandler HP, Danylchuk K et al. (1990) Blood gas and cirulatory changes during total knee replacement. Role of the intramedullary alignment rod. J Bone Joint Surg (Am) 72:19–26

Figgie HE, Goldberg VM, Heiple KG, Moller HS, Gordon NH (1986) The influence of tibialpatellofemoral location on function of the knee in patients with the posterior stabilized condylar knee prosthesis. J Bone Joint Surg (Am) 68:1035

Figgie HE, Goldberg VM, Figgie MP et al. (1989) The effect of alignment of the implant on fractures of the patella after condylar total knee arthroplasty. J Bone Joint Surg (Am) 71:1031–1039

Freeman MAR (1984) Surgical pathology of arthritis. In: Insall JN (ed) Surgery of the knee. Churchill Livingstone, New York, pp 505–526

Freeman MAR, Hammer A (1978) Patellar fracture after replacement of the tibialfemoral joint with ICLH prosthesis. Arch Orthop Traumat Surg 92:63

Galinat BJ, Vernace JV, Booth RE, Rothman RH (1988) Dislocation of the posterior stabilized total knee arthroplasty. A report of two cases. J Arthroplasty 3(4):363

Goldberg VM, Figgie HE, Inglis AE et al. (1986) Patellar fracture type and prognosis in condylar total knee arthroplasty. Clin Orthop 236:115

Goldberg VM, Figgie MP, Figgie HE, Heiple KG, Sobel M (1988) Use of a total condylar knee prosthesis for treatment of osteoarthritis and rheumatoid arthritis. J Bone Joint Surg (Am) 70:802–811

Grace JN, Sim FH (1986) Fracture of the patella following total knee arthroplasty. Orthop Trans 10:496

Grace JN, Sim FH (1988) Patellar fracture complicating total knee arthroplasty. Complic Orthop [Nov/Dec]: 149–155

Hood RW, Vanni M, Insall JN (1981) The correction of knee alignment in 225 consecutive total condylar knee replacements. Clin Orthop 160:94

Hood RW, Wright TM, Burstein AH (1983) Retrieval analysis of total knee prosthesis: a method and its application to 48 total condylar prostheses. J Biomed Mater Res 17:829–842

Hozack WJ, Booth RE, Balderston RA, Rothman RH (1988) The patellar "clunk" syndrome. Clin Orthop 231:79

Insall JN (1984) Total knee replacement. In: Insall JN (ed) Surgery of the knee. Churchill Livingstone, New York, pp 587–696

Insall JN (1986) Infection of total knee arthroplasty. AAOS Instructional Course Lectures, pp 319–324

Insall JN, Dethmers DA (1982) Revision of total knee arthroplasty. Clin Orthop 170:123–129

Insall JN, Tria AJ (1979) The total condylar knee prosthesis type II. Presented at the Annual Meeting of the AAOS, San Francisco

Insall JN, Scott WN, Ranawat CS (1979a) The total condylar knee prosthesis. J Bone Joint Surg (Am) 61:173–180

Insall JN, Tria AJ, Scott WN (1979b) The total condylar knee prosthesis: the first 5 years. Clin Orthop 145:68–77

Insall JN, Lachiewicz PF, Burstein AH (1982) The posterior stabilized condylar prosthesis: a modification of the total condylar design. J Bone Joint Surg (Am) 64:1317

Insall JN, Binazzi R, Soudry M, Mestriner LA (1985) Total knee arthroplasty. Clin Orthop 192:13

Kayler DE, Lyttle D (1988) Surgical interruption of patellar blood supply by total knee arthroplasty. Clin Orthop 229:21

Laskin RS, Turtel A (1989) The use of an intramedullary tibial alignment guide in total knee replacement arthroplasty. Am J Knee Surg 2:123–130

Laskin R, Rieger M, Schob C, Turen C (1988) The posterior-stabilized total knee prosthesis in the knee with a severe fixed deformity. Am J Knee Surg 1:199

Leblanc AU (1989) Patellar complications in total knee arthroplasty. Orthop Rev 18:296–304

Levai JP, McLeod HC, Freeman MAR (1983) Why not resurface the patella? J Bone Joint Surg (Br) 65:448

Lombardi AV, Sydney SV, Mallory TH et al. (1988) Six year survivorship analysis of the Insall-Burstein posterior stabilized knee: a clinical and radiographic evaluation. Orthop Trans 12:711

Merkow RL, Soudry M, Insall JN (1988) Patellar dislocation following total knee arthroplasty. J Bone Joint Surg (Am) 67:1321

Mochizuki PM, Schurman DJ (1979) Patellar complications following total knee arthroplasty. J Bone Joint Surg (Am) 61:879

Moreland JR, Bassett LW, Hanker GJ (1987) Radiographic analysis of the axial alignment of the lower extremity. J Bone Joint Surg (Am) 69:745–749

Peterson CD, Hillberry BM (1985) Measurement of contact between the femoral cam follower and the tibial stabilizing post of the Insall-Burstein posterior stabilized condylar knee prosthesis using the Purdue knee simulator. Unpublished. School of Mechanical Engineering, Purdue University, West Lafayette, Indiana, September 25

Pettine KA, Bryan RS (1986) A previously unreported cause of pain after total knee arthroplasty. J Arthroplasty 1:29–33

Ranawat CS, Brigham L (1977) Preliminary evaluation of stabilo-condylar arthroplasty. Orthop Trans 1:92

Ranawat CS, Hansraj KK (1989) Effect of posterior cruciate sacrifice on durability of the cement bone interface: a nine year survivorship study of 100 total condylar knee arthroplasties. Orthop Clin N Am 20:63–70

Ranawat CS, Rose HA, Bryan WJ (1984) Replacement of the patellofemoral joint with the total condylar knee arthroplasty. Int Orthop 8:61

Ritter MA, Campbell BS (1987) Postoperative patellar complications with or without lateral release during total knee arthroplasty. Clin Orthop 219:163

Ritter MA, Stringer EA (1979) Predictive range of motion after total knee replacement. Clin Orthop 143:115

Roffman M, Hirsh DM, Mendes DG (1980) Fracture of the resurfaced patella in total knee replacement. Clin Orthop 148:112–116

Scapinelli R (1967) Blood supply of the patella. J Bone Joint Surg (Br) 49:563

Scott RD (1979) Prosthetic replacement of the patellofemoral joint. Orthop Clin N Am 10:129

Scott RD (1982) Duopatellar total knee replacement: the Brigham experience. Orthop Clin N Am 13:89–102

Scott RD, Reilly DT (1980) Pros and cons of patellar resurfacing in total knee replacement. Orthop Trans 4:328

Scott RD, Turoff N, Ewald FC (1982) Stress fracture of the patella following duopatellar total knee arthroplasty with patellar resurfacing. Clin Orthop 170:147

Scott WN, Rubinstein M (1986) Posterior stabilized knee arthroplasty. Six years' experience. Clin Orthop 205:138

Scott WN, Schosheim P (1982) Posterior stabilized knee arthroplasty. Orthop Clin N Am 13:131

Scott WN, Rozbruch JD, Otis JC et al. (1978) Clinical and biomechanical evaluation of patella replacement in total knee arthroplasty. Orthop Trans 2:203

Scott WN, Rubinstein M, Scuderi G (1988) Results after knee replacement with a posterior cruciate-substituting prosthesis. J Bone Joint Surg (Am) 70:1163

Scuderi GR, Insall JN (1989) The posterior stabilized knee prosthesis. Orthop Clin N Am 20:71

Scuderi GR, Scarf SC, Meltzer LP, Scott WN (1987) The relationship of lateral releases to patella viability in total knee arthroplasty. J Arthroplasty 2(3):209

Scuderi GR, Insall JN, Windsor RE, Moran MC (1989) Survivorship of cemented knee replacements. J Bone Joint Surg (Br) 71:798–803

Shoji H, Yoshino S, Kamagamine M (1987) Improved range of motion with the Y/S total knee arthroplasty system. Clin Orthop 218:150–163

Shoji H, Yoshino S, Kajino A (1989) Patellar replacement in bilateral total knee arthroplasty. A study of patients who had rheumatoid arthritis and no deformity of the patella. J Bone Joint Surg (Am) 71:853

Simison AJM, Noble J, Harding K (1986) Complications of the Attenborough knee replacement. J Bone Joint Surg (Br) 68:100

Sneppen O, Gudmundsson GH, Bunger C (1985) Patellofemoral function in total condylar knee arthroplasty. Int Orthop 9:65

Soudry M, Binazzi R, Johanson NA, Bullough PG, Insall JN (1986a) Total knee arthroplasty in Charcot and Charcot-like joints. Clin Orthop 208:199

Soudry M, Mestriner LA, Binazzi R, Insall JN (1986b) Total knee arthroplasty without patellar resurfacing. Clin Orthop 205:166

Stern S, Insall JN (1989) Total knee arthroplasty in patients with psoriasis. Clin Orthop 248:108–111

Stern S, Scuderi GR, Bowen MK, Insall JN (1990) Total knee arthroplasty in gonarthrosis patients less than 55 years old. Clin Orthop (in press)

Thompson FM, Hood RW, Insall JN (1981) Patellar fractures in total knee arthroplasty. Orthop Trans 5:490

Vernace JV, Rothman RH, Booth RE, Balderston RA (1989) Arthroscopic mangement of the patellar clunk syndrome following posterior stabilized total knee arthroplasty. J Arthroplasty 4:179

Vince KG, Dorr LD (1987) Surgical technique of total knee arthroplasty: principles and controversy. Techn Orthop 4:69–83

Vince KG, Insall JN, Kelly MA et al. (1988a) Long term assessment of joint line position and motion in a cruciate sacrificing knee arthroplasty. Orthop Trans 12:710

Vince KG, Insall JN, Bannerman CE (1988b) Total knee

arthroplasty in patients with Parkinson's disease. J Bone Joint Surg (Br) 71:51–54
Vince KG, Kelly MA, Insall JN (1988c) Posterior stabilized knee prosthesis: follow-up at five to eight years. Orthop Trans 12:157
Vince KG, Kelly MA, Insall JN (1988d) Posterior stabilized and total condylar knee arthroplasties: comparative long-term survivorship analysis. Presented at the annual meeting of the American Academy of Orthopedic Surgeons, Atlanta, Georgia, February 5
Vince KG, Insall JN, Kelly MA (1989) The total condylar prosthesis. J Bone Joint Surg (Br) 71:793–797
Walker PS, Ranawat C, Insall JN (1976) Fixation of the tibial components of condylar replacement knee prostheses. Biomech 9:269
Wetzner SM, Bezreh JS, Scott RD, Bierbaum BE, Newberg AH (1985) Bone scanning in the assessment of patellar viability following knee replacement. Clin Orthop 199:215
Windsor R, Insall JN, Vince KG (1988) Technical considerations of total knee arthroplasty after proximal tibial osteotomy. J Bone Joint Surg (Am) 70:547–555
Wright TM, Bartel DL (1986) The problem of surface damage in polyethylene total knee components. Clin Orthop 205:67
Wright TM, Rimnac CM, Faris PM, Bansal M (1988) Analysis of surface damage in retrieved carbon fiber-reinforced and plain polyethylene tibial components from posterior stabilized total knee replacements. J Bone Joint Surg (Am) 70:1312
Yoshino S, Shoji H (1987) Yoshino-Shoji total knee system: its features and postoperative results. In: Niwa S, Pau JP, Yamamoto S (eds) Total knee replacement. Springer-Verlag, Tokyo, pp 221–225
Zelicoff SB, Scuderi GR, Vince KG et al. (1988) Total knee arthroplasty in posttraumatic arthritis. Orthop Trans 12:547–548

Chapter 9

Experience with the Sledge Prosthesis

D. Stock, R. Fabisiak and A. Niezgoda

Introduction

The knee is the human body's most complex joint. Failure of this joint is very common. The selection of the proper therapeutic measure for a "failed knee joint" presupposes many years of prior experience with a wide variety of methods (Müller 1982).

Clinical and radiological signs often do not fully describe the functional performance of the knee (Charnley 1979; Ranawat and Rose 1985; Stuhlberg et al. 1988). Radiographic evidence of destruction does not always correlate with pain or with limited ability to ambulate. We do not know what are the effects of a localized articular disturbance on the kinetic chain of motion and what feedback mechanisms are involved. We do not know how to assess nutritional supply disturbances of the cartilage and how to relate them to the mechanical irritation of the knee. We have some basic ideas but still cannot fully describe the complete interactions between muscles, ligaments and the articular surface geometry.

Degenerative changes can develop at any time, however their incidence increases with age (Wagenhäuser 1969). Advanced gonarthrosis normally can be treated using a variety of surgical modalities. Synovectomy, debridement and proximal tibial osteotomy all are excellent procedures in properly indicated patients (Windsor et al. 1988). If these methods have already been carried out or do not hold out any promise of success, and the patient is still seriously disabled by pain, we then consider the use of an endoprosthesis.

We continue to use a variety of different types of endoprosthesis for our patients. The non-axial surface prostheses as described by Freeman et al. (1972, 1973), Insall et al. (1979) and Laskin (1981) are our most commonly used implants. The patients in whom we insert these prostheses have tricompartmental disease with mild to moderate instability or deformity. These implants are usually inserted using acrylic cement for fixation. For patients under the age of 60, we are concerned about the long term stability of bone cement and have begun to use similar implants that do not rely upon acrylic cement. This is based upon the work of Blaha et al. (1982), Hungerford et al. (1983), Laskin (1988) and Laskin et al. (1984).

For patients with marked instability, or for those with an extensor lag greater than 20° or a fixed angular deformity greater than 20° we used a linked implant. The linked implant we favor is the cemented GSB.

Finally, in knees with unicondylar arthrosis, minimal instability, minimal angular deformity, a range of motion greater than 120°, and only mild retropatellar chondromalacia we use a modular sledge prosthesis. This chapter will describe our results using this prosthesis.

Our experience with sledge prostheses dates back to 1971. These implants have not supplanted but rather complemented our use of the high tibial osteotomy. Our personal results using the osteotomy (Fabisiak and Stock 1989) parallels that reported on by Coventry (1979), Bauer et al. (1969), Insall et al. (1984) and Giebel et al. (1985).

The most significant advantages of the modular sledge type prostheses are that they permit retention of the cruciate ligaments, and allow immediate weight bearing and early mobilization.

Early in the 1960s Charnley introduced the principle of "low friction arthroplasty" for artificial hip joints. This led to a rapid series of successful developments in the entire field of prosthetic replacement of joints including the surface replacement, or sledge prosthesis.

Relevant Biomechanics

The articular surface of the knee is eccentrically placed to the longitudinal axis of the leg in the sagittal plane. The articular surfaces are both located dorsal to this axis, the femur more so than the tibia. No two points on the joint surfaces show the same radius of curvature. The femoral articular surfaces are polyradial with their axis of curvature forming an evolute tangent to all radii of curvature. The joint itself is stabilized by the ligaments as well as by the interaction of the muscles spanning the joint.

The menisci act as movable cushions distributing condylar pressure onto the tibial articular surfaces. They increase the elasticity of the joint and allow for a smooth concentric range of motion. It is the elasticity of these menisci that adapts the movements continually to the stiffness of the articular ligaments controlling the joint motion.

The collateral ligaments prevent the joint from springing open under valgus or varus stress. They are supported by the muscles of the pes anserinus group and semimembranosis medially and by the iliotibial tract and biceps femoris muscles laterally. The cruciate ligaments provide support in the horizontal and rotatory planes. Some portion of the cruciate is taut during every position of the knee joint.

The force exerted by the quadriceps is three times that of the knee flexors. This force is further increased by the lever effect of the patellar tendon and patella.

The kinematics of the knee joint were first described by the Weber brothers in 1836. The concept of rolling and gliding was elaborated upon by Groh (1955), Kapandji (1970), Frankel (1971), Menschik (1974) and Goodfellow and O'Connor (1978). The four bar linkage concept which combined torsional sliding with rolling was further elucidated by Kapandji and Menschik.

The Sledge Prosthesis at Our Clinic

In our clinic we continue to use the Modular-I Sledge prosthesis (Richards Medical Company, Memphis, Tenn. USA) as initially designed by Marmor (1976, 1985, 1987). This prosthesis consists of a sliding femoral runner with a polycentric axis and an almost flat tibial bearing surface. This configuration results in prostheses with little built-in constraint. Consequently there must be considerable stability in the collateral ligaments if the arthroplasty is to succeed. Small amounts of instability can be compensated for, however, by using tibial components of varying thicknesses. The femoral component is fitted with a keel-like lug to help withstand shearing forces at the bone–cement interface. The tibial component is inset into the metaphysis.

Anatomical approximation can be achieved with a choice of four different femoral implant sizes and 12 different tibial plateau sizes. The femoral components are made of a stainless steel alloy (Type 316L) and the plateaus of an ultra high molecular weight polyethylene.

The major indications for a sledge prosthesis as well as the corresponding indications for an osteotomy, an arthrodesis and a total replacement prosthesis are listed in Table 9.1. For us, the main diagnostic indications for a sledge prosthesis are chronic polyarthritis with knee joint destruction, idiopathic gonarthrosis, post-traumatic arthrosis and in some cases, fresh fracture of the tibial plateau. Although two sledge prostheses can be used together (one medially and one laterally) we will limit our further discussion to those cases in which only one compartment has been resurfaced using the sledge implant.

In our hands, absolute contraindications to use of this implant are a history of previous infection in the knee, florid dermatitis about the knee, massive bone resorption and lack of patient motivation. We consider osteoporosis or

Table 9.1. Criteria used in choice of prostheses

	Sledge	Osteotomy	Arthodesis	Total knee replacement
Age				
50	–	++	++	–
50–60	+/–	+	+	+/–
60	++	+/–	+/–	++
Arthrosis				
Mild	–	++	–	–
Moderate	–	+	–	–
Severe	++	–	++	++
Axial deviation				
20°	++	+	n/a	n/a
20°	–	+	n/a	n/a
Stability				
Stable	++	++	n/a	n/a
Unstable	–	–	n/a	n/a
Total flexion				
120°	++	++	n/a	n/a
120°	–	–	n/a	n/a
Flex control				
20°	++	++	n/a	n/a
20°	–	–	n/a	n/a

osteomalacia and the diagnosis of rheumatoid arthritis to be relative contraindications. Obviously for all patients, severe medical disease may preclude this as well as any other surgical procedures.

The Surgical Procedure

Patients are usually seen in the preoperative period by an internist in order to stabilize any medical problems. X-rays of the knee as well as of the entire leg are taken so as to evaluate the bony structures and the axis of the leg. We also take tangential radiographs of the patella in 30°, 60°, and 90°, of flexion of the knee in order to rule out any significant arthrosis in the patello-femoral articular surface.

The operation is carried out under general or peridural anesthesia. Perioperative short term antibiotic prophylaxis is given using Cefazedene, 2 g ½ hour before surgery and then 8 hours thereafter.

We use low dose heparin for all patients. Until 1982 we administered 5000 IU of heparin three times daily. We subsequently changed to 5000 IU twice daily, and most recently to 1500 IU of low molecular weight heparin supplemented by 0.5 g dihydroergotamine-mesilate give daily until the wound healed. We perform all our surgery in an ultrasterile operating theater. The patient is placed in the supine position and a tourniquet used for all cases.

For teaching purposes we use the parapatellar Payr incision for a sledge prosthesis (for all other prostheses we prefer a midline anterior incision). Before the joint is exposed, the patella is mobilized by separating the vastus muscle from the quadriceps tendon on the side of implantation (i.e. vastus medialis muscle from the quadriceps tendon for a medial compartment replacement). We then dissect subperiosteally elevating the soft tissue from the tibial metaphysis and preserve the retropatellar fat pad. We then dislocate the patella laterally as we flex the knee to 90°. If this is not possible, it may be necessary to release further the quadriceps proximally. At this point we sew Betadene soaked sponges to the fascial edges on both sides of the wound.

The meniscus is removed and the posterior aspect of the femoral condyle is resected. The femoral component is fitted using templates, retaining as much of the subchondral bone as possible. The front end of the femoral component should lie slightly under the level of the articular surface in order to avoid a step in the patellar bed. Several holes are drilled into the femur to enchance the anchoring with cement.

The tibia is prepared so as to allow inlaying of the tibial component. After the proper template had been applied the recess is created using small chisels, the oscillating saw and a micromill (Fig.9.1). The correct size trial plateau is inserted. The implant should follow the normal 5° posterior slope of the normal tibial plateau. The thickness of implant chosen depends on the amount of defective bone stock as well as the degree of insufficiency of the collateral ligaments. In principle we do not subscribe to a full or overcorrection of the arthrotic deviation in the weight bearing axis as suggested by Miculicz, because this results in too much load stress on the implant and stretching of the collateral ligament.

Before cementing the permanent implants, the trial implants are tested by repeatedly flexing and extending the knee. The proper position of the implants, the gliding of the femoral component on the tibial prosthesis, and the stability of the ligaments can all then be assessed.

Obstructive peripheral osteophytes are removed and the intra-articular space irrigated.

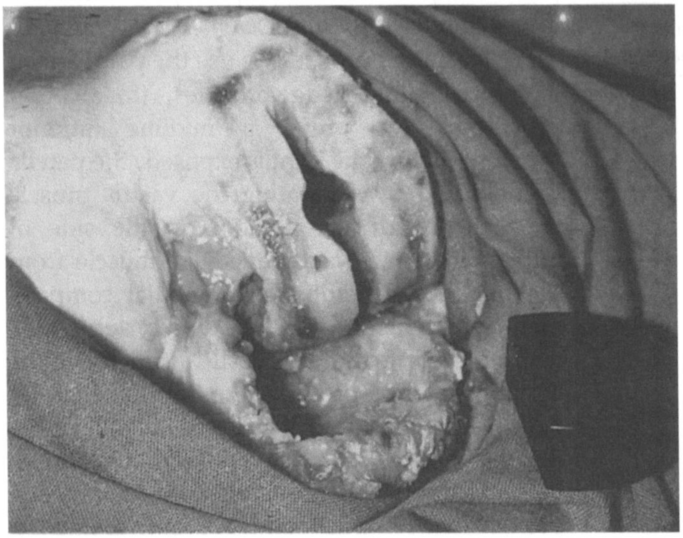

Fig.9.1. Preparation of the tibial and patellar recesses.

We generally do not perform synovectomies on arthrotics but do perform them in cases of considerable synovial changes as seen in rheumatoid arthritic patients. The implant bed is rinsed and dried following which the femoral and then the tibial components are implanted. When the cement has cured, articular motion and patellar tracking are rechecked (Fig. 9.2).

The tourniquet is released and after hemostasis is secured, 2 Redon drains are inserted. The capsule is closed in a single layer using #2 suture material. During suturing, repeated 90° flexion maneuvers are performed to prevent capsular tension. A final subcutaneous Redon drain is placed and the skin closed using the atraumatic button technique. The leg is wrapped with elastic bandages to prevent thrombosis.

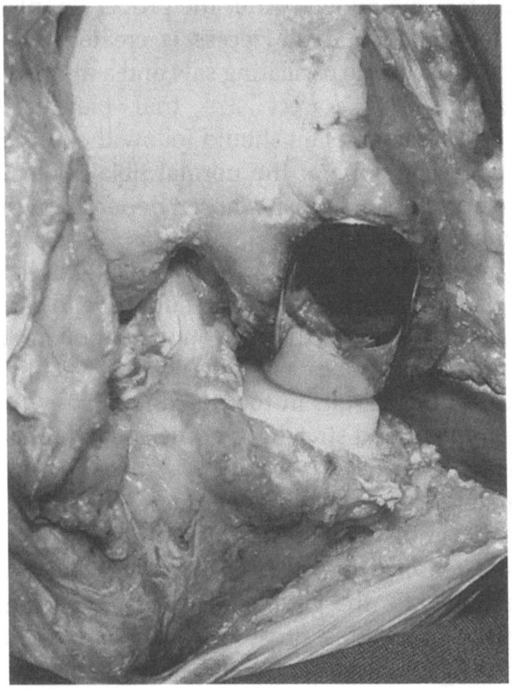

Fig.9.2. Permanent implants cemented in place.

Postoperative Treatment

The leg is laid on a raised splint. Physiotherapeutic mobilization begins on the first postoperative day to the patient's pain limit. The Redon drains are removed on the second postoperative day, following which the knee joint is passively moved twice a day for 30 minutes at a time using a continuous passive motion machine.

The patient first ambulates under full weight bearing load using a walker. After one week the walker is exchanged for crutches. The patients are first assisted in isometric muscle training, and are then encouraged to do them on their own. On the 12th day, the sutures are removed and the patient started on kinotherapeutic baths and forced ambulatory exercises including climbing stairs.

The patient is released from the hospital as soon as the range of motion of the knee has

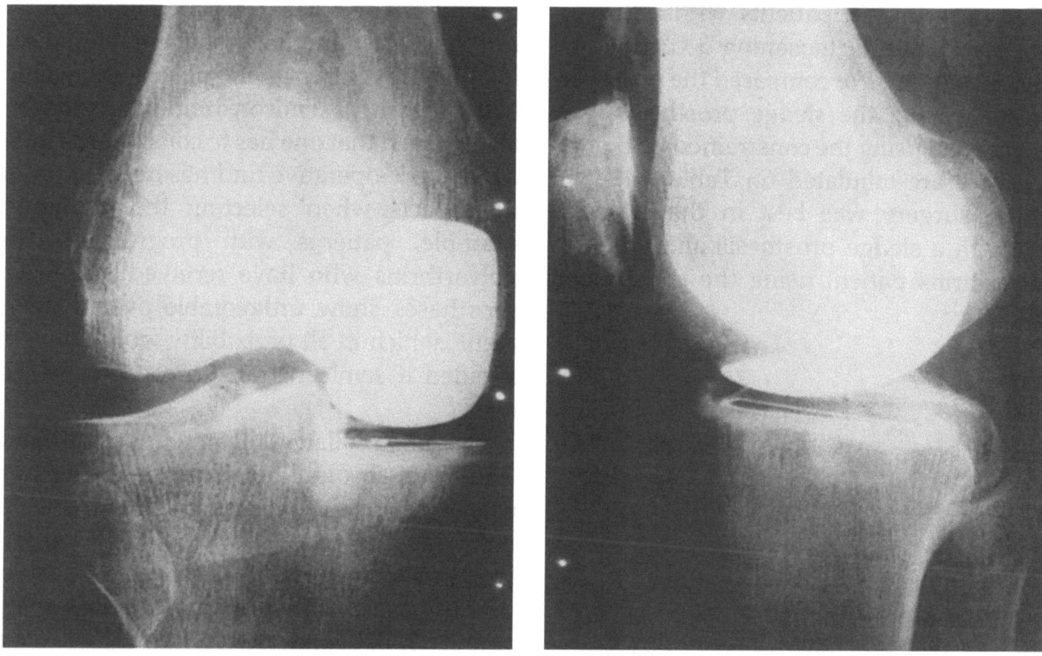

a b

Fig. 9.3. a,b. Radiographs one year after a unicompartmental replacement. **a** Posteroanterior radiograph demonstrating implant at 90° to the anatomical axis of the tibia. **b** Lateral radiograph demonstrating slight posterior tilting of the tibial implant and proper positioning of the femoral component posteriorly on the femoral condyles.

reached at least 90°, the knee is free of discomfort, and the patient can bear weight without pain (Fig. 9.3a,b). Physical therapy is continued for a further 8–12 weeks on an outpatient basis. Radiological and clinical check-ups are then carried out after 3 months and 1 year postoperatively.

Demographic Data and Results

From 1980 to 1984, 324 endoprosthetic knee joint replacements were performed. Of these procedures 90 patients (104 knee joints) received a sledge prosthesis. The demographic data is summarized on Table 9.2. Most patients were women, and over 85% had idiopathic arthrosis as their etiology. Over 90% of the sledge procedures were for medial compartment disease, the operation taking usually about 1.5–2 hours to complete.

Overall there were 5 cases in which there were postoperative complications (Table 9.3). The immediate postoperative complication rate was

Table 9.2. Demographic data

Average age at surgery	
Women	69
Men	21
Range	54–81
Etiology	
Idiopathic arthrosis	89 (85.6%)
Rheumatoid arthritis	6 (6.0%)
Post-traumatic	5 (4.8%)
Other	4 (3.8%)
Sledge procedures	
Total	104
Right	53
Left	51
Bicondylar	2

Table 9.3. Complications

	No.	%
Early		
Secondary wound healing	2	2.2
Deep infection	1	1.1
Pulmonary embolism	1	1.1
Deep vein thrombosis	1	1.1
Late		
Septic loosening	3	3.3[a]
Aseptic loosening	1	1.1[b]

[a] All the patients with late septic loosening had idiopathic arthrosis as their original etiology for surgery.
[b] The one patient with aseptic loosening had rheumatoid arthritis as the original etiology for surgery.

4.5%. There were three cases of late septic loosening occurring in patients with arthrosis, and one case of aseptic loosening occurring in a rheumatoid patient. We compared the postoperative results using the sledge prosthesis with results obtained using the constrained GSB prosthesis. These are tabulated on Table 9.4. Pain relief after surgery was best in the arthrosis patients with a sledge prosthesis and worst in the polyarthritis patient using the constrained implant.

Table 9.4. Results

Section 1		
Was the pain after surgery less than before surgery?	PA IA	83.8% 95%
Could you walk further after surgery than before?	PA IA	75.7% 81.7%
Did you have to rely less upon external walking supports after surgery than before?	PA IA	83.2% 85.8%
Section 2		
The functional score was derived from a quantification of pain, use of ambulatory aids, ability to stand from a chair, ability to climb stairs, and knee joint swelling.		
Very good (28–25 pts)		47.4%
Good (24–19 pts)		43.0%
Satisfactory (18–13 pts)		9.6%
Unsatisfactory (13 pts)		0.0%
Section 3. Total Amount of Flexion after Surgery		
80°	PA	0
	IA	0
80–100°	PA	52.9%
	IA	54.7%
100°	PA	29.4%
	IA	37.7%

PA, primary arthrosis.
IA, inflammatory arthritis.

Discussion

Using a variety of endoprostheses leads naturally to a search for a diagnostic indication for each. It is precisely in this restricted indication range that we see one reason for our success. Individual analysis of the poorer results seen with some knee replacement procedures showed that the success of the operation is particularly dependent on the preoperative findings. While it is true that knee instability caused by the collateral ligaments can be fully compensated by unicondylar and bicondylar sledge prostheses, this is not the case with central instabilities of the cruciate ligaments. We learned early on that a patient with cruciate insufficiency discovered at surgery would be better off with a semiconstrained prosthesis. We also learned that one has to consider not only the current pre-operative findings but also prognostic aspects when selecting the implant. For example, patients with progressive chronic polyarthritis who have received sledge endoprostheses show unfavorable overall development, which in all probability would have been avoided if semiconstrained implants had been used.

Too much collateral ligament tension can later lead to an absolute deficit in the ability to fully extend the knee that may be irreparable. Ligament insufficiency, on the other hand, if left largely uncompensated can cause an instability which may severely limit the patient's ability to ambulate. Both of these conditions have resulted in our developing a surgical technique that involves selecting the tibial implant thickness so as to result in no more than a 5°–10° block to full extension when the patient is under anesthesia. We feel that postoperative therapy can gradually stretch out a contracture such as this. It is for these same reasons that we do not attempt to achieve complete correction of the mechanical axis at surgery.

We feel that the inlay technique of placing the tibial implant results in longevity of the prosthesis since the cortical rim can absorb some of the shearing forces exerted during weight bearing. Likewise the inlay technique prevents impingement between the implant and the surrounding soft tissues.

Much to our surprise it appeared that exact positioning of the femoral component in the anatomical position on the femur was not crucial to obtaining a good result after surgery. The sliding of the two components one against another appeared to compensate for differences in positioning of the femoral component.

The cementing technique employed in our hospital in Braunschweig seems to be a significant factor in avoiding malposition of the tibial component. We cement in the tibial component only after the femoral component has been cemented in place and do not extend the knee while the tibial cement is curing. We feel that by extending the knee there is a definite risk that the implant will be forced deeply into the bone and result in knee joint instability.

We had a low incidence of wound complications after surgery. We feel that this is the result of an atraumatic closure performed without the tissues being under tension. Likewise we feel that peri-operative antibiotics have a beneficial effect in the prevention of wound infection for these patients.

Various pathological processes can lead to radiolucent lines on radiographs. The exothermic reaction involved in acrylic bone cement polymerization as well as the toxic effect of the residual monomer (Willert et al. 1974) can result in a localized necrosis that may not become visible until the necrotic bone is reabsorbed. True lysis of bone occurs at a considerably later time as a reaction to foreign bodies, metalosis, and early and late infections. Their extent also depends on the reaction of the individual patient.

According to Gschwend et al. (1987) a lysis seam of 2–3 mm is insignificant as long as it does not extend to the articulating surfaces of the endoprosthesis. Radiolucent lines near the implant are thus not tantamount to a diagnosis of loosening of the implant. Loosening should be suspected, however, when the line occurs in combination with weight-bearing pain. We have interpreted radiolucent lines between the undersurface of the implant and the bone cement as an indication that the mechanical connection is not solid. If, however, there is a good mechanical interlock between the cement and the bone, the only effect will be to increase the stress in the bone–cement mass. Such a radiolucent line is significant inasmuch as it has a negative influence on the mechanical anchoring situation and probably will lead to a premature wearing down of the cement and a shorter life expectancy for the implant.

Our results support the contention that the occurrence and extension of radiolucent lines increase with time if the implant is not properly positioned and if it is not properly supported by bone. Since, in our series, an asymptomatic radiolucent line up to 1 mm in width was practically the rule along the cement–bone interface, we feel that it should be considered "physiological". It should be consider "pathological" only if it undergoes change and is associated with pain during weight bearing.

In the past, the old endoprostheses available offered no prosthetic replacement for the patellofemoral compartment of the knee. At that time we were more generous with the diagnostic indications for the sledge prosthesis. Nowadays, however, we only implant the sledge components when the retropatellar area shows no macroscopically degenerative processes upon radiological or intraoperative inspection.

The results of follow-up knee examination cannot be considered in isolation since the ability to walk is also influenced by impairment in other joints. Ambulation ability is subjectively improved in approximately 80% of the patients undergoing surgery with the sledge prosthesis. The same improvement in walking without necessity for support aids has been seen.

The ability to stand up from a chair depends on the knee's range of motion as well as the strength of the gluteus maximus and quadriceps muscles. Patients with chronic polyarthritis tended to assist themselves with their arms, even through there was no serious diminution in muscle strength or range of motion in the legs. This is possibly a protective reaction habit incurred in the many pre-operative years they have spent living with their handicap. The patients who were able to stand up with the greatest ease were those with idiopathic arthrosis in just one leg.

The ability to negotiate stairs of normal height requires 85° of knee flexion. In addition, the quadriceps muscle must have sufficient strength and the knee joint must be stable. More of our patients with a sledge prosthesis were able to negotiate stairs normally than were patients with total knee replacements. We feel, however, that this was due to the more normal physiology in their knees as well as the better condition of their thigh musculature in the pre-operative period.

The structural limits to freedom of movement inherent in endoprotheses are of course a major factor in determining general functional suitability. Constrained or semiconstrained endoprostheses fulfill a different purpose from a sledge prosthesis. The former types are intended to restore stability to the joint in cases where the knee's ligamentous apparatus is slack, whereas the sledge prostheses are intended only to replace the bearing surfaces. If the knee capsule ligaments are already destroyed or are inadvertently destroyed at surgery, a restricted range of motion will have to be accepted as a matter of course in connection with a constrained endoprosthesis. This would not be the case for a sledge prosthesis.

Preoperative mechanical axis deviations greater than 20° proved difficult, if not impossible, to correct surgically with sledge implants. The same held true for those knees with severe preoperative laxity. Since these problems are often found in patients with chronic polyarthritis, we usually are now hesitant to prescribe a sledge prostheses in these cases.

Summary

The advantage of a unicondylar prosthesis over a total joint replacement is that a large amount of the "natural joint structure" is left intact. The contracompartmental cartilage and meniscus, as well as the cruciate ligaments and patellofemoral joint are able to retain their functions without limitation imposed by foreign materials.

During a 5–7 year follow-up significant pain reduction as well as increase in walking distance and range of motion have been reported not only by our group but also by Mackinson et al. (1988), Goodfellow et al. (1987), Knutson et al. (1986), Engelbrecht et al. (1976) and Marmor (1987). The cumulative survival rate after 7 years is above 95%.

Based upon a nearly identical diagnostic spectrum, the results of a high tibial osteotomy for a varus deformity in the osteoarthritic patient are equally as good (Coventry 1985; Insall et al. 1984; Giebal et al. 1985). These results, however, also parallel those with cementless total joint replacement as reported by Laskin et al. (1984); Freeman and Railton (1985); Hungerford and Kenna (1983) and Stock et al. (1990). It is thus a matter of choice between a potential of long service from a cementless total joint prosthesis and long service from a unicondylar prosthesis, or from a high tibial osteotomy.

Are there any difficulties doing a high tibial osteotomy or a sledge procedure as a first procedure, and if that fails with time then performing a total knee replacement? Katz et al. (1987) have shown that total knee replacement performed in a patient with a prior high tibial osteotomy has a greater chance of complications and never achieves the functional status of total joint replacement performed as the original definitive procedure. The results in our clinic seem to demonstrate that the results of a total knee replacement performed after a sledge prosthesis, however, is as good as a primary total knee replacement (Fabisiak and Stock 1989; Stock et al. 1990).

The orthopaedic surgeon must therefore decide individually for each patient which method will achieve the best long term results. The patient's activity level, body weight, physiological age, and accompanying pathological conditions in other joints must all be considered. Just as important is the status of the ligaments, cartilage, and soft tissues in the affected knee.

References

Blaha JD, Insler HP, Freeman MA, Revell PA, Todd RC (1982) The fixation of a proximal tibial polyethylene prosthesis without cement. J Bone Joint Surg (Br) 64:326–335

Charnley J (1979) Low friction arthroplasty of the hip. Springer-Verlag, Berlin Heidelberg New York

Coventry MA (1979) Upper tibial osteotomy for gonarthrosis. The evaluation of the operation in the last 18 years and long term results. Orthop Clin N Am 10:191

Coventry MA (1985) Osteotomy of the upper portion of the tibia for degenerative arthritis of the knee. J Bone Joint Surg (Am) 47:984–990

Engelbrecht E, Siegel A, Roettger J, Buchholz HW (1976) Statistics of total knee replacement, design St. George: A review of a four year observation. Clin Orthop 120:54–64

Fabisiak R, Stock D (1990) Die gelenknahen Knieosteotomien in der Behandlung der Fehlstellungsarthrose. Mittel-u. Langzeitresultate. Z. Orthop

Frankel VH (1971) Biomechanics of the knee. Orthop Clin N Am 2:175–190

Freeman MAR, Railton GT (1985) Die zementlose Verankerung in der Endoprothetik. Orthopäde 16:206–219

Freeman MAR, Swanson SVA, Zahin A (1972) Total knee replacement of the knee using a metal-polyethylene two part prosthesis. Proc R Soc 65:374–380

Freeman MAR, Swanson RC, Todd RC (1973) Total replacement of the knee using a Freeman-Swanson knee prosthesis. Clin Orthop 94:153–170

Freeman MAR, Samuelson KM, Bertin KC (1985) Freeman-Samuelson total arthroplasty of the knee. Clin Orthop 94:153–170

Giebel G, Tscherne H, Daiber M (1985) Die Tibiakopfosteotomie zur Behandlung der Gonarthrose. Orthopäde 14:144–153

Goodfellow J, O'Connor J (1978) The mechanics of the knee and prosthesis design. J Bone Joint Surg (Br) 60:358–369

Goodfellow JW, Tibrewal SB, Sherman MA, O'Connor J (1987) Unicompartmental Oxford meniscal knee arthroplasty. J Arthroplasty 2:1–9

Groh W (1955) Kinematische Untersuchungen des menschlichen Kniegelenkes und einige Prothesen-Kniekonstruktion, die als "physiologische Kniegelenke, bezeichnet werden". Arch Orthop Unfall-Chir. 47:637–645

Gschwend N, Iosevic-Radovanovic D, Scheier H, Bäher A, Munzinger U (1987) Langzeitergebnisse der GSB-I Prothese. In: Primar- und Revisionsalloarthroplastic Hüft und Kniegelenk. Springer-Verlag, Berlin Heidelberg New York

Hungerford DS, Kenna (1983) Preliminary experience with a total knee prosthesis with porous coating used without cement. Clin Orthop 176:95–107

Insall JN, Scott WN, Ranawat CS (1979) Total condylar prosthesis. J Bone Joint Surg (Am) 61:173–180

Insall JN, Joseph DH, Msika C (1984) High tibial osteotomy for varus gonarthrosis. A long term follow-up study. J Bone Joint Surg (Am) 66:1040–1048

Kapandji IA (1970) The physiology of joints, vol II. Churchill Livingstone, Edinburgh

Katz, MM, Hungerford DS, Krackow KA, Lennox DW (1987) Results of total knee arthroplasty after failed proximal tibial osteotomy for osteoarthritis. J Bone Joint Surg (Am):69:225–233

Knutson J, Lindstrand A, Lindgreen L (1986) Survival of the knee arthroplasties. A nationwide multicentre investigation of 8000 cases. J Bone Joint Surg (Br) 68:795–803

Laskin RS (1981) Total condylar knee replacement in rheumatoid arthritis. J Bone Joint Surg (Am) 63:29–35

Laskin RS (1988) Tricon-M uncemented total knee arthroplasty. A review of 96 knees followed for longer than two years. J Arthroplasty 3:27–38

Laskin RS, Denham R, Apley AG (1984) Replacement of the knee. Springer-Verlag, London

Mackinson J, Young S, Baily RAJ (1988) The St. George sledge for unicompartmental replacement of the knee. J Bone Joint Surg (Br) 70:217–222

Marmor L (1976) The modular (Marmor) knee. Case report with a minimum follow-up of two years. Clin Orthop 120:86–90

Marmor L (1985) Unicompartmental and total knee arthroplasty. Clin Orthop 192:75–81

Marmor L (1987) Unicompartmental knee arthroplasty. Ten to 13 year follow-up study. Clin Orthop 226:14–20

Menschick A (1974) Mechanik des Kniegelenkes. Z Orthop 112:481–495

Müller W (1982) Das Knie. Form, Funktion und ligamentäre Wiederherstellungschirugie. Springer-Verlag, Berlin Heidelberg New York

Ranawat CS, Rose HA (1985) Clinical and radiographic results of total condylar knee arthroplasty. A three to eight year follow up. In: Ranawat CS (ed) Total knee arthroplasty, technique, results and complications. Springer-Verlag, Berlin Heidelberg New York

Stock D, Czosnowsky W, Fabisiak R (1990) Zementfreier Kniegelenkersatz mit der Tricon-M Prothese. Kongreßband of Polish Orthopkongress 09/90 Stettin Poland (in press)

Stuhlberg SD, Stuhlberg BN, Bauer TW, Manley M (1988) Four-year follow up of a porous coated unicompartmental total knee replacement. Correlation with animal model. Presented as a Scientific Paper at the 55th Annual Meeting of the American Academy of Orthopaedic Surgeons, Atlanta, Georgia

Wagenhäuser FJ (1969) Die Rheumamorbidität. Hans Huber Verlag, Bern

Willert HG, Ludwig J, Semlitsch J (1974) Reaction of bone to methacrylate after hip arthroplasty. J Bone Joint Surg (Am) 65:1368–1382

Windsor RE, Insall JN, Vince KG (1988) Technical considerations of total knee arthroplasty after proximal tibial osteotomy. J Bone Joint Surg (Am) 70:547–554

Chapter 10

Uncemented Total Knee Replacement: The Tricon-M and Genesis Prostheses

Richard S. Laskin

Introduction

Both the short and long term results of total knee replacement arthroplasty performed using acrylic cement for fixation have been excellent (Goldberg et al. 1988; Insall et al. 1983; Laskin 1990a; Ranawat and Boachie-Adjei 1988). Methylmethacrylate, when used in a low viscous state and when pressure injected into properly prepared and cleansed bone, can be an excellent luting agent for obtaining an interference fit between the implants and the host bones. The use of methylmethacrylate carries with it, however, several potential problems including fragmentation, thermal necrosis of adjacent bone, and immunological defects in leukocytes (decreased leukotaxis and phagocytotic rates) (Petty 1978). In view of these inherent problems associated with methylmethacrylate, we embarked in 1981 on a program of designing and testing a series of total knee prostheses that would not require acrylic for fixation. This chapter will discuss our results with those prostheses.

The Tricon-M Prosthesis

The Prosthesis: Configuration and Design Rationale

Our first uncemented prosthesis, designed by Dr Hugh Cameron and myself, was designated the Tricon-M. It has been used extensively both in the United States and Europe since 1982. The Tricon-M is a tricompartmental replacement implant with cobalt-chrome-molybdenum alloy metallic components and ultra high molecular weight polyethylene components.

The undersurfaces of all the components were covered with a multilayered surface of sintered cobalt-chrome beads (Fig. 10.1). The average pore size formed by these beads on the tibial, distal femoral, and patellar undersurfaces is 250 μm. The average pore size on the anterior and posterior femoral undersurfaces is 75 μm. The average surface porosity is 30%.

The rationale for this two-sized porous surface was based upon the experimental work of

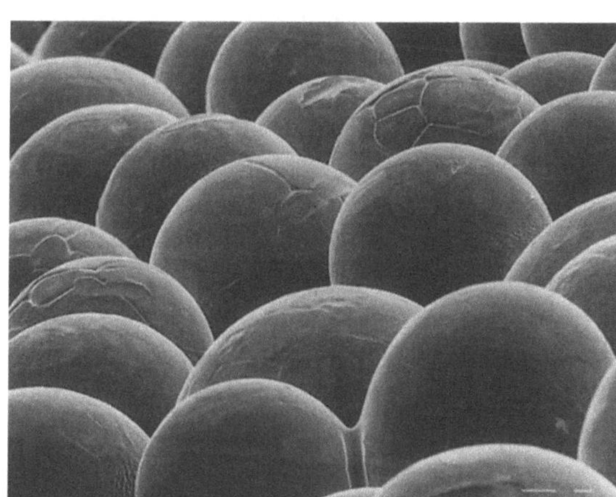

Fig. 10.1. Beaded undersurface of the tibial component. The pores enclosed between the beads are 250 μm in diameter.

Cameron et al. (1974) and Bobyn et al. (1980). They had shown that in the dog model, bone would grow into a metallic implant that was covered with a 250 μm porous surface, while only fibrous tissue would grow into an implant with a surface of 75 μm pores. They also showed that if a femoral total knee was lined completely with a 250 μm porous surface, there would be extensive bone ingrowth and that this ingrowth anteriorly and posteriorly caused marked stress shielding of the entire distal femur. It was for these reasons that we decided to place 250 μm pores only on the inner distal surface, and restricted bony ingrowth anteriorly and posteriorly by lining those surfaces with a 75 μm porous surface. We did not consider leaving the anterior and posterior inner surfaces smooth (i.e. without any pores at all), since experimentally this configuration resulted in cortical bone atrophy.

Each of the components is fixed to the bone at surgery by its flanged polyethylene pegs. Each of these pegs has a root diameter of 9 mm and a flange diameter of 13 mm. They were obtained, under license, from the British Technology Group and were identical to those that had been devised by Freeman and subsequently evaluated by Bobyn, et al. (1980) and Blaha et al. (1982).

The Tricon-M tibial component articular surface is identical to that on the cemented, central-stemmed RMC tibial component that we had previously used for many years. We experimentally implanted both types of tibial components into both foam beam and cadaveric tibiae. We subsequently measured strain distribution patterns in these two media and found that the Tricon-M components with the two flanged uncemented pegs distributed the overlying stresses more evenly across the cut tibial surface than did a tibial component with just a cemented tibial stem (Laskin et al. 1984).

The femoral component (Fig. 10.2) has both condylar and trochlear surfaces. The medial condylar surface is larger than the lateral, as in the normal knee. The trochlear facet is wide and shallow for articulation with the prosthetic polyethylene patellar implant. The two flanged polyethylene pegs are each 20 mm long. There are five different sized femoral components, differing in both anteroposterior and medial-lateral dimensions. All have the same 12 mm distal thickness.

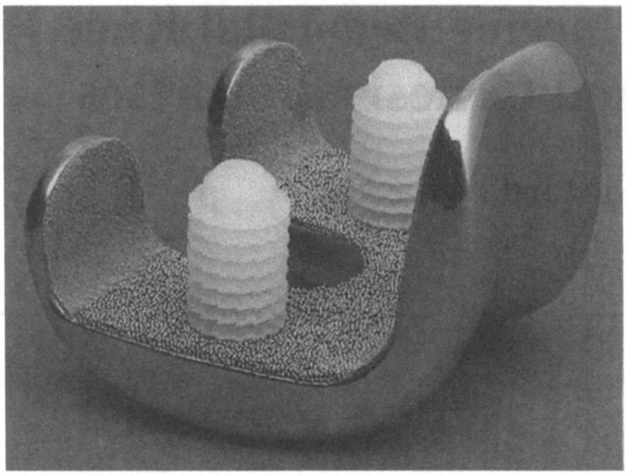

Fig. 10.2. Tricon-M femoral component. Note smaller bead size posteriorly and flanged polyethylene pegs.

The high density polyethylene tibial component (Fig. 10.3 a,b) has a 60/40 articular asymmetry to match that of the femoral component. There is an interspinous eminence to help prevent mediolateral translation of the prosthetic knee, a posterior recess to permit retention of the posterior cruciate ligament and a 10° posterior articular slope. There are four different sized tibial components each available in thicknesses from 6 to 22 mm in 4 mm increments. The undersurface of each of the tibial components is supported by a metal base covered with a 250 μm porous surface. There are two flanged polyethylene pegs, each 20 mm in length.

The high density patellar component is symmetrical, has a metal base covered with a 250 μm porous surface, and has one 6 mm flanged polyethylene fixation peg (Fig. 10.4). At the time this study was performed there was only one size patellar implant available.

Materials and Methods

In 1983 we began a clinical study of this prosthesis at our institution. The study was approved by the Institutional Review Board of our medical center and all patients enrolled met the strict criteria of that board. A multicenter multisurgeon study was started the following year, under the regulations of the Food and Drug Administration with the primary investigators being Dr Hugh Cameron in Toronto, Canada, and myself in New York. In all there were 19 surgeons in the study.

a 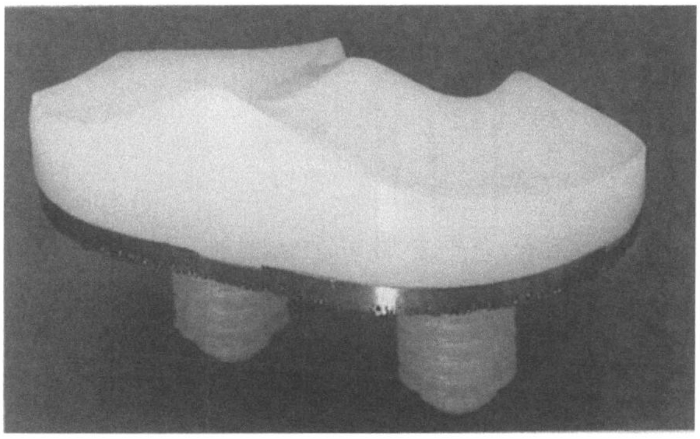 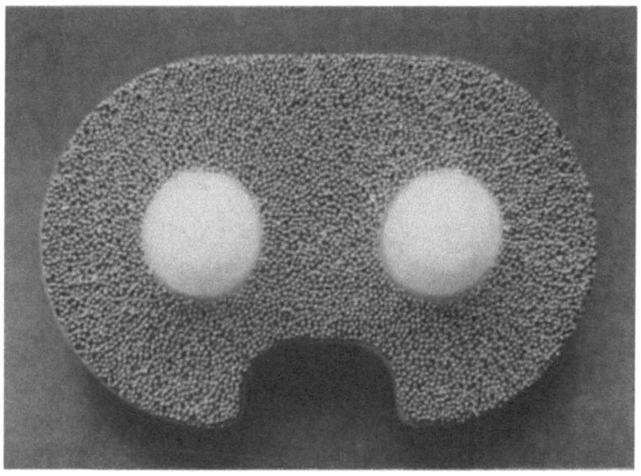 b

Fig. 10.3 a,b. Tricon-M tibial component. **a** Articular surface. **b** Undersurface.

The Tricon-M prosthesis was inserted without cement in all patients undergoing a primary total knee replacement with the following exceptions:

1. Knees with large bony cysts which encroached on the recess holes made for the flanged polyethylene pegs.
2. Knees with such severe osteoporosis that the cut bone surface could be indented with a finger.
3. Patients who did not wish to be a part of an investigative study.
4. Patients with a severe flexion/angular deformity which required resection of the posterior cruciate ligament in order to obtain ligament balancing.

In the first three situations, a posterior cruciate-retaining cemented total knee prosthesis was implanted. In the fourth case, a cemented Posterior Stabilized implant was used. No patients were excluded from the study based solely on body weight, diagnosis, or age. As per the requirements of our Institutional Review Board and the Food and Drug Administration Protocol, all patients were carefully advised of the investigative nature of the procedure, as well as its potential risks and benefits.

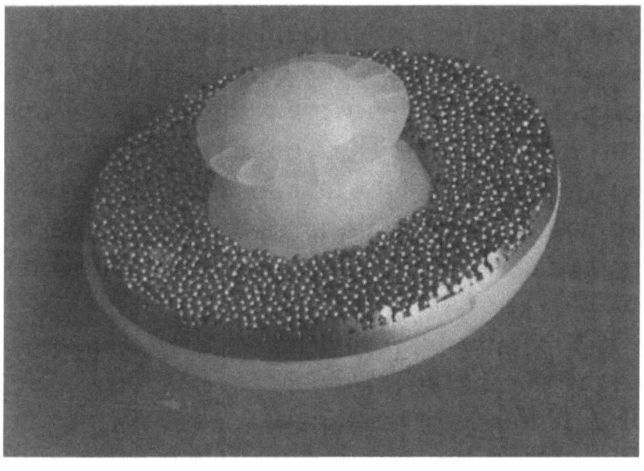

Fig. 10.4. Tricon-M patellar component.

Five hundred and forty uncemented Tricon-M knee replacements were performed in the entire study. At our institution we implanted 102 prostheses in 82 patients. Over half of our patients had inflammatory arthritis (rheumatoid arthritis, psoriatic arthritis, and other seronegative spondyloarthropathies). Two patients had post-traumatic arthritis, while the remainder had osteoarthritis. Overall in the entire 19 surgeon clinical series, about 80% of the patients had osteoarthritis and the remainder inflammatory arthritis. This difference in etiology between our patients and the other investigators did not lead to any statistical difference in the results that we obtained using the implant.

All patients were evaluated before operation, at 6 weeks, 3 and 12 months after surgery, and then yearly. Roentgenographic studies at each visit included a weight bearing posterioranterior and lateral views, as well as a patellar skyline view. At our institution, the P/A and lateral X-rays were taken using an image intensifier to assure parallelism between the X-ray beam and the interface between the prosthesis and the bone. The X-rays were measured using a computerized digitizing program (Orthographics) and all the data was then statistically analyzed using the Student *t*-test sampling distribution.

The surgical technique that we used for implantation of the Tricon-M prosthesis in this

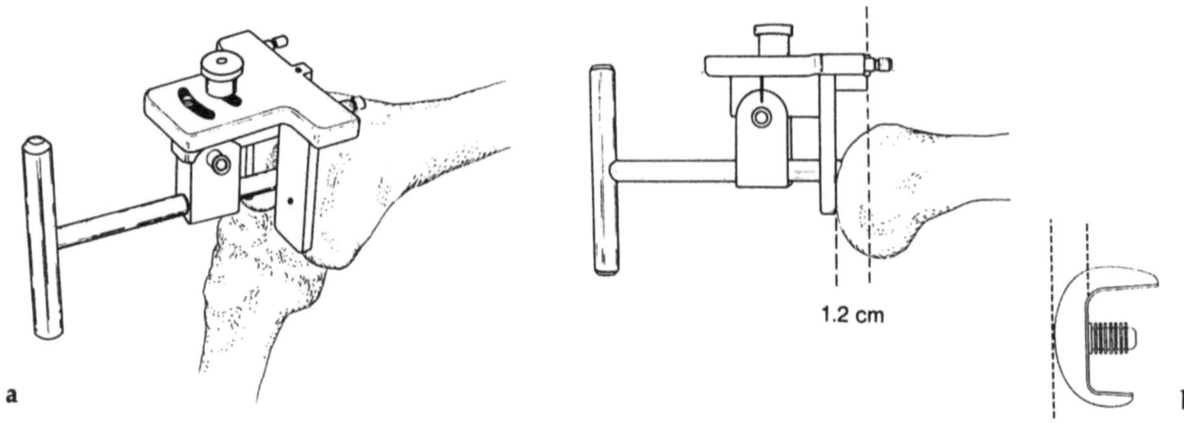

Fig. 10.5 a, b. Resection guide for cutting distal femur. **a** The guide is aligned by an intramedullary rod. **b** The guide is seated so that 1.2 cm of bone will be removed. This equals the distal thickness of the femoral component.

study followed the general guidelines that we have used for total knee replacement for the past 15 years (see Chaps. 3 and 4). Angular deformities were corrected by soft tissue releases so that the capsular sleeve could be balanced and the limb restored to a normal femoral-tibial alignment of 7° of valgus. An attempt was made to cover as much of the resected bony surfaces as possible with the prosthetic implants. Implants of sufficient thickness were used so as to fill the flexion and extension spaces properly.

An intramedullary femoral alignment rod was used to position the distal femoral cutting guide. The guide was set at 7° to the anatomical axis of the femur in the coronal plane and at 90° to the anatomical axis of the femur in the sagittal plane. Twelve millimeters of bone were removed from the distal femur so as to restore the joint line to its normal height (Fig. 10.5 a, b). The cutting block used to guide the resection was affixed to the femur in the proper orientation prior to the bone being resected (Fig. 10.6 a–d).

Although we presently use an intramedullary tibial alignment rod for positioning of the tibial cutting jig (Laskin and Turtel 1989), during the period of this study we used an extramedullary reference system (Fig. 10.7). We resected the tibia at 90° to its anatomical axis in the coronal plane. Since the articular surface was itself sloped posteriorly 10°, the tibial resection was made at 90° in the lateral plane (Fig. 10.8).

The anterior and posterior femoral resections were guided by jigs that assured that the femoral cortex was not notched anteriorly, and that the amount of posterior condylar bone removed equaled that of the femoral component (Fig. 10.9 a–c). A patellar clamp and depth guide were used to make the recess hole for the patellar implant. An attempt was made, using the depth guide, to replace the prosthetic patella at the "normal" anatomical height (Fig. 10.10).

Immediate fixation at the time of surgery was obtained by impacting the flanged polyethylene pegs into undersized recess holes in each of the bones (Fig. 10.11). We did not use any supplemental screws in any patient. If, because of technical problems in forming the peg recess holes, the implant demonstrated gross motion after impaction, it was removed and cement used for fixation. These cases were not included in the statistical analysis.

All the operations were performed in a horizontal laminar flow operating theater with the operating personnel using body exhaust suits. The patients were started on Coumadin beginning the night before surgery and on prophylactic antibiotics, just prior to the onset of anesthesia. The antibiotics were continued until the closed suction drains were removed, 48 hours after the operation. The Coumadin was continued until the end of the first postoperative week. The aim was to obtain a prothrombin time of approximately 3–4 seconds greater than the control.

Postoperatively, patients were allowed to bear weight on the affected leg several days after surgery. Range of motion exercises were begun early during the first postoperative week and

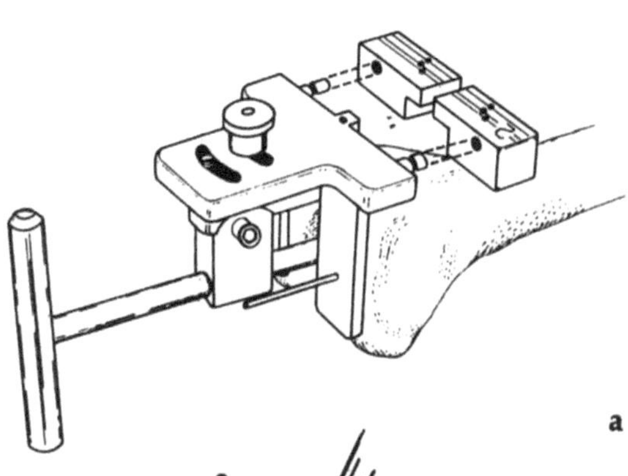

a

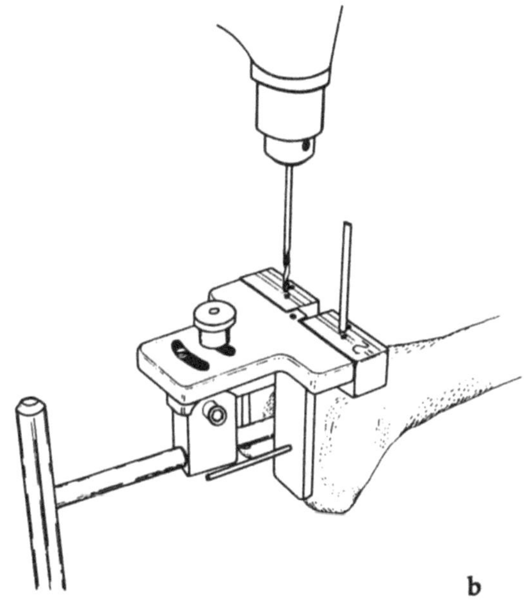

b

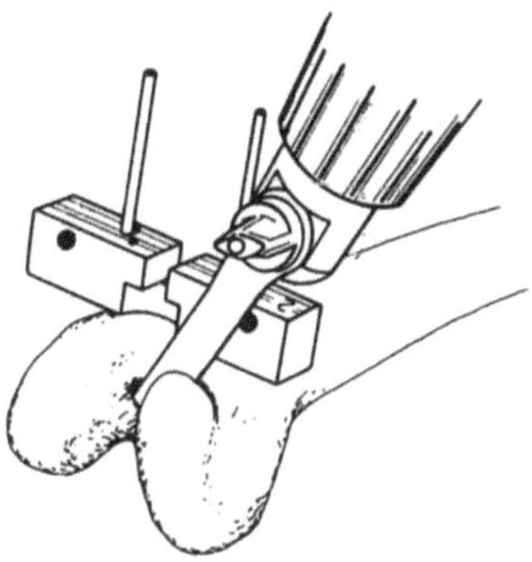

c

Fig. 10.6 a–d. Resection of the distal femur. **a** The cutting block is affixed to the cutting guide. **b** The block is affixed to the femur. **c** The distal femur is resected. **d** The saw blade may be held against the block with a surgical peanut.

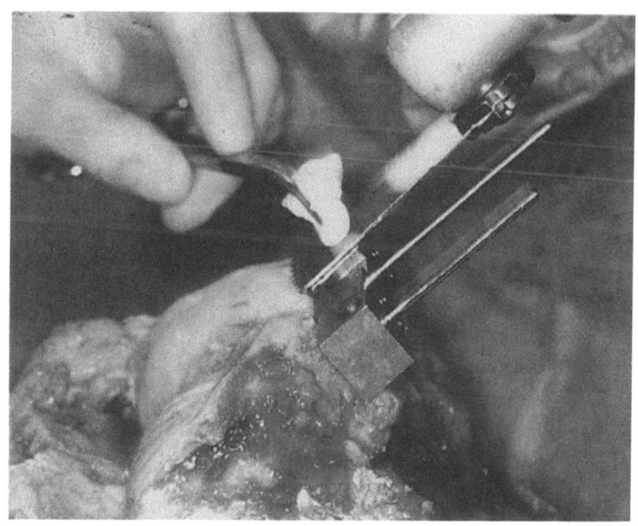

d

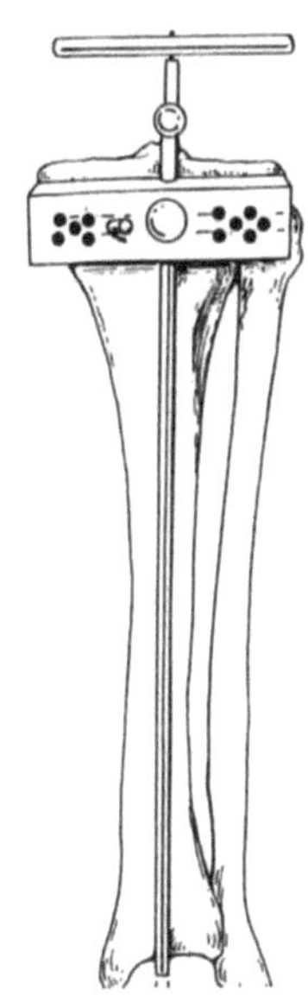

Fig. 10.7. Extramedullary tibial alignment guide and cutting jig.

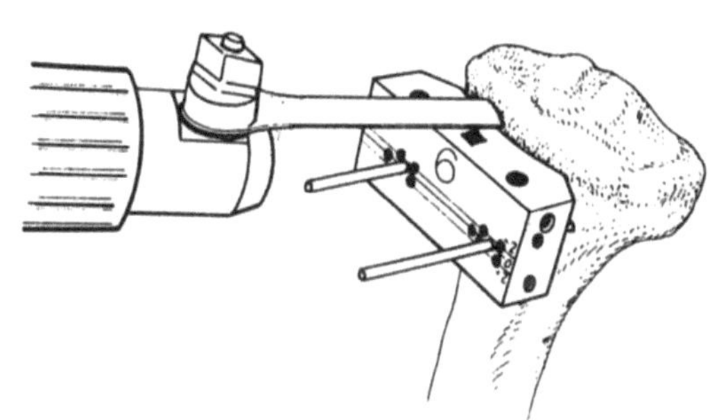

Fig. 10.8. Tibia resected at 90° in lateral plane retaining the insertion of the posterior cruciate ligament.

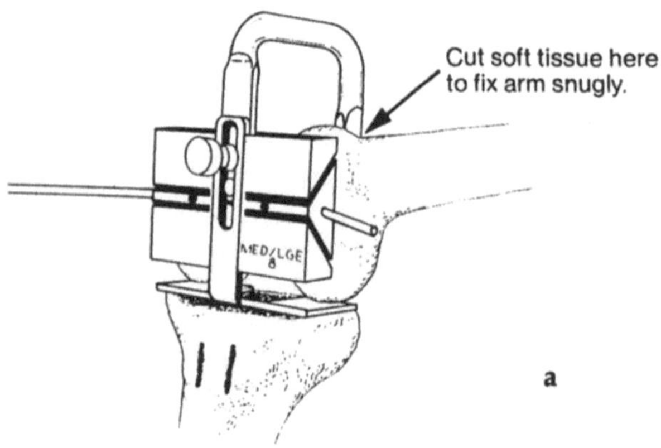

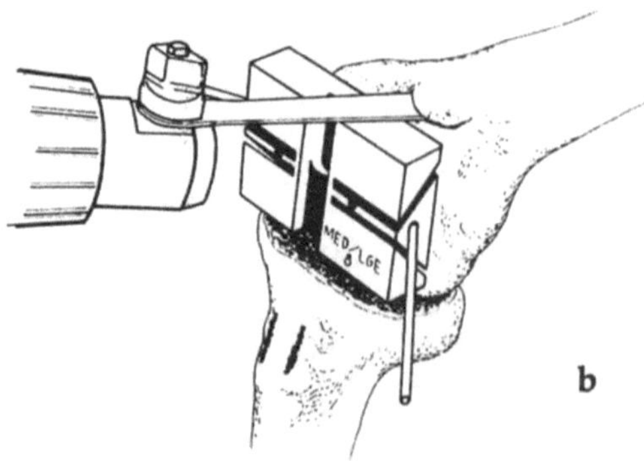

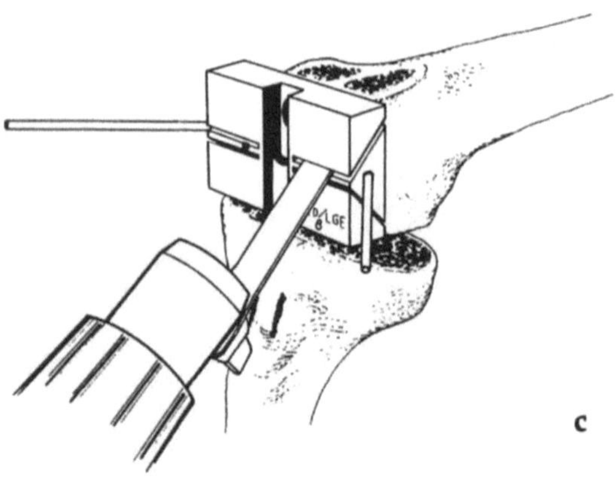

Fig. 10.9 a–c. Resection of the anterior and posterior femur. **a** The anterior indexing arm assures that the femoral cortex will not be notched. **b** Resection of the anterior femur. **c** Resection to accommodate the chamfers on the implant.

continued during the hospitalization. The patients used two Løfstrand canes for support for 6 weeks after surgery and then one cane in the contralateral hand for a subsequent 6 weeks.

Results

The Hospital for Special Surgery (HSS) rating system was used to evaluate the clinical results

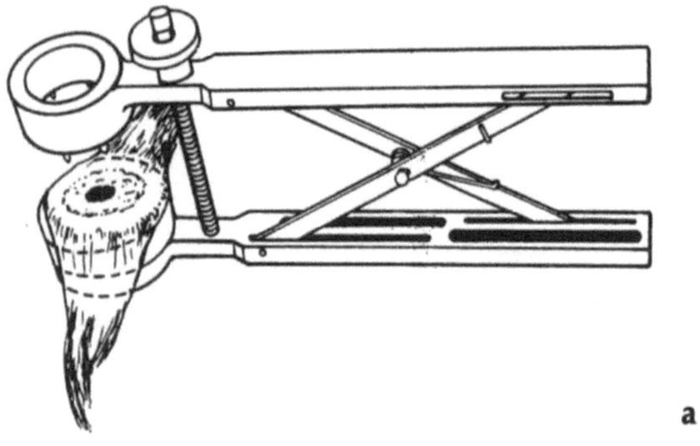

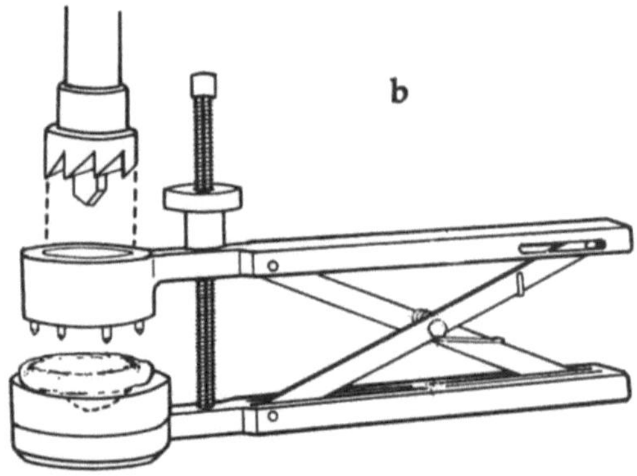

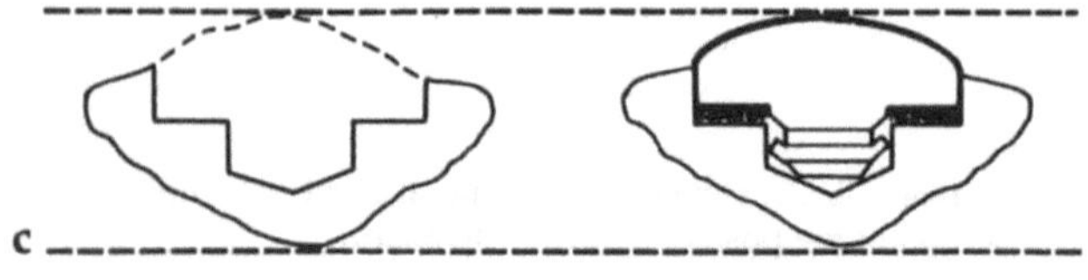

Fig. 10.10 a–c. Patellar resection to restore patellar height. **a** A patellar clamp is used centered on the mid-point of the patella. **b** The recess hole is drilled through the clamp. **c** The aim is restore patellar height with the implant.

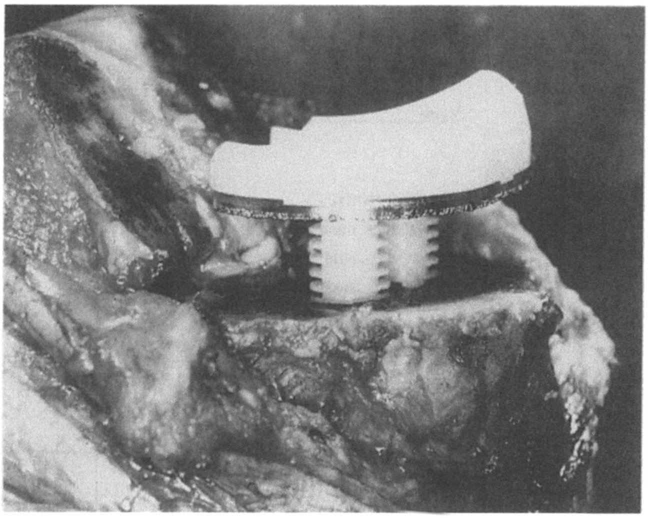

Fig. 10.11. Flanged pegs give immediate fixation to bone.

in the patients in this series. With this system, points are assigned for pain, function (walking, stair climbing, transferring ability), knee motion, muscle strength, flexion deformity, instability, use of external support, and leg deformity (Fig. 10.12). The total HSS score can, unfortunately, become unreliable in the presence of systemic neurological or cardiovascular problems or of localized disease in adjacent joints. A patient who cannot walk more than one block due to severe angina pectoris, immediately loses 8 points from the total rating, despite the fact that his limited walking has no relationship to his knee. Likewise, ability to ascend or descend stairs, or transfer from a chair without support may be compromised not by any problem with the knee but rather by severe arthritis in the adjacent hip or upper extremity. Despite these flaws, this system, however, has been widely used for the past 15 years, and therefore allows data from various series, including ours, to be directly compared.

The results that I will describe are those that were obtained in our patients. I have chosen this group because, being the primary investigatory center, we have a large number of patients who have passed the 5 year evaluation period. One should note, however, that the shorter term results (up to 3½ years) obtained from the other investigators in this series have matched those seen in our institution. Preoperatively 98% of all the patients had severe or moderate pain while bearing weight. At the 5 year evaluation, 81% had no pain, while another 13% had only mild barometric discomfort (Fig. 10.13). Pre-operatively 79% of the patients had severe or moderate pain while at rest. After surgery 88% were completely pain free, while another 7% had mild barometric pain. Whereas before surgery only 14% of the patients could walk more than 5 blocks, at the time of the 5 year evaluation 82% could walk this far or further. The ability to walk distances was directly correlated with the absence of pain.

The mean range of motion pre-operatively was 105° while that at 5 years was 113°. This difference was not statistically significant (Fig. 10.14). Patients who had a markedly limited flexion arc pre-operatively tended to gain some motion after surgery but never reach those levels achieved by patients whose motion was over 90° before surgery.

Before surgery only 11% of the patients were able to get out of chair without using their arms for support. After surgery, 70% were able to do so. Likewise before the operation 46% were able to ascend stairs foot over foot, while after surgery 71% could climb stairs in this manner.

At our institution we performed a statistical analysis of the Tricon-M patients comparing them to a comparable group of patients who had a cemented RMC (Smith and Newphew Richards Inc.) total knee prosthesis implanted (the articular surface of the RMC and the Tricon-M

THE HOSPITAL FOR SPECIAL SURGERY
KNEE SERVICE
Knee Rating Sheet

Name__________ HSS #________ Preoperative date__________

	Score	LEFT						RIGHT					
		pre	6 mo	1yr	2yr	3yr	4yr	pre	6 mo	1yr	2yr	3yr	4yr
PAIN (30 points)													
Walking: none	15												
mild	10												
moderate	5												
severe	0												
At rest: none	15												
mild	10												
moderate	5												
severe	0												
FUNCTION (22 points)													
Walk:													
walking & standing unlimited	12												
5-10 blocks, standing >30 min	10												
1-5 blocks, standing 15-30 min	8												
walk <1 block	4												
cannot walk	0												
Stairs: normal	5												
with support	2												
Transfer: normal	5												
with support	2												
ROM (18 points) each 8° = 1 point													
MUSCLE STRENGTH (10 points)													
cannot break quadriceps	10												
can break quadriceps	8												
can move through arc of motion	4												
cannot move through arc of motion	0												
FLEXION DEFORMITY (10 points)													
none	10												
5°-10°	8												
10°-20°	5												
>20°	0												
INSTABILITY (10 points)													
none	10												
0°-5°	8												
6°-15°	5												
>15°	0												
TOTAL													
SUBTRACTIONS:													
one cane	1												
one crutch	2												
two crutches	3												
extension lag of 5°	2												
10°	3												
15°	5												
Deformity (5° = 1 point) varus													
valgus													
TOTAL SUBTRACTIONS													
KNEE SCORE													

Fig. 10.12. Hospital for Special Surgery rating system.

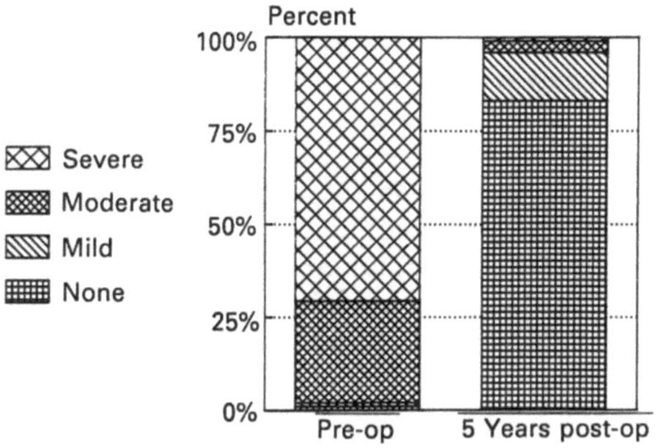

Fig. 10.13. Pain with weight bearing before and 5 years after surgery (Tricon-M).

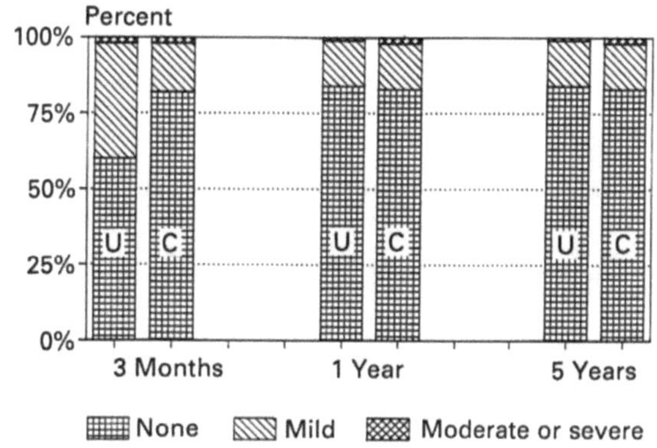

Fig. 10.15. Comparison of pain after surgery between uncemented (U) Tricon-M and cemented (C) RMC arthroplasties.

are identical). Each Tricon-M patient was categorized as to age decade, diagnosis, and body habitus. A match in all three categories for each was sought in the RMC group and the pair then compared for pain, walking ability, range of motion, and patient satisfaction. At the 3 month evaluation, more patients in the uncemented group had mild pain and less had no pain as compared to the cemented group. At all points after 3 months, the groups were statistically indistinguishable in all respects (Fig. 10.15).

At the 5 year follow-up examination, no subsidence of the tibial component was found in 36% of the knees (Fig. 10.16), while subsidence <1 mm was found in 55%. Seven per cent had subsidence between 1 and 2 mm and 2% had greater than 2 mm of subsidence.

Ryd (1986) using spectrophotogrametric analysis, has demonstrated subsidence in all tibial components, cemented or uncemented (see Chap. 14). He did not find that body weight, the use of steroids, or the amount of coverage of the tibial plateau was related to the degree of such subsidence. Although we could not demonstrate in our series that any one of these factors increased the incidence of subsidence, a combination of two or more of these factors led to an 85% incidence of subsidence of the implant ($P<0.01$).

In our patients evaluated at the 5 year follow-up period, 76% scored excellent, 18% good, 5% fair and 1% poor. The mean total HSS score was 94 (Fig. 10.17). For the entire group of 540 knees evaluated after 3 years, 79% scored excellent, 14% good, 4% fair, and 3% poor; the mean total score was 93 (Fig. 10.18 a c). The difference between these scores for the entire clinician's group at 3 years, and our data at 5 years was not statistically significant. Furthermore the difference between these scores and the two year

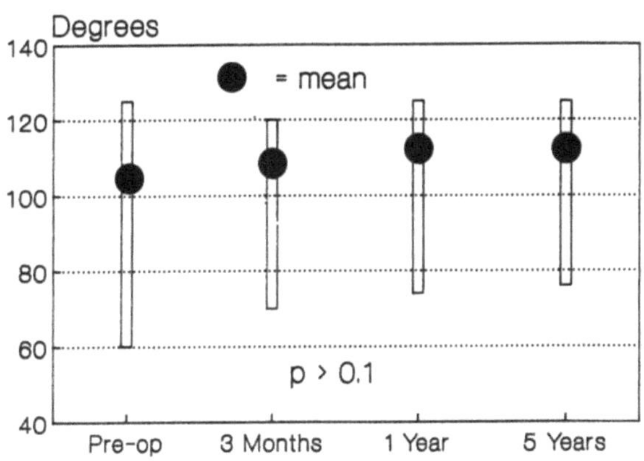

Fig. 10.14. Range of motion before and after surgery (Tricon-M).

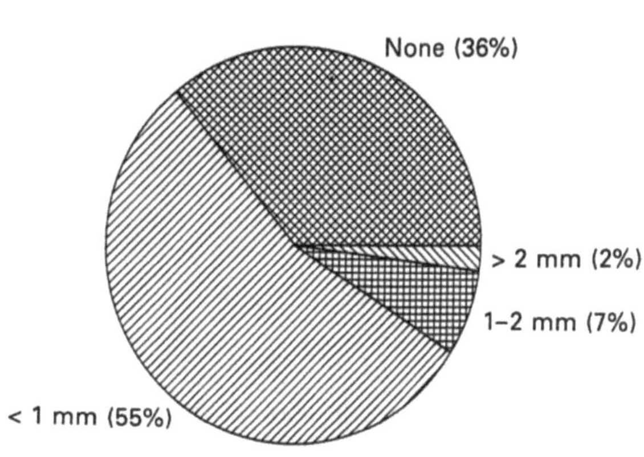

Fig. 10.16. Subsidence of tibial component 5 years after surgery (Tricon-M).

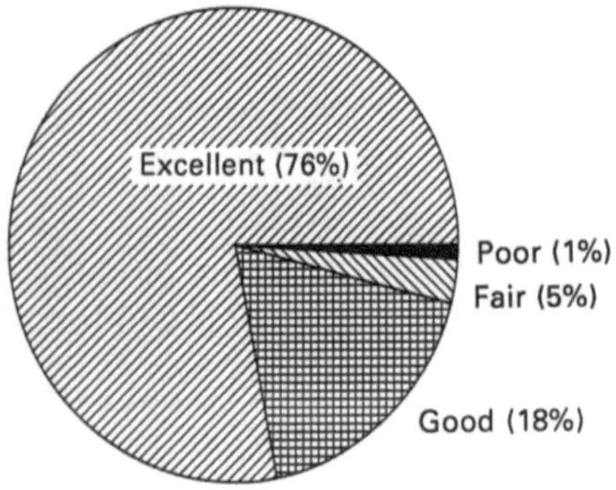

Fig. 10.17. Total Hospital for Special Surgery rating score 5 years after surgery (Tricon-M).

follow-up scores (Laskin 1988) were not statistically significant. These scores compared very favorably with HSS scores of 90, 92 and 96 found evaluating cemented Total Condylar (Insall et al. 1983), Insall-Bernstein Posterior Stabilized (see Chap. 6 and 7) and the LCS Meniscal Bearing knees (all cemented) and the PCA Knee (Hungerford et al. 1987) (uncemented).

A survivorship analysis was performed according to the Kaplan and Meier system (1958). The cumulative survivorship after 5 years was 94.5% (Fig. 10.19).

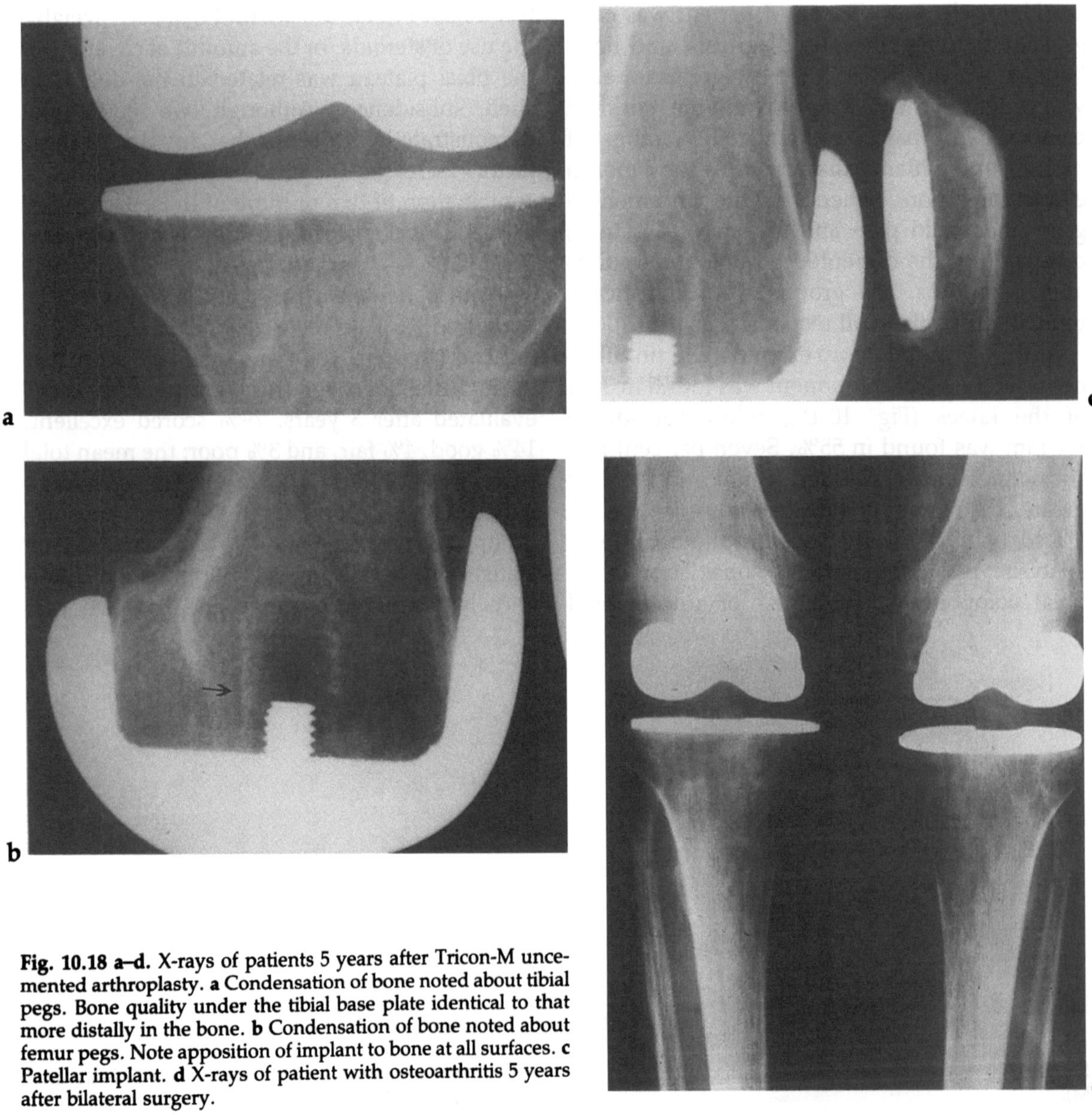

Fig. 10.18 a–d. X-rays of patients 5 years after Tricon-M uncemented arthroplasty. **a** Condensation of bone noted about tibial pegs. Bone quality under the tibial base plate identical to that more distally in the bone. **b** Condensation of bone noted about femur pegs. Note apposition of implant to bone at all surfaces. **c** Patellar implant. **d** X-rays of patient with osteoarthritis 5 years after bilateral surgery.

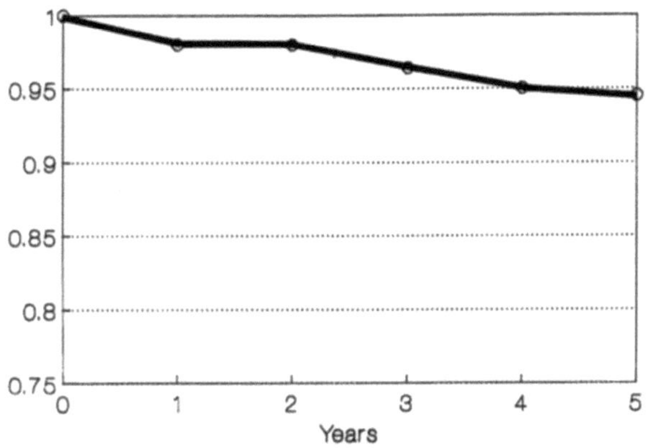

Fig. 10.19. Survivorship analysis (Tricon-M).

The Tricon-M Central Stem Tibial Prosthesis

The Prosthesis: Configuration and Design Rationale

The Tricon-M Central Stem Tibial Prosthesis was a modification of the original Tricon-M design. The tibial component maintained the articular surface, porous coated metal-backed undersurface, and flanged polyethylene pegs of the original Tricon-M. It differed in that it also incorporated an 8 cm central I-beam metallic stem as part of the base plate. The stem was bevelled so as to permit its approximation to the inner posterior wall of the proximal tibia (Fig. 10.20 a–c).

Walker (1981) demonstrated that a central stem assisted in preventing toggling of the tibial component, in a manner analogous to a long keel on a sailing vessel. Freeman has suggested that the stem should be cylindrical and long enough so as to obtain firm purchase in the isthmus of the tibia. Scott has preferred a shorter rounded stem with lateral fins to augment rotatory stability. Insall et al. (1979) designed a more rectangular stem, placed slightly posterior so that it could contact the inner posterior cortex of the femur.

The I-Beam cross-sectional configuration for the Tricon-M Central Stem tibial component permitted preservation of bone stock between the stem hole and the holes made for the flanged pegs. The pull-out strength of the implant in both cadaveric bones and foam composites was equal to that of cemented central stemmed implants in similar materials.

A clinical study was undertaken using the uncemented stemmed Tricon-M tibial component combined with the standard Tricon-M femoral and patellar components. The prosthesis was used prospectively for all patients undergoing total knee replacement except for those with marked angular deformities, severe

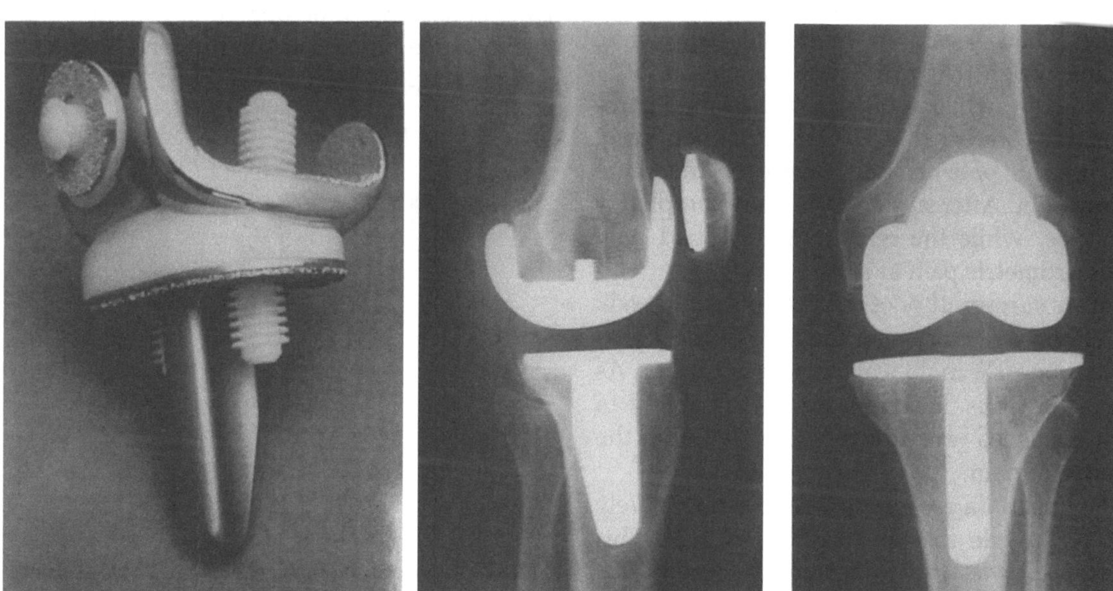

a b,c

Fig. 10.20 a–c. Tricon-M Central Stem Tibial prosthesis. **a** Implants. **b** Posterior bevel of stem abuts against inner tibial cortex. **c** Complete coverage of the tibial plateau by the implant.

osteoporosis or large bony cysts (the same caveats as in the original Tricon-M study).

Materials and Methods

Sixty-seven knee replacements using the uncemented Tricon-M Central Stem Tibial component were performed in 61 patients. Sixty-four per cent of the patients had rheumatoid arthritis, while the remainder all had osteoarthritis. The average age at the time of surgery was 58 in the rheumatoid group and 63 in the osteoarthritic group.

The surgical technique differed from that in the Tricon-M series only in the preparation of the proximal tibia. After the holes for the flanged polyethylene pegs were drilled, a guide was used to position the punch that created the recess for the central stem. If the bone between the stem hole encroached upon either of the peg holes the implant was inserted using acrylic cement for fixation. Those few knees were excluded from this analysis.

Results

The Hospital for Special Surgery rating system was again used to evaluate the clinical results in this series. Pre-operatively 97% of all the patients had severe or moderate pain while bearing weight. At the 2 year evaluation, 84% had no pain, while another 13% had mild barometric discomfort (Fig. 10.21). Pre-operatively 41% of the patients had severe or moderate resting pain. After surgery 90% were completely pain free, while the remaining 10% had only mild barometric pain at rest.

Before surgery 10% of the patients could walk more than five blocks. At the time of the 2 year evaluation 80% could walk this far or further. As in the previous Tricon-M study, the ability to walk distances was directly correlated with the absence of pain.

The mean range of motion pre-operatively was 108° while that at 2 years was 112°. This difference was not statistically significant. Again, as in the previous study, patients with severe restriction of motion pre-op never obtained the same flexion ability as those patients who had a pre-operative flexion of at least 90°.

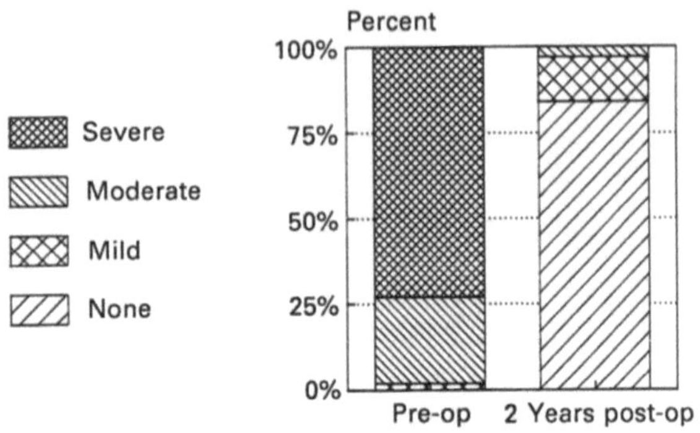

Fig. 10.21. Pain with weight-bearing before and 2 years after surgery (Tricon-M Central Stem Tibial prosthesis).

Before surgery only 7% of the patients were able to get out of a chair without using their arms for support. After surgery, 65% were able to do so. Likewise before the operation 43% were able to ascend stairs foot over foot, while after surgery 73% could climb stairs in this manner.

We performed a matched pain evaluation of patients using this uncemented prosthesis compared with those that had a cemented RMC prosthesis. We again evaluated pain, walking ability, range of motion, and patient satisfaction. We found no difference evaluating any parameter at any evaluation point between the two groups. Of special interest was the fact that these patients had the same degree of complete pain relief at three months as did the cemented RMC patients (Fig. 10.22).

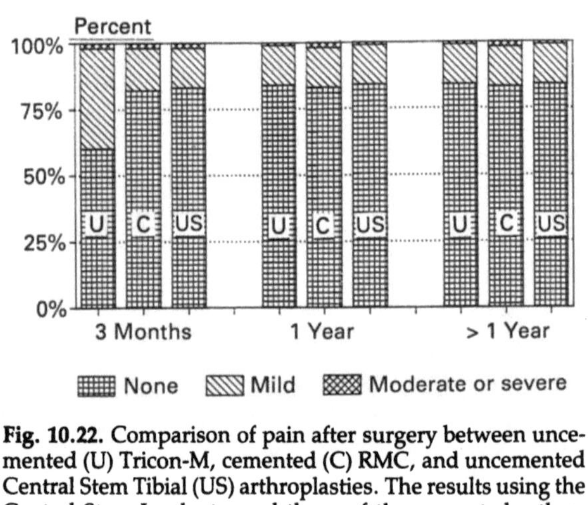

Fig. 10.22. Comparison of pain after surgery between uncemented (U) Tricon-M, cemented (C) RMC, and uncemented Central Stem Tibial (US) arthroplasties. The results using the Central Stem Implant equal those of the cemented arthroplasties.

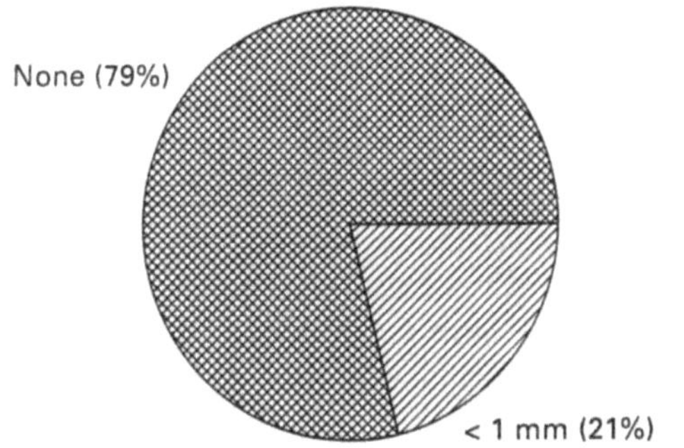

Fig. 10.23. Subsidence two years after surgery (Tricon-M Central Stem Tibial prosthesis).

At the 2 year follow-up examination, no subsidence of the tibial component was found in 52 of the 66 knees evaluated. There were 14 knees in which subsidence occurred and in all cases this was less than 1 mm. This compared to a subsidence rate of approximately 50% in the tibial component without a central stem discussed previously (Fig. 10.23).

Of the 66 knees evaluated at 2 years, 84% scored in the excellent range, 15% scored good, and 1% scored fair. The one knee scoring only fair at 2 years was artificially in that lower category due to severe rheumatoid involvement of both hips and the opposite knee as well as marked interstitial pulmonary restrictive disease all of which severely limited her function.

Based upon this study we have concluded that the addition of a central stem to the prosthesis further stabilized it against subsidence. We feel that this was the probable cause for the excellent immediate relief of pain that was seen.

The Genesis Uncemented Total Knee Prosthesis

The Prosthesis: Configuration and Design Rationale

Encouraged by what we had learned from the previous studies using the two types of Tricon-M uncemented prosthesis, we now progressed to a new prosthesis that further incorporated many recent ideas in metallurgy and instrumentation. This prosthesis was designed in cooperation with Dr. James Rand of the Mayo Clinic, Dr. Raymond Gustillo of the University of Minnesota, and Dr. James Howe of the University of Vermont. The prosthesis was named the Genesis Uncemented Total Knee, and is the implant we are presently using for our total knee patients.

The Genesis femoral component (Fig. 10.24) is fabricated of cobalt-chrome-molybdenum alloy (CoCrMo) and maintains the asymmetry of the femoral condyles that had existed in the Tricon-M, with the medial condyle having a 20% greater surface area than the lateral condyle. The trochlear facet is wider than that of the Tricon

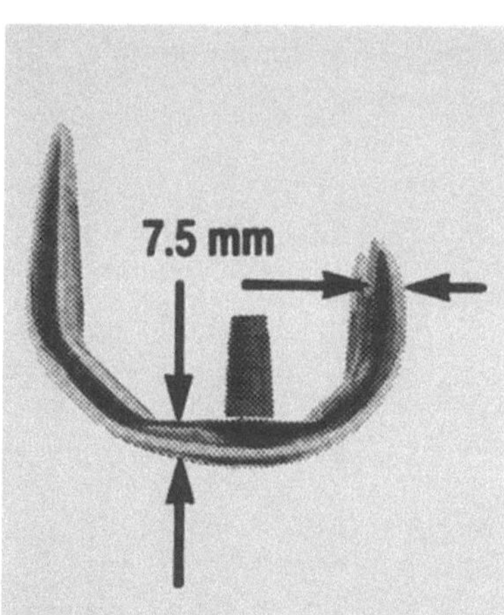

a

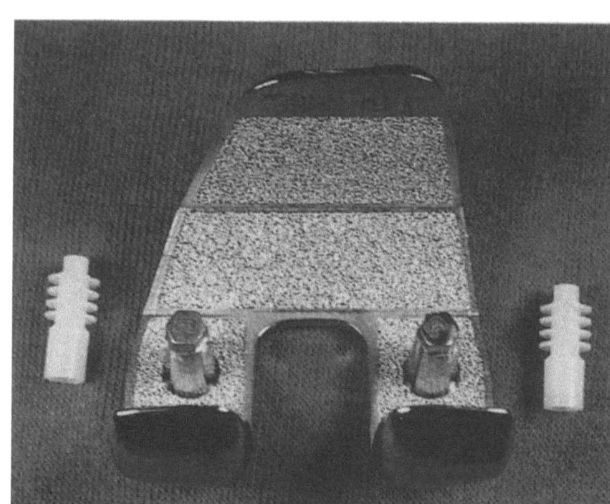

b

Fig. 10.24 a–b. Genesis femoral component. **a** The distal and posterior surfaces have a thickness of 10.5 mm. **b** The inner surface is covered with beads of sintered cobalt-chrome-molybdenum forming pores of 250 μm in diameter.

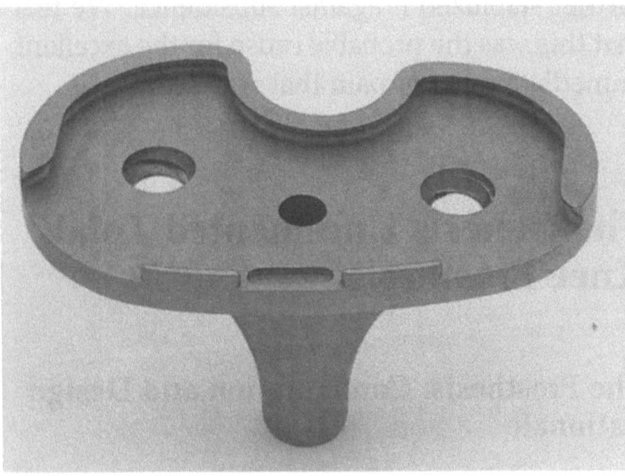

Fig. 10.25. Genesis tibial component has an asymmetric baseplate.

and is prolonged more distally to allow a broader contact area with the prosthetic patellar implant, especially in flexion. The posterior condyles are likewise longer than those on the Tricon so as to completely cap the resected bone surface. There are five femoral component sizes (mediolaterally and anteroposteriorly), all have the same 10.5 mm distal thickness. Having such a small distal thickness minimizes the amount of bone that needs be resected, an important consideration especially in small-statured rheumatoid patients. The static and fatigue strength of such a thin component has been shown to be more than sufficient for the stresses imparted to it.

The entire undersurface of the femoral component is covered with a multilayered surface of sintered cobalt-chrome-molybdenum beads forming pores of 250–300 μm in diameter. Based upon Cameron's canine model we had previously felt that by covering the entire implant with a porous ingrowth medius such as this might lead to stress shielding of the femoral condyles. When, however, we reviewed the long-term data from other investigators who used a one pore surface, we came to the conclusion that this was not a true problem in humans. There are two flanged polyethylene pegs on the implant that are impacted into undersized recess holes when the femoral component is seated on the femur.

The tibial component retains the mediolateral asymmetry of the articular surface found in the Tricon implants. There is as well an asymmetry to the entire contour of the metal base plate of the Genesis tibial component (Fig. 10.25). The medial portion of the implant projects further posteriorly than does the lateral portion to allow more accurate and complete coverage of the tibial cut surface. The base plate is fabricated of titanium-aluminum-vanadium alloy and has an undersurface of sintered pure titanium beads enclosing pores of 250–300 μm in diameter. The base plates come in a variety of sizes, and the corresponding bearing inserts in numerous thicknesses (Fig. 10.26). This modularity reduces the storage and inventory problem that had existed with one piece tibial components. The central stem of the base plate will accept intramedullary extension rods if they are necessary in a particular clinical situation. The metal base plate is affixed to the tibia either by flanged polyethy-

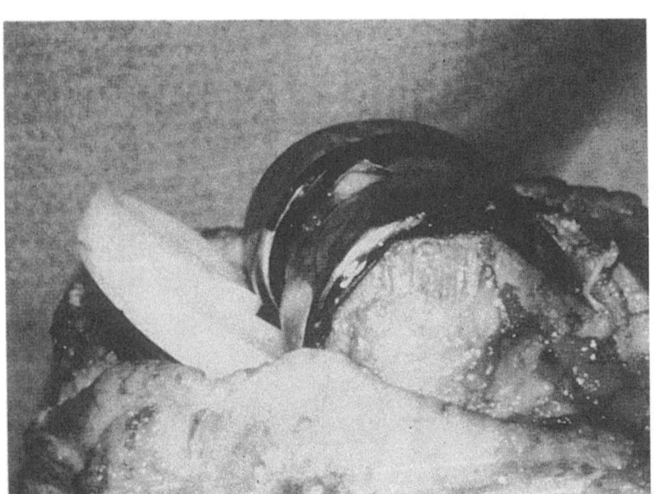

Fig. 10.26. Polyethylene inserts for Genesis tibial component.

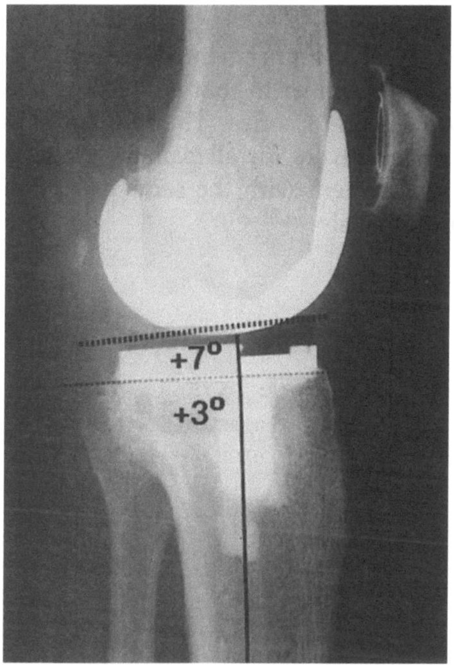

Fig. 10.27. X-ray demonstrating posterior sloping of articular surface. The proximal tibia has been resected with a 3° backslope. The polyethylene has a 4° backslope. Overall this results in the articular surface being sloped posteriorly 7°.

lene pegs, as in the Tricon-M, or by large cancellous screws. The bearing surfaces have a 4° posterior slope (Fig. 10.27). Since the tibia is resected at a 3° posterior slope, the overall joint surface is sloped posteriorly at 7°.

The unfacetted polyethylene patellar implant (Fig. 10.28) has a titanium-aluminum-vanadium base plate covered with a multilayer surface of titanium beads enclosing 250–300 μm pores. There is a short flanged polyethylene peg on its undersurface for bony interlock. The articular surface of the implant is a mate for the femoral component trochlear surface. There are two sizes of patellar implants available.

The decision to use a sintered pure titanium beaded surface for the patellar and tibial implants was based upon experience using this material in an investigatory total hip protocol, Optifix Total Hip (Smith and Newphew Richards Inc). The biocompatibility of titanium is superior to any other implant metal and its modulus of elasticity is closer to bone than that of CoCrMo or stainless steel. There has been some evidence to show that ingrowth may occur more reproducibly in such a surface than in a CoCrMo construct.

Although porous titanium is a good ingrowth material, titanium alloy is not a good choice for a bearing surface. Agins and his co-workers (1988) at the Hospital for Special Surgery demonstrated that the passivating layer of titanium oxide on the surface of a titanium alloy implant can be rubbed off by constant motion with polyethylene, releasing titanium alloy particles into the soft tissue. Furthermore polyethylene wears at an increased rate when it articulates with a unpassivated titanium alloy surface. It is for these reasons that the femoral component of this implant is fabricated of cobalt-chrome-molybdenum alloy rather than titanium alloy. The

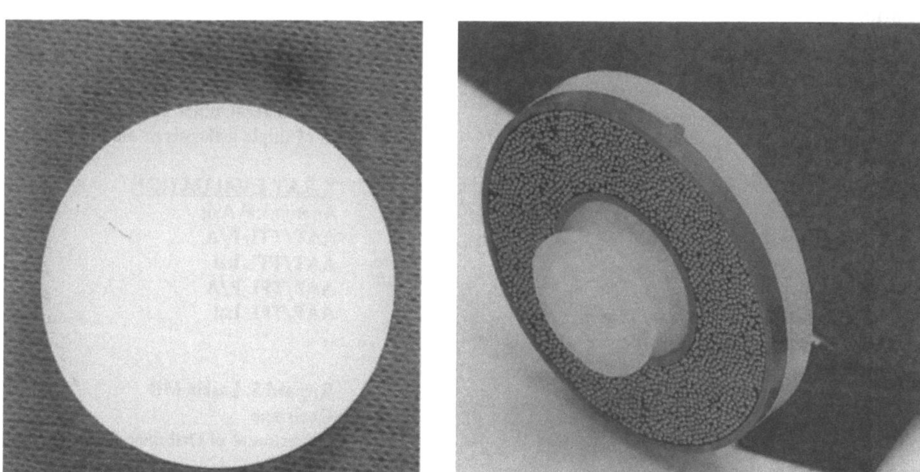

a b

Fig. 10.28 a,b. Genesis patellar component. **a** Articular surface of the Genesis patellar implant. **b** Undersurface of the Genesis patellar implant.

theoretical hybrid of a CoCrMo implant with a titanium porous surface is difficult to fabricate because of the differences in sintering temperatures between the different alloys. Work is presently under way to elucidate whether a more effective and long-lasting passivation process may be possible so as to allow titanium alloy to be used as a bearing surface.

Materials and Methods

The study of the uncemented Genesis Porous Prosthesis is similar to that which was used in the two Tricon-M series. The implant is being used prospectively for all patients undergoing knee replacement with the same exceptions as noted previously.

KNEE SCORE

LAST NAME____________ FIRST NAME____________
DATE _/_/_ KNEE _ PRE:_ 3 MOS:_ 1 YR:_ 2 YR:_ 3 YR:_ 4 YR:_ 5 YR:_
DIAGNOSIS _

Pain	Points
None	50
Mild/occasional	40
Stairs only	40
Walk + Stairs	30
Moderate	
Occasional	20
Continual	10
Severe	00
Range of Motion	
(5° = 1 pt)	
Stability	
A/P	
< 5mm	10
5-10mm	05
> 10mm	00
Mediolateral	
$<5^o$	15
$6\text{-}9^o$	10
$10\text{-}14^o$	05
$> 15^o$	00
SUBTOTAL	___
Deductions (minus)	
Flex.Contracture	
$5\text{-}10^o$	2
$10\text{-}15^o$	5
$16\text{-}20^o$	10
$>20^o$	00
Extension lag	
$<10^o$	05
$10\text{-}20^o$	10
$>20^o$	15
Alignment	
$5\text{-}10^o$ valgus	00
$0\text{-}4^o$ valgus	3 pts/ degree
$11\text{-}15^o$valgus	3 pts/degree
Other	20
Total Deductions	___
KNEE SCORE	___

(if score is a minus #, score = 0

Function	
Walking	
Unlimited	50
> 10 blocks	40
5-10 blocks	30
<5 blocks	20
Household	10
Unable	00
Stairs	
Norm. Up/Down	50
Norm. Up/Rail Down	40
Up/Down with Rail	30
Up Rail/Unable Down	15
Unable	00
Subtotal	___
Deductions (minus)	
Cane	05
Two canes	10
Crutches/walker	20
Total Deductions	___
FUNCTION SCORE	___

Patient category ___
A: Unilateral or bilateral (opposite knee successfully replaced)
B: Unilateral, other knee symptomatic
C: Multiple arthrosis or medial infirmity

X-RAY EVALUATION	
Anatomical Axis	___
AAT/TTL P/A	___
AAT/TTL Lat	___
AAF/TFL P/A	___
AAF/TFL Lat	___

Richard S. Laskin MD
Chairman
Department of Orthopaedic Surgery

Fig. 10.29. Knee Society rating system.

The patient data is being evaluated using the Knee Society rating system (Fig. 10.29). This sytem separates those parameters that are attributable specifically to the knee, from those that result from general function in the entire patient. The knee parameters being evaluated are pain, range of motion, and stability in both the anteroposterior and mediolateral planes. There are deductions from the knee score for the presence of a flexion contracture, extensor lag, and malalignment of the leg. The general function parameters are walking and stair climbing, with deductions for the use of external supportive devices.

The rating system separates the patients into three classes. Class A patients are those with monoarticular arthritis in the knee being operated upon. Class B patients have arthritis in the opposite knee as well. Class C patients are those with arthritis in multiple weight bearing joints including the knee. This separation of patient types and of factors related to the knee from general function factors allows a better comparison of patients and their results than had been obtained using the Hospital for Special Surgery System. The result for any particular patient is a letter, followed by two numbers, one for knee function, and one for general function (i.e. A,20,60).

The surgical technique again follows the guidelines set down earlier in Chaps. 4 and 5. An intermedullary rod, fluted so as to avoid pressurization of the marrow elements, is used to position the distal femoral resection block (Fig. 10.30). The distal femoral resection is made at 95° to the femoral anatomical axis in the coronal plane and 90° to the femoral anatomical axis in the sagittal plane and removes 10.5 mm of bone (Fig. 10.31).

The level for cutting the tibia is determined by external spacer blocks which are positioned after the ligaments are balanced and the soft tissues tensed with laminar spreaders. The cutting block is positioned by an 8 mm intramedullary tibial alignment rod (Laskin and Turtel 1989) (Fig. 10.32). The tibia is resected at 90° to its anatomical axis in the coronal plane and at 93° to its anatomical axis in the lateral plane (a slight downward slope) (Fig. 10.33).

The anterior and posterior femoral cuts are made in 2° external rotation to accommodate for the 90° cut of the proximal tibia (Fig. 10.34) (see Chap. 4). In this manner a rectangular flexion space is created for the implant. Chamfer cuts are made on the femur to accommodate for the internal structure of the femoral component.

A tibial template is used to position the component (Fig. 10.35). Through it the center hole for the stem is drilled (Fig. 10.36) and then punched (Fig. 10.37). A cutting guide is then used for preparation of the slots for the fins on

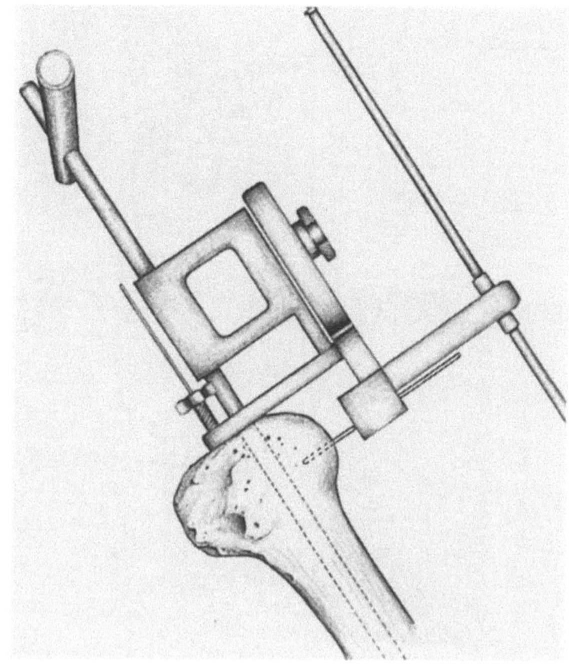

Fig. 10.30. Intramedullary alignment jig and guide for resection of distal femur.

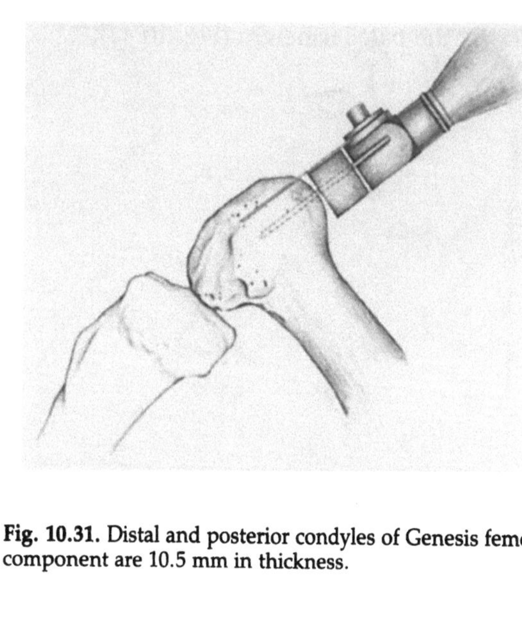

Fig. 10.31. Distal and posterior condyles of Genesis femoral component are 10.5 mm in thickness.

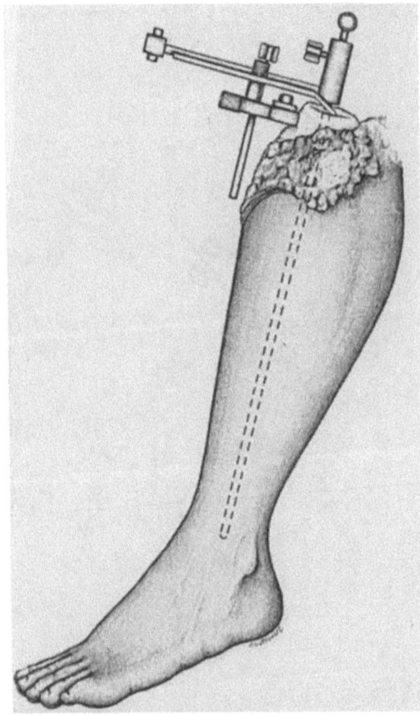

Fig. 10.32. Tibial intramedullary alignment rod and cutting guide (Genesis).

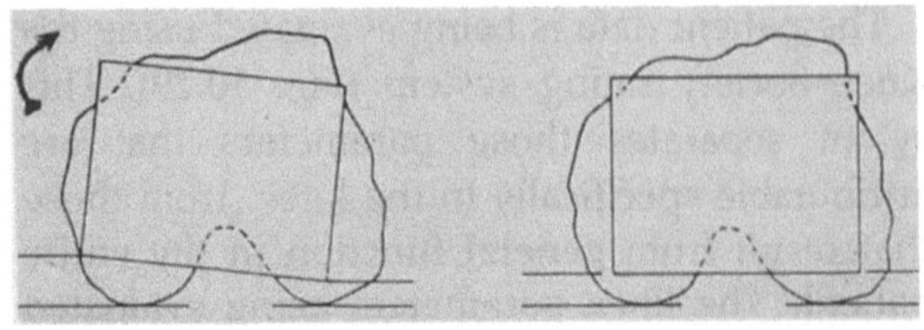

Fig. 10.34. External rotation of the anterior and posterior femoral cuts to establish a rectangular flexion space.

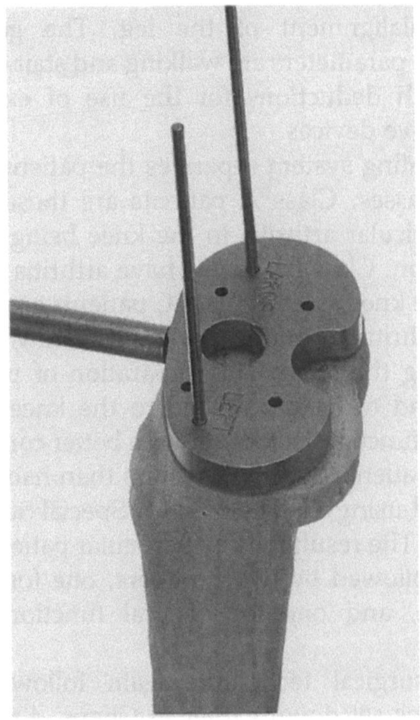

Fig. 10.35. Template placed for positioning of the tibial component compression screws.

the component (Fig. 10.38 a–c). Either large compression screws (Fig. 10.39 a–e) or flanged polyethylene pegs (Fig. 10.40) are used to obtain initial fixation of the base plate to the tibia. The proper sized bearing surface is then inserted manually and seated using an insertion tool (Fig. 10.41).

The patellar prosthesis is inset into the patella with instruments similar to those used in the Tricon study. A depth guide assures that sufficient bone is reamed so as not to increase artificially the patellar height (Fig. 10.42).

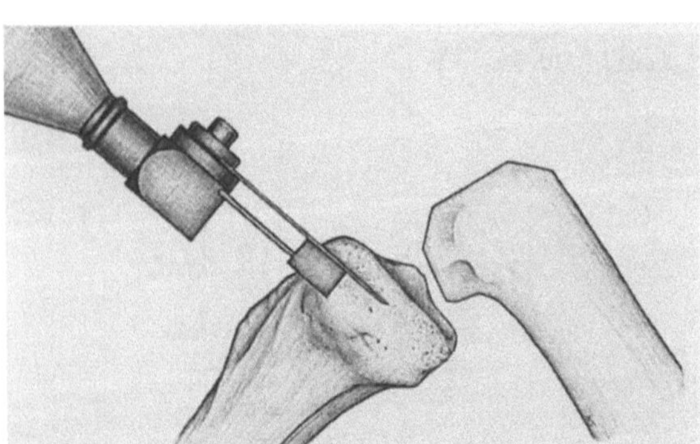

Fig. 10.33. Resection of proximal tibia for Genesis implant.

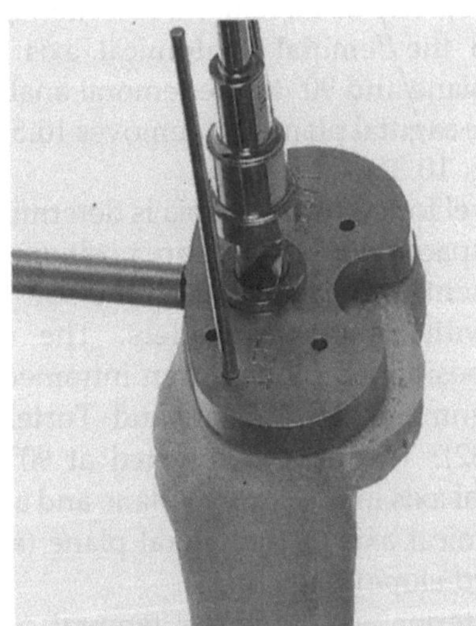

Fig. 10.36. The hole for the central stem is drilled.

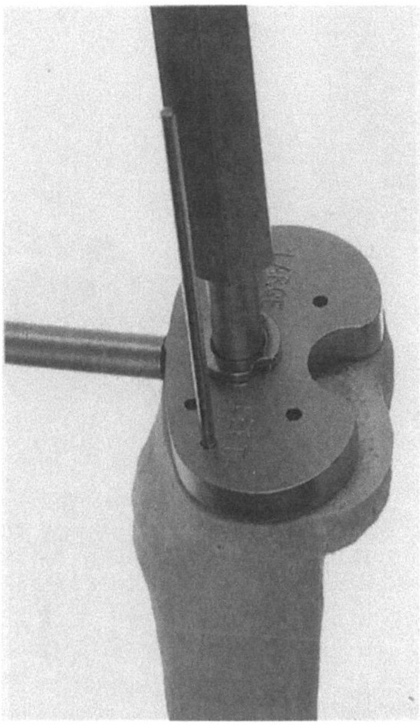

Fig. 10.37. The hole is deepened with a punch.

Results

The early results that we have obtained using this prosthesis have been excellent in parallel with those seen in the Tricon-M Central Stem tibial component study. Pain relief, motion, stability, and muscle strength have been equal to that found in our cemented total knee studies.

A biomechanical study is presently under way to determine in which clinical situations the compression screws are most applicable, and in which situations the flanged polyethylene pegs are indicated. Through a combination of hardness testing at the operating table, and preoperative CT densitometry readings the indications for both methods of fixation are being clarified. In our experience, the use of both of these fixation techniques has all but eliminated the use of acrylic cement, except in those cases of marked osteoporosis.

Conclusions

Based upon our results in these series it would appear that a noncemented total knee prosthesis can give clinical results equal to those found in cemented total knees. We feel, however, that certain criteria must be met before these types of excellent results are obtained.

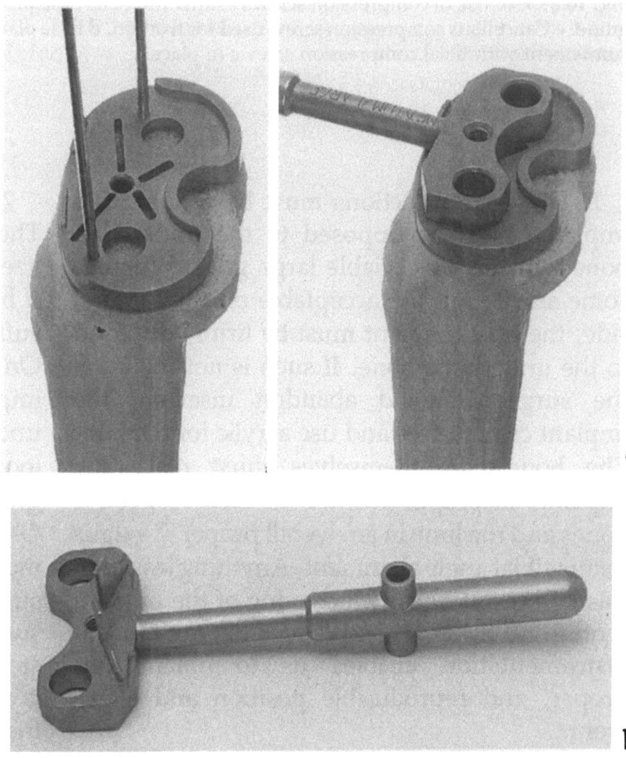

a c b

Fig. 10.38 a–c. Preparation of the slots for the derotation fins of the tibial component. a Placement of the guide. b Fin punch/guide. c Guide/punch seated in position.

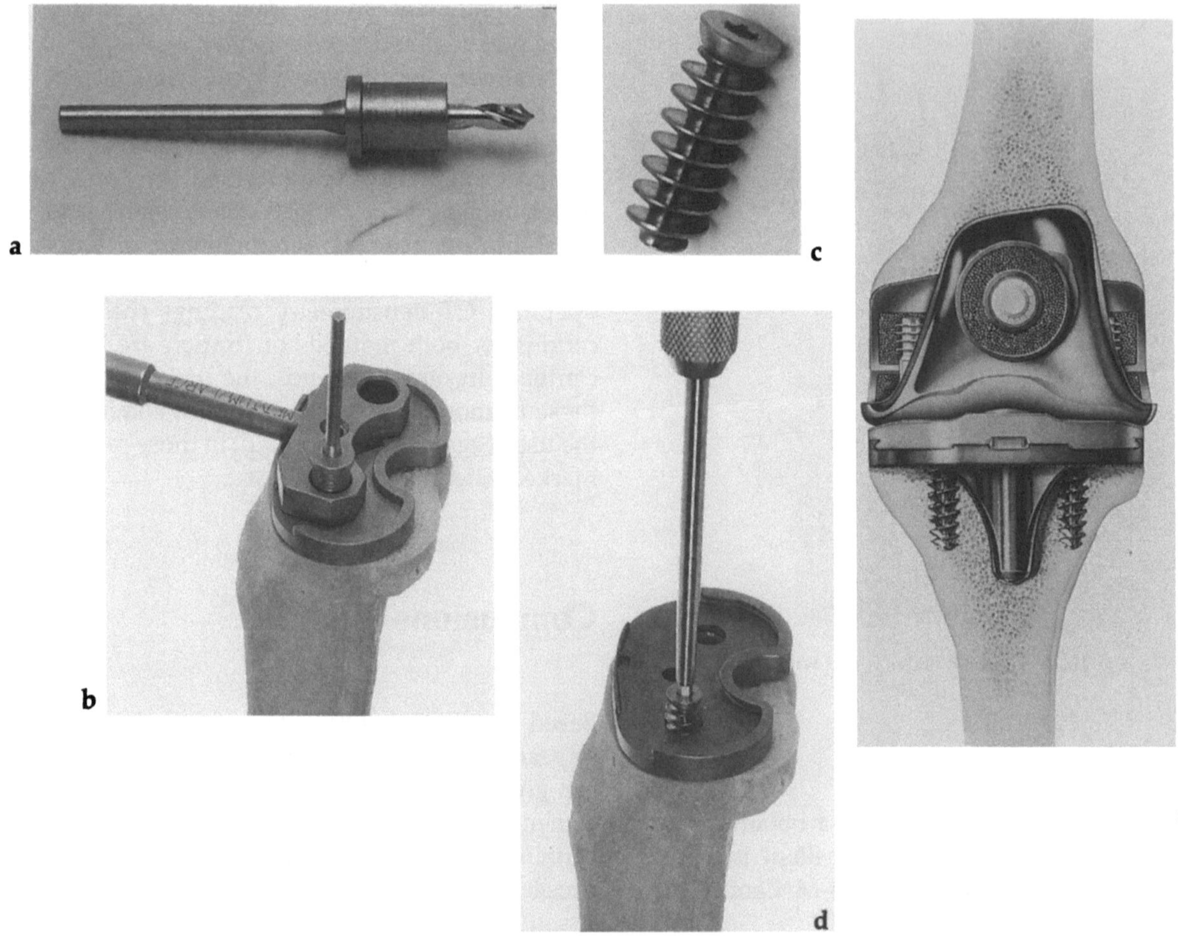

Fig. 10.39 a–e. Use of compression screws to affix the tibial base plate. **a** Drill for compression screws. **b** Drilling through the guide. **c** Cancellous compression screw used for fixation. **d** Base plate being affixed to the proximal tibia. **e** Uncemented tibial component with tibial compression screws in place.

1. The bone resections must be proper. The implants must be opposed to the underlying bone with no appreciable large gaps. Whereas some small gaps are acceptable on the femoral side, the tibial implant must be firmly opposed to the underlying bone. If such is not the case, the surgeon should abandon inserting the implant cement-free and use acrylic for fixation. The bone cuts themselves must place the implants in proper position to their respective bones and the limb in an overall proper 7° valgus femur-tibial angle alignment. Anything less than this will result in early loosening of the implant (Lotke and Ecker 1977). We feel that our current instrumentation enables us to obtain this proper, and reproducible position and alignment.

2. The design of the implant must be proper. The initial fixation must be sufficient to immobilize the implant until biological ingrowth occurs. If biological ingrowth does not occur it must be sufficient to immobilize the implant long-term. On the femoral side this is rarely a problem. The implant is fixed by the multiple shapes of its undersurface, and indeed, femoral component loosening has been reported only in cases of gross malalignment or surgical technical error. On the tibial side we must attempt to achieve the most rigid fixation possible since the plateau surface of the implant is supported on a planar surface. This implant should include a central stem, and lateral pegs or screws. Since the bone is cancellous we feel that if screws are to be used they should have large threads and allow lag-

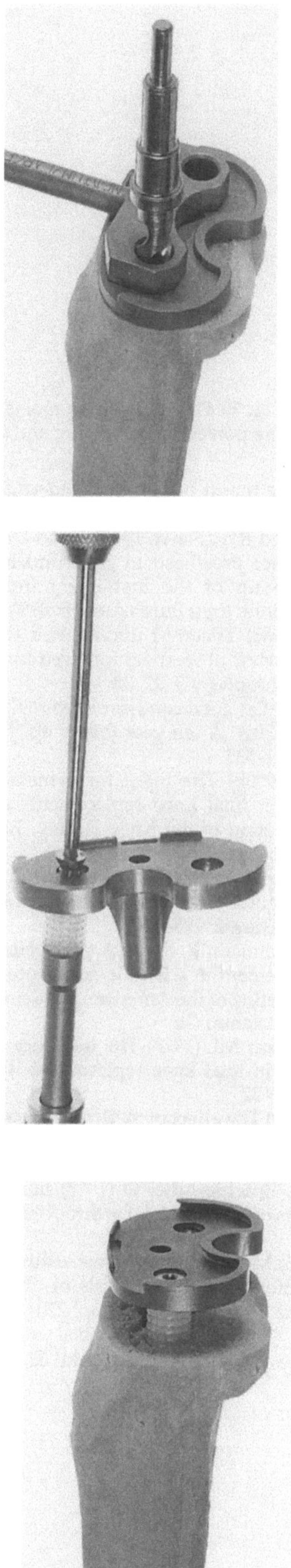

a

b

c

Fig. 10.40. Use of flanged polyethylene pegs to affix the tibial base plate.

ging of the implant to the bone. We do not feel that cortical screws extending back through the cortex distally are proper. Fixation of the patellar implant is possible and is maximized if it is inset in the patellar bone. We do not feel that onset patellar implants can be sufficiently fixed to the bone without the use of acrylic cement.

3. The consistency of the bone must be proper. If the bone is too soft, an initial press fit will not be obtained. If in such a case, micromotion of a degree greater than 50% the diameter of the pores on the implant, will obviate any long lasting bone ingrowth. Hvid et al. (1984) have described the use of an osteopenetrometer in an attempt to quantify bone strength with the ability to fix a noncemented component. Our study, as described above, should help clarify this situation. If we can somehow determine in advance which bone is best for an uncemented implant we will now doubt increase our success rate significantly.

4. The undersurface of the implant must be proper so as to facilitate biological ingrowth. This means pores of the proper dimension (75–350 μm in diameter). We feel that the porous surface should be fabricated of pure titanium since this type of surface appears to be most conducive to ingrowth. We are not sure that one can expect bone ingrowth into all the pores. Indeed, ours and other studies appear to indicate that this is not the case. We feel that possibly more rigid fixation of the implant (especially the tibial implant) with compression screws may permit further ingrowth by diminishing micromotion. We feel that one can use an uncemented implant and get excellent clinical results without bone ingrowth but with a solid press fit (Ryd 1986 and Chap. 14). The advantage of ingrowth is that such bone helps resist tensile stresses; fibrous tissue and cement are notoriously weak in tension.

5. We feel that a metal-backed patellar component can be used if it is inset in the bone and has a thick polyethylene surface (Laskin 1990b). Indeed the Tricon-M metal-backed patella is presently the only one available in the United States in which wear through and metal on metal wear of the backing has **not** been reported. Our new Genesis patellar design is a direct outgrowth of our success with the Tricon-M.

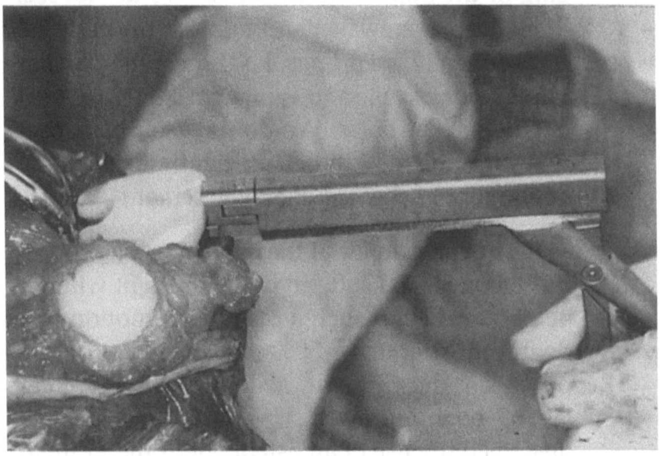

Fig. 10.41. An insertion tool is used to seat the polyethylene bearing surface.

Bearing all these factors in mind we have found that an uncemented total knee is a viable procedure which is standing the test of time well. We feel that further enhancements of our surgical technique, in implant materials, and in the exact design of the implants will further increase the applicability to a large number of patients undergoing total knee replacement.

References

Blaha JD, Insler HP, Freeman MAR (1982) The fixation of a proximal tibial polyethylene prosthesis without cement. J Bone Joint Surg (Br) 64: 326–331

Bobyn JD, Pilliar RM, Cameron HU (1980) The optimum pore size for fixation of a porous surfaced metal implant by ingrowth of bone. Clin Orthop 12: 239–241

Cameron HU, Pilliar RM, McNab I (1974) Porous vitallium in implant surgery. J Biomed Mater Res 8:283–290

Goldberg VM, Figgie MP, Figgie HE, Heliple KHG, Sobel M (1988) Knee arthroplasty in rheumatoid arthritis. Four to six years follow-up study. J Arthroplasty 2: 233–239

Hungerford D, Krackow K, Kenna R (1987) Two to five year experience with a cementless porous-coated total knee prosthesis. In: Rand J, Dorr L (eds) Total knee arthroplasty. Aspen, Rockville, MD

Hvid I, Anderson K, Olesen S (1984) Cancellous bone strength measurements with the osteopenetrometer. Eng Med 13: 2–15

Insall J, Scott W, Ranawat CS (1979) The total condylar knee prosthesis: a report of two hundred and twenty cases. J Bone Joint Surg (Am) 61: 173–180

Insall JN, Hood RW, Flawn IB, Sullivan DJ (1983) The total condylar knee prosthesis in gonarthrosis. A five to nine year follow up of the first one hundred consecutive patients. J Bone Joint Surg (Am) 65: 619–627

Laskin RS (1988) Tricon-M uncemented total knee arthroplasty. A review of 96 knees followed for longer than two years. J Arthroplasty 3: 27–38

Laskin RS (1990a) Total condylar knee replacement in rheumatoid arthritis. A ten year follow up. J Bone Joint Surg (Am) 72: 529–535

Laskin RS (1990b) The place for a metal-backed patellar prosthesis in total knee replacement. Presented at the Annual Meeting of the Knee Society, New Orleans, La. Clin Orthop 260:52–55

Laskin RS, Turtel A (1989) The use of an intramedullary tibial alignment guide in total knee replacement arthroplasty. Am J Knee Surg 2: 123–130

Laskin RS, Lohmann R, Sinha A (1984) Non-cemented total knee replacement. A scientific exhibit presented at the 51st Annual Meeting of the American Academy of Orthopaedic Surgeons, Atlanta, Ga

Lotke PA, Ecker ML (1977) The influence of positioning of prostheses in total knee replacement. J Bone Joint Surg (Am) 55: 77–82

Petty W (1978) The effect of methylmethacrylate on bacterial phagocytosis and killing of human polymorphic leukocytes. J Bone Joint Surg (Am) 60: 752–758

Ranawat C, Boachie-Adjei O (1988) Survivorship analysis and results of total condylar arthroplasty. Clin Orthop 226: 6–13

Ryd L (1986) Micromotion in knee arthroplasty: a roentgen stereophotogrammetric analysis of tibial component fixation. Acta Orthop Scand (Suppl 220)

Walker PS (1981) Fixation of tibial components of knee prostheses. J Bone Joint Surg (Am) 63: 258–267

Chapter 11

Results of Uncemented Total Knee Arthroplasty using the PCA System

Kenneth A. Krackow, David S. Hungerford and Robert V. Kenna

Introduction

Total knee arthroplasties evolved from the placement of implants which were true, fixed mechanical hinges and conservative interpositional metallic wafers to a variety of "condylar" resurfacing implants, which model the anatomic knee quite accurately. The PCA* total knee prosthesis can reasonably be considered the forerunner of the latest changes in total knee implant design. These changes are most conspicuously characterized by the introduction of porous surfaces to permit biologic fixation. These surfaces are evident in addition to the more anatomic shapes and considerations which began to appear in the late 1970s as prostheses provided for preservation of the posterior cruciate ligament and right–left differences on the femoral components.

Despite a significant clinical experience over time, and despite the design changes occurring in the 1960s and 1970s, specific problems have plagued the field of total knee arthroplasty. As a minimum, such problems have included component loosening, various limits to postoperative range of motion, small groups of patients with persistent stiffness and/or pain, and delayed postoperative infection. To this list may be added problems with component wear, patellar stability and fracture, as well as others.

In examining these problems then, as well as now, there has been great emphasis placed upon the issue of component loosening. This fact probably derives from a feeling that loosening is ultimately under the surgeon's control together with the fact that it is so significant – being accompanied by substantial periprosthetic bone loss. While many are familiar with reports of superb intermediate to almost long term results with the original cemented total condylar prostheses, the commercial success of newer designs implies less "community" satisfaction with these implants which were most popular in the middle 1970s. Furthermore, the proliferation of uncemented total knee designs speaks to a widespread suspicion of methylmethacrylate, even in the presence of improved cementing technique/technology.

It was within this context that the PCA system was developed starting in the late 1970s and introduced to the US orthopaedic community in 1981. A "seconding" of the concerns mentioned above is evident by the proliferation of similar designs up to this very date.

Experience with total knee arthroplasty has taught us that prosthetic constraint, especially as evidenced at the extremes inherent in true and rotating hinges, is plagued with problems of component loosening and subjacent bone loss. Furthermore, inconsistency of component placement as it relates to axial alignment, and, as mentioned above, problems with specific component fixation, have also evolved as clear concomitants of prosthetic loosening. Combining all of these considerations, the system detailed in

*PCA and PCA-Modular are trade marks.

this chapter was created with the following main objectives: (1) the reproducible recreation of normal anatomic alignment, (2) the provision of prosthetic kinematics as close to normal knee movements as possible, and (3) improvement of component fixation, both when methylmethacrylate would be used, as well as with the possibility of uncemented biologic fixation.

PCA Knee Prosthesis

The prosthesis implanted in this longer term group of patients has undergone some modifications over the total 9+ year life span of the system. Most obvious were the recent changes which led to the redesignation of this system as the PCA-Modular in February 1988. Such changes may raise immediate questions or suspicions as to the existence of certain major problems with the original design reported here.

Upon reviewing the specific changes, which are described later in this chapter, it should be clear that these were made in an effort to effect various small and moderate improvements in outcome and to address issues of inventory and component cost. These changes were not made, as should be clear from the clinical data which follow, to address major design or conceptual flaws in the original system.

A relatively detailed description of this system follows and is viewed as appropriate in this source. It is material which is commonly not included in peer review journal publications, and involves a commentary which may have not been evident at the time the original manufacturer's literature was produced. In consideration of the major position that this system has occupied in the area of total knee arthroplasty in the United States, the documentation of these points in this format seems appropriate.

Component Surfaces

Essentially all surfaces of PCA knee prostheses used in this study which are apposed to bone are metal (vitallium-chrome-cobalt alloy) backed and porous coated. Porous coating is comprised of a double layer of sintered chrome cobalt beads yielding an average pore size of 450 μm with 35% porosity. Each component's beaded surface is surrounded by a smooth margin which serves to contain the beads during the sintering process and provides marginal surfaces for labeling. This fact is mentioned, as characteristically a fibrous interface develops at the junction of bone with such smooth metal, while it does not typically develop at the specific interfaces of bone and beads.

Also of note with respect to the porous beaded surface was a manufacturing change in the cold quenching aspect of the sintering process which provided an average 35% increase in the bead to bead and bead to substrate bond strength.

Femoral Component

The PCA femoral component, available in four sizes, is characterized by differences in medial and lateral condylar dimensions as well as a laterally directed trochlear groove. There are varying radii of curvature within each condyle in addition to differences from medial to lateral. This geometry relates to re-creation of a passive internal and external rotation of the femur with respect to the tibia during flexion and extension. It provides for relative relaxation of the collateral ligaments in flexion, which is necessary for such passive rotation to occur, and favors relaxation and greater femoral rollback in the lateral compartment, thereby directing a more normal internal rotation of the tibia during flexion, and external rotation with extension. In addition, the intercondylar "edges" of the femoral component are shaped at the notch's most proximal anterior aspect, as well as at its distal most posterior aspect, to articulate against the medial and the lateral borders of the tibial spine aspect of the tibial component and to further facilitate passive external rotation with extension and internal rotation with flexion.

A somewhat detailed description of this design aspect is made not as a "pitch" for its superiority, but to foster understanding of what might otherwise be very subtle differences among systems. A "two-ligament" more "classical" total condylar knee design very specifically seeks to create flexion and extension spaces with essentially equal ligamentous tension. This tension provides good anterior-posterior stability from the interaction of femoral component curvature, i.e. tibial component dishing, especially in flexion. Such collateral ligament features and tibial femoral conformity can be seen quite obviously to be inconsistent with the development of significant passive internal/external rotation during ordinary flexion and extension. Whether such constraint represents a significant factor in the development of the component loosening has not been demonstrated. However, the understanding of this issue is important if the nature of the differences among prostheses are to be understood.

Tibial Component

The combined polyethylene articular surface and metal baseplate of the tibial component were supplied routinely as a unit. With experience, we developed the ability to exchange plastic "inserts", but this was not an original part of the design considerations. The component is available in four different area sizes and overall thicknesses of 7, 9, 11, 13, and 16 mm routinely. The intercondylar eminence of the component is present not only to provide general medial-lateral stability, but is also shaped at its anterior-posterior aspects to permit the automatic screwhome rotation with respect to the femoral component. The tibial component of this system was possibly the first in the field to distinguish medial and lateral plateaus, hence to be supplied in specific right and left forms.

In particular, the lateral plateau was formed with a longer "flat" portion in comparison with the medial aspect. The component was therefore less constrained in the lateral compartment to model the arrangement present in the normal knee and to provide the normal screwhome rotation features.

For "uncemented" use, only one of the two available forms of the tibial component was viewed by the designers as appropriate. This was the component designated as the "resurfacing" form. It is characterized by slanted medial and lateral porous coated pegs and an anterior hole which receives a fixation screw. The second, central stemmed component, was intended only for implantation with methylmethacrylate. It was not viewed as sufficiently stable, in the presence of asymmetrical component loading and normal femoral rollback, to be used in the uncemented mode.

A similar point is that the resurfacing component, which was intended for optional use without cement, was only intended to be so used in combination with the anterior fixation screw. These points are emphasized strongly because we have seen over the years many examples of lack of adherence to these directions – occasionally with the undesirable result of early loosening.

The existence, even regularity, of asymmetric loading due to normal femoral component rollback, was anticipated, and the anterior fixation screw was used to prevent anterior lift off with posterior loading. The posterior slant to the fixation pegs was included to decrease posterior lift up with relative anterior loading and with asymmetric medial lateral loading. In addition, the posterior direction to these pegs facilitates component placement as it is not necessary to have total anterior displacement of the tibia or an excessively large flexion space to get the component in and properly seated.

The tibial component has a centrally located posterior cutout for preservation of the posterior cruciate ligament. While the overall prosthesis was viewed as a posterior cruciate ligament sparing implant, we initially judged that it would in many, if not most, cases be sufficiently stable in the absence of a posterior cruciate ligament. Relative to the total condylar prosthesis, which seemed to be the most widely used at the time, the specific anteriorposterior dimension of the PCA tibial component and the existence of reasonably deep anterior and posterior slopes suggested this would be safe.

Patellar Components

The series of patients presented all had "anatomic" styled PCA patellas. These implants, placed on a flat prepared bed of patellar bone, had a central ridge, a larger lateral facet, a smaller medial facet, and a quite small medial edge "odd" facet. Two porous coated pegs, medially and laterally positioned, were provided for rotational and translational fixation stability.

Early in the clinical experience with this implant, the length of the fixation pegs was

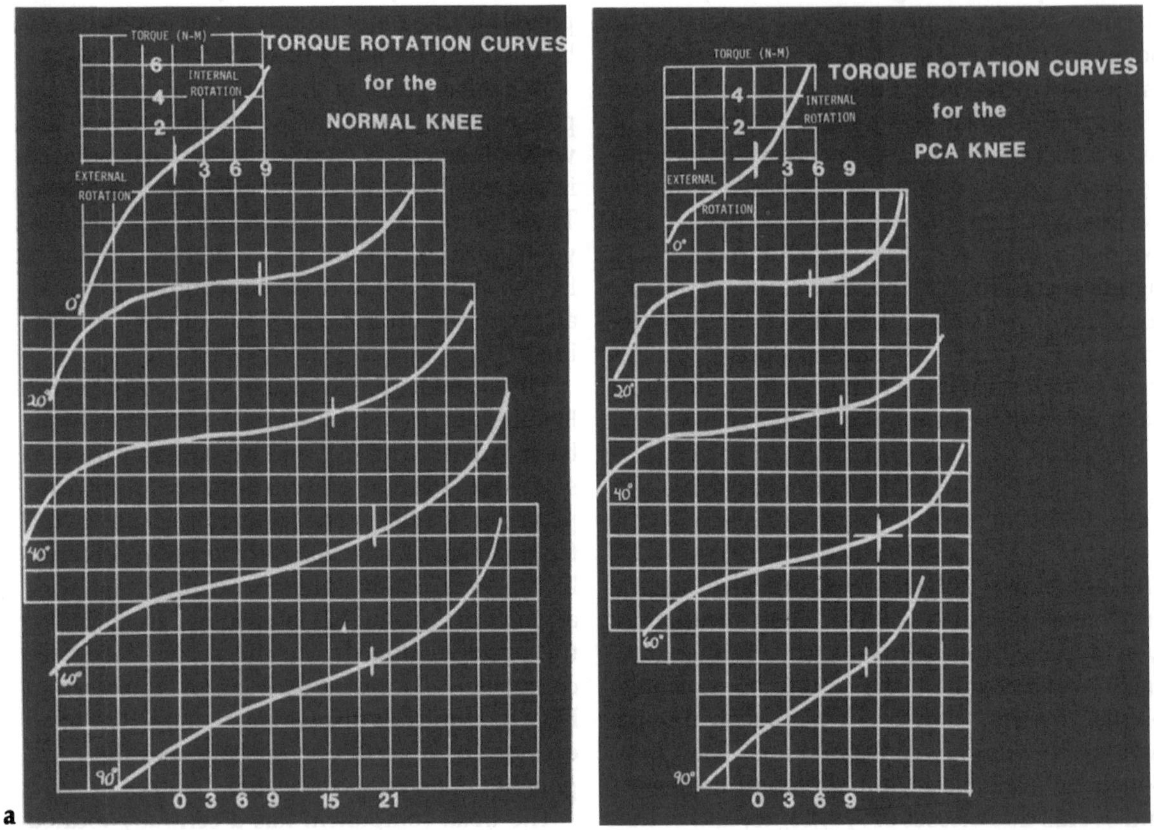

a b

Fig. 11.1. a Torque rotation curves for normal knee – anatomic specimen. Each curve is a sampling or study at the specified flexion angle 0°, 20°, 40°, 60° and/or 90°. The vertical mark on each sigmoid curve represents the starting or resting position which is assumed as the knee is flexed or held at that degree of flexion by quadriceps tension. The more "horizontal" form of the curve for 40° compared to 0° indicates greater freedom of internal and external rotation. The vertical mark at approximately 16° of internal rotation for the 40° curve indicates the passive internal rotation of the tibia equal to 16° when the joint is flexed 40°. **b** Torque rotation curves for a PCA prosthesis implanted in a cadaver knee and studied in similar fashion to the normal situation of **a**. Note the generally similar form of the curves.

increased to provide better initial fixation stability. This move was in response to a small but nonetheless concerning number of component dissociations in the early postoperative course.

The "anatomic" form of this patellar component was seen to embody specific design features. Its patellofemoral contact was seen as more extensive then that of typical single point touching with the classical dome design. Furthermore, the minimal convexity and more uniform thickness evident in sagittal section were seen to provide a joint reaction force which was more nearly normal or perpendicular to the bone–prosthesis interface.

In summary, regarding the design features of these femoral, tibial, and patellar components, care was taken to provide adequate initial fixation and very nearly anatomic surfaces with an adherence to the notion that replacing normal anatomy would lead to re-creation of normal kinematics. It has been felt that these goals were achieved as evidenced by the graphs displayed in Fig. 11.1 a,b. These torque rotation curves depict a passive or automatic internal and external rotation which occur with flexion and extension. They also show at the individual lines the relative freedom for elective internal and external rotation which is possible at points in the 0–90° range of flexion. The obvious similarity in plots for the normal and prosthetic knee is clearly distinguished from what results with the study of other condylar knees. They differ principally in displaying greater constraint to rotation, as well as a total or nearly total absence of passive/automatic rotation.

Instrumentation

The Universal Total Knee Instrumentation System used for implantation of the original PCA knee was undoubtedly one of the most attractive developments in the system and was eagerly and widely accepted. The instruments sought to eliminate in three basic ways much of the "eyeball", "Kentucky-windage" aspect of total knee arthroplasty previously present:

1. Use of relatively long and very specific alignment instrumentation.
2. Attention to specific femoral component placement position with a measured resection technique.
3. Introduction of cutting block instrumentation sufficiently accurate routinely to create close interfacial apposition at the femoral component and allow placement of that component without cement.

Two aspects of this instrumentation were fundamentally new. They are: (1) the introduction of what is here designated as "anatomic" axial alignment in comparison to "classical" arthroplasty alignment and (2) the above mentioned issue of femoral component positioning by "measured resection".

Classical arthroplasty alignment, due mostly to M.A.R. Freeman and J.N. Insall, is an arrangement in which the prosthetic joint line is reconstructed to be perpendicular to the re-created mechanical axis (the line from the center of the femoral head through the knee and to the center of the ankle). Normal or "average" anatomic situations differ slightly from classical alignment as regards rotation of the joint line. In the "anatomic" case the joint line is rotated 2–3° such that the lateral compartment positions closer to the femoral shaft axis while the medial is closer to the tibial shaft axis by 2–3°. While in classical arthroplasty alignment the joint line can be described as being at 0° or perpendicular with respect to the tibia, in the anatomic situation, it is in 2–3° of varus sloping "down" on the medial side. At the same time, the femoral joint line in classical arthroplasty is perpendicular to the femoral portion of the mechanical axis and forms approximately a 6° valgus angle relative to the femoral shaft. In "anatomic" alignment, the femoral joint line is at typically 9° valgus. In either case, the resulting tibiofemoral angle is approximately 6° valgus. However, the specific joint line orientation with respect to the shafts is different by the 2–3° factor. In two-legged stance, this anatomic joint line tends to parallel the ground when the subject's feet are held close together, and during the weight-bearing phases of gait it may be viewed as more level during the times that anatomic internal and external rotation are occurring.

Our purpose in this description is to characterize the differences which exist between what is described here as "anatomic" alignment as it contrasts with "classical arthroplasty" alignment. It is not the intention to argue the merits of this arrangement. However, this concept of anatomic alignment at arthroplasty, while not universally accepted over the past eight to nine years, has been employed by a large number of orthopaedic surgeons.

The second fundamental and new aspect of the Universal Total Knee Instrumentation System is the method of femoral component positioning by "measured resection". It is, in all total knee arthroplasty cases, necessary for one to position properly the femoral component in an anteriorposterior and cephalad-caudad or proximal-distal sense. Such positioning will most obviously impact upon the relative ligament tension across the joint in flexion versus extension. A femoral component which is positioned more distally tends to produce relative tightness in extension; one that is excessively proximal or cephalad leads to relative laxity in extension. As an isolated maneuver, anterior positioning of a given femoral component tends to increase posterior space (flexion space) and lead to relative laxity in flexion, while abnormal posterior positioning of the component tends to lead to relative tightness in flexion.

The more typical approach to addressing the issue of flexion/extension ligament balance was, prior to the introduction of the Universal Total Knee Instrumentation System, what may be referred to as a flexion/extension gap balancing technique. A minimum thickness tibial cut was made; a seemingly appropriate posterior femoral condylar resection was made; and these together created a flexion space when the knee was held at 90° with the tibia distracted downward. The tibia was then brought to 0° full extension with respect to the femur and was held taut, that is pulled in a caudad direction. Sufficient distal femoral bone was then removed so that the resulting extension space would be the same size as the previous flexion space. One therefore had theoretically equal ligament and soft tissue balance in flexion (at least at 90° flexion) and at full extension.

The measured resection technique of the Universal Total Knee Instrumentation System directs the surgeon to remove specific amounts of distal femoral and posterior femoral bone and then to replace those resected surfaces with a prosthetic component of appropriate, corresponding size. The rationale behind this approach is that such specific resection and replacement will result in reconstitution of the prosthetic joint surface with the ligament origins on the femur and, in the majority of cases, address problems of proper femoral component position, as it relates to flexion/extension ligament balance in just this way. It is the relative relationship of the femoral joint surface to ligament origins which affects the length, separation, and behavior of the ligaments as the knee ranges through flexion/extension because the instant centers and/or axes of rotation lie at or close to the ligament origins.

The measured resection and flexion/extension gap balancing techniques may lead to similar component positioning in many cases and different results in others – particularly those with moderate to severe flexion contracture. Again, it is the concepts and issues of difference which are important in this presentation, not the relative merits of one versus the other technique.

Surgical Technique

The surgical exposure and techniques utilized in the patient series reported here are relatively standard and can be found in a variety of more detailed sources. Relatively straight, very slightly medially positioned parapatellar skin incisions were used in combination with a very standard median parapatellar capsular incision. The patella was everted and retracted laterally. The anteromedial and anterolateral tibial regions were cleaned subperiosteally. Moderate to partial patellar fat pad resection was routinely performed by one of the surgeon authors and total sparing of the fat pad was done by the other.

Most varus and valgus deformities were corrected by release of "tight" soft tissue on the concave side of the deformity – this was from the medial tibia in varus cases and the lateral femur in valgus cases. It is the practice on our service to tighten ligaments on the originally convex side of the deformity in those cases where adequate release of the concave side tissues is viewed or found to be impractical and/or impossible.

Postoperatively patients were managed in CPM (continuous passive motion) or without CPM, according to circumstances of equipment availability, whether the patients possessed flexion contractures, and whether their extremities would appropriately fit into CPM apparatuses. CPM was just being introduced during the time of this patient group. No specific attempts to analyze our ultimate range of motion results regarding CPM versus no CPM are made.

Patient Selection

The cases reported here, being the very first of our cementless series, show mixed selection features. They were, in all cases, viewed as suitable candidates for total knee arthroplasty due to joint surface wear felt not satisfactorily manageable with proximal tibial osteotomy, distal femoral osteotomy, or unicompartmental arthroplasty. A detailed description of the fine points of patient selection on this group is beyond the scope of this presentation. Suffice it to say that all of these alternative procedures are performed by our service and were considered for any appropriate candidate.

The most basic requirement of implantation of uncemented components was apparent mechanical stability of the elements at the time of implantation. If such stability could not be achieved because of severe, profound osteoporosis, unmanageable bone defects, or other unmanageable aspects of bone quality, then cemented arthroplasties were performed. We could not document any case in this time period in which cement was used when it otherwise would not have been because of inaccuracy of bone cuts and a general inability to achieve stability in that type of situation.

The basic feature for selection of the uncemented options were, in addition to issues of bone quality and stability, the factors of age and activity. However, there was not strict adherence to this as a consideration. The average age for this group of patients may seem a few years lower than some groups of total knee arthroplasties and is approximately 3–4 years younger than a parallel cemented group on our service done at the same time. However, as one notes, the oldest entry who was 81 years of age at the time of surgery shows that strict allotment of the uncemented technique to "younger" patients was not adhered to.

Clinical Results and Case Material

This section reports our experience with the first 50 cementless PCA total knee units implanted in our center from the time 6 May 1980 to 27 April 1982. As an overview, the surgical authors (KAK, DSH) have performed in excess of 1225 PCA total knee arthroplasties from January 1980 to May 1989. Seven hundred and seventy-seven of these were performed as cementless cases. Seventy-two total knees were placed in 63 patients (nine bilaterals) between 29 April 1980 and 27 April 1982 of whom 17 patients with 22 prostheses are currently deceased. We, therefore, present below 50 knees in the 46 surviving patients.

The mean age of these patients is 59 years (range 20–81). Thirty-four were cases of osteoarthrosis, 13 rheumatoid arthritis, and 3 avascular necrosis. Average length of follow-up is 74 months, ranging from 9 months to 8 years 11 months. The patient with 9 months' follow-up was fused at 10 months post-operation, as will be discussed below. There was one other patient revised at 10 months; otherwise, all other patients have greater than or equal to 5-year follow-up with a distribution of follow-up as follows: 14 at 5–6 years, 16 at 6–7 years, 12 at 7–8 years, and 6 at over 8 years.

All patients have been followed with data management according to a specifically planned protocol consisting of a 100 point functional score, tabulation of range of motion, pain level, ligamentous stability, overall alignment, muscular strength, walking aids, walking distances, location and amount of lucent lines at the interfaces.

The 100 point functional score has been published and described previously. It assigns 50 points for pain, 20 points for range of motion, and 10 points each for deformity, ligamentous stability, and quadriceps strength. Its scores are independent of overall general activities which might be compromised by conditions of generally poor health or problems with other aspects of the neuromuscular locomotion system. Patients scoring 90–100 are declared or classified as excellent, 80–89 good, 70–79 fair, and below 70 poor.

Pre-operative scores averaged 45 points with a range of 0–70. The postoperative score improved an average of 43 points to 88 with a range of 0–100. Pre-operative range of motion averaged 7–97° (arc = 91°). (Range: 0–130°, 35–40°; arc range: 30–130°.) Postoperative was 1–104° (arc = 103°). (Range: 0–140°, 30–60°; arc range: 55–140°.)

Using our original external alignment system, the mean tibia femoral angle at 1–2 year follow-up was 3.5° valgus (± 2.9°) and the average tibia femoral angle at mean follow-up of 6 years was 3.75° valgus (±3.12°). While frequency and extent of interface lucencies were recorded, tabulation is less revealing than examination of represented postoperative X-rays, as offered below. Excluding the two patients described below who required revision fusion, the remaining 48 knees demonstrated a 94% good and excellent result, 4% of fair, and 2% poor outcomes.

Re-operations for specific component loosening involved only one tibia, no femurs, but three patellar components. The one patient with a total three component revision was operated upon elsewhere solely for pain without evidence of gross loosening and has not had significant improvement after placement of a cemented total condylar type of implant. Two additional patellar components were changed in re-operations for patellar subluxation problems. The one patient who was re-operated upon receiving a knee fusion had a long history of unsatisfactory knee procedures and was fused for persistent pain which was basically unexplainable.

There was only one case of recognized and treated deep venous thrombosis, no cases of deep infection, and one patient treated with oral antibiotics for temporary wound drainage.

X-rays and Figs. 11.2 – 11.5 have been chosen to demonstrate particular relevant points. Fig. 11.2a and b shows the one patient with complete three component revision for pain without clear

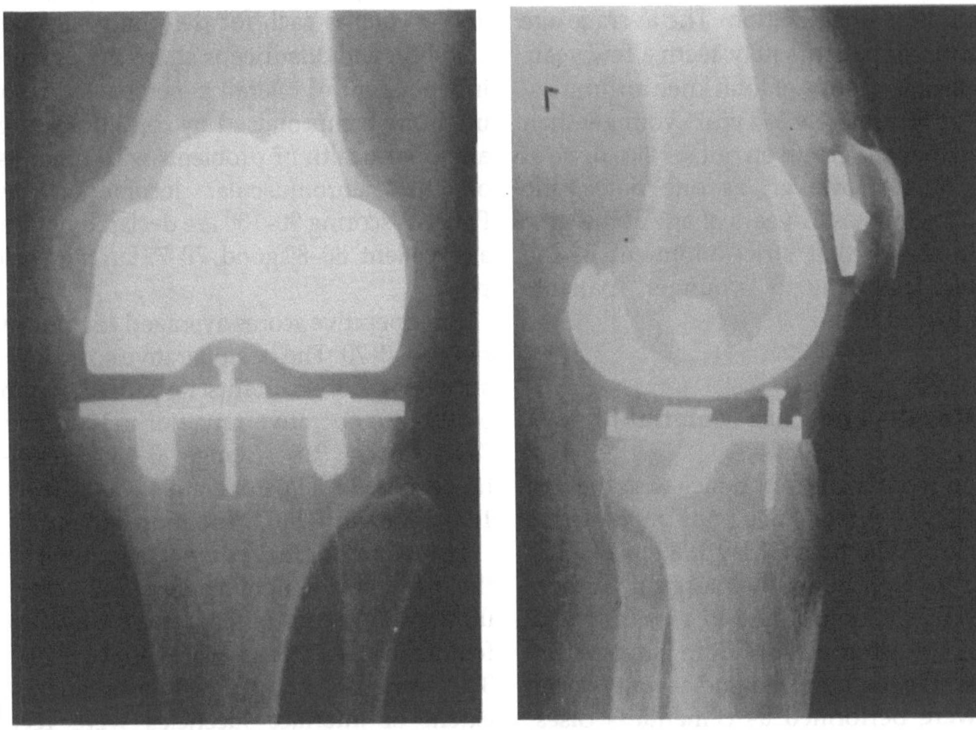

a b

Fig. 11.2 a,b. AP and lateral postoperative radiographs of the one patient with a persistent pain who was revised elsewhere to a Total Condylar type of prosthesis. No radiographic problems are evident, and the patient's clinical course was not improved with the cemented Total Condylar prosthesis.

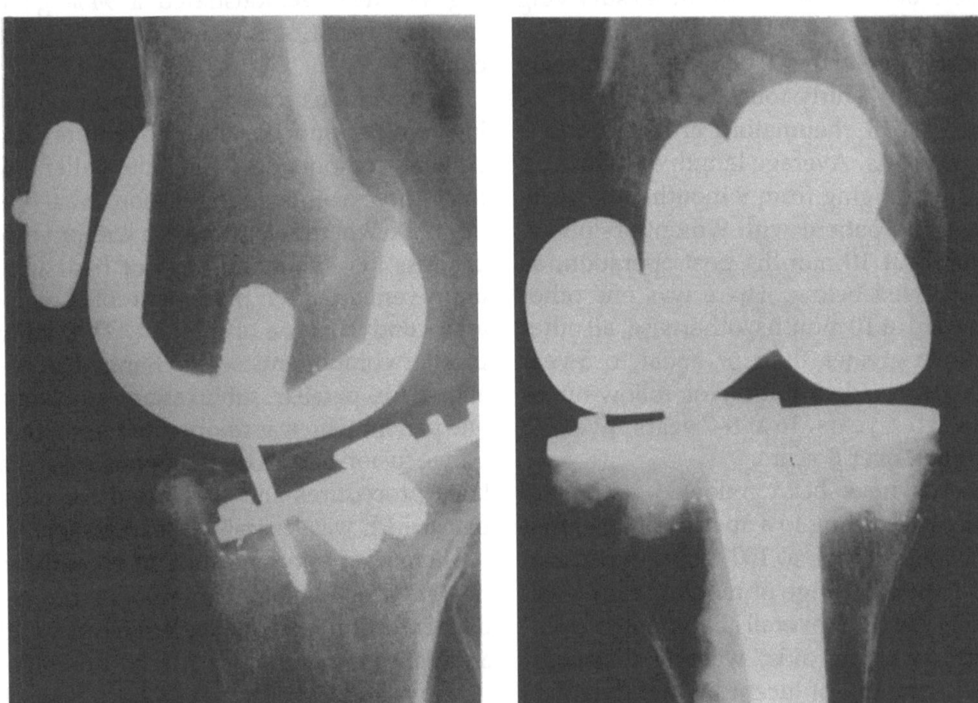

a b

Fig. 11.3. a Five year follow-up lateral X-ray showing tibial component subsidence and loosening. Suboptimal fit to the anterior cortex was a possible cause in this rheumatoid patient. b AP postoperative revision X-ray.

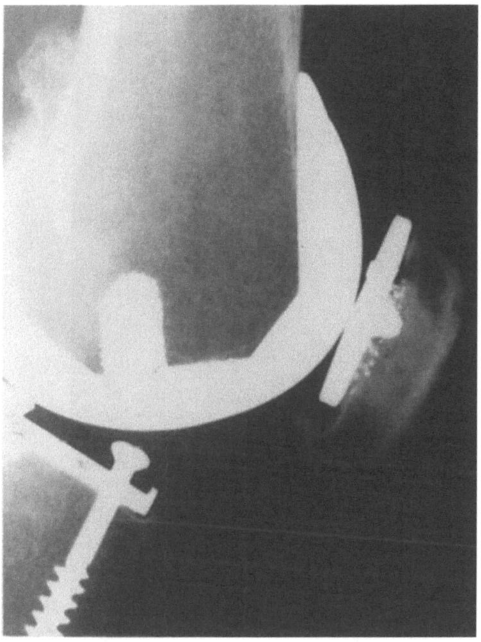

Fig. 11.4. Lateral view of a loosened patellar component.

loosening. Fig. 11.3 shows X-rays for the one patient with tibial component loosening. An example is also shown of a loosened patellar component (Fig. 11.4). Fig. 11.5a and b shows a fairly typical postoperative X-ray with essentially no lucent lines visible even on fluoroscopically positioned views. When lucent lines are present, their appearance is typified by specific areas in Fig.11.5b and c.

Discussion

The patient group presented is a small subset of our total experience but represents a more significant group in consideration of the intermediate to long term follow-up which we do have. Furthermore, follow-up on the surviving patients, excluding the three component revision done elsewhere and the fusion case, which are now out of the series, has been total.

This group, as regards issues of component loosening, demonstrates early problems with maintenance of patellar fixation. Some of this has been addressed with design changes of longer fixation pegs and, later, an increased number of pegs. Whether these changes will prove to be totally adequate and productive of results comparable to those with cemented patellar buttons remains to be seen. Candidly, one of the operating authors (KAK) has, for the time being, elected to use all polyethylene non-metal-backed patellar components secured with methylmethacrylate cement. This move was first made because of concerns over polyethylene wear and patellar base plate damage to the femoral surface – a problem not seen in our series or very frequently with this particular system. However, this has been seen to a significant degree in other systems and is bound to occur in all. An additional concern has been a small but occasional instance of uncemented patellar component loosening despite the design changes noted.

That only one tibial component has been revised in this group, for loosening, is encouraging, especially as the tibial component is the one for which intermediate and long term fixation is so problematic. The originally hoped for occurrence of complete bony ingrowth, however, is probably not as frequent as some of us may have wished. It is encouraging, however, that these interfaces appear stable. Also, histologic sections from well functioning interfaces from other series have shown a highly organized soft tissue attachment at fibrous regions different from that seen in cemented cases and at soft tissues adjacent to smooth metal implants.

Conclusion

This chapter has presented features of the prosthesis and instrumentation rationale for the PCA total knee system. This system has been an undisputed forerunner regarding useful improvements in sophisticated instrumentation and also developments in the application of biologic fixation of porous coating of total knee components.

While the cases reported here demonstrate that consistent perfection has not been achieved, our results both functionally and radiographically are indeed consistent with the high quality of total knee outcomes being observed fairly routinely over the past 5–7 years. That such can be said about this very first group of patients

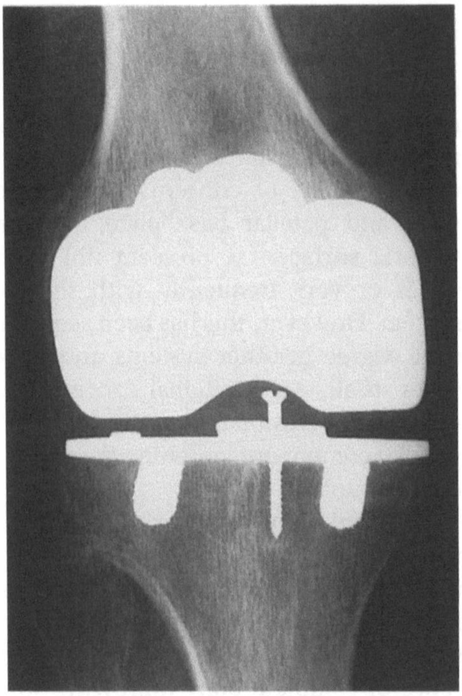
a

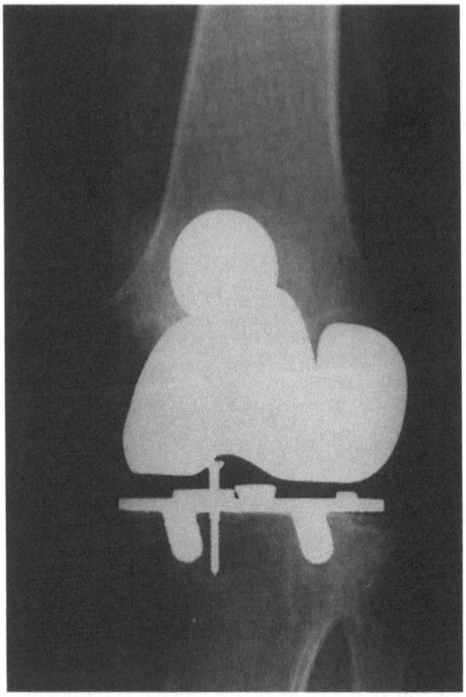
c

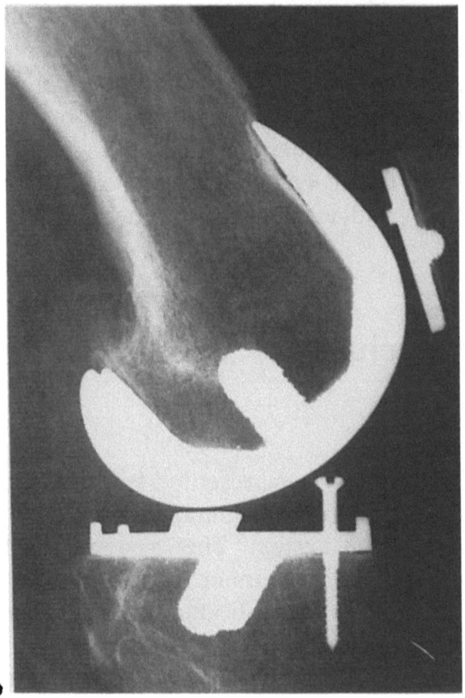
b

Fig. 11.5. a Well positioned AP X-ray showing no lucencies at the tibia. **b** Well positioned lateral X-ray shows no significant lucency at the femur or tibia. However, the anteriormost area at the tibial base plate, anterior to the screw has a small lucency as well as the one at the cephalad aspect of the anterior flange. These are both areas of metal surface without porous coating. The cephalad one-third of the posterior femoral surface may be described as having a small lucent line. **c** A small lucent line is seen at the lateral aspect of the tibial base plate – lateral to the peg.

with a new and technically challenging technique used during the developers' early experience is particularly encouraging.

Uncemented total knee arthroplasty is, as hinted, a technically challenging, patient selection sensitive procedure, which finds continued acceptance around the world and is most likely here to stay in one form or another for selected patients until something more promising is introduced.

Section IV

Problem Areas in Total Knee Replacement

Chapter 12

The Painful Total Knee Replacement

Thomas P. Sculco

Introduction

The goal of the surgeon performing a total knee arthroplasty is to effect a painless, functional knee joint which is freely movable and allows comfortable ambulation. The orthopaedic literature is replete with reports of successful long term results in total knee arthroplasty in 85%–90% of patients (Aglietti and Buzzi 1988; Bourne et al. 1988; Donaldson et al. 1988; Ecker et al. 1987; Goldberg et al. 1988; Insall et al. 1982; Scott et al. 1988). Improvements in operative technique, instrumentation and prosthetic design have led to a more reproducible end result after total knee arthroplasty. Even so, patients with painful total knee replacements continue to occur and they present diagnostic and treatment challenges to the operating surgeon. The cause of knee dysfunction may be obvious and amenable to treatment. At other times its etiology may be more clandestine and exhaust evaluative tools without a firm explanation or treatment plan being obtained. This chapter will discuss some of the causes of the painful knee replacement and present an algorithmic approach to the painful knee replacement. An attempt will be made to provide a problem-solving flow sheet to the operating surgeon which demonstrates pathways leading to the diagnosis of the pain after the knee replacement.

Causes of Pain in Total Knee Arthroplasty

The general symptom of knee pain after a total knee replacement should alert the surgeon to a variety of possible etiologies. As a rule, these etiologies can be placed in several categories. These general categories include infection, mechanical failure, patellofemoral dysfunction, soft tissue problems and, pain from sources distant to the knee.

Infection

Deep periprosthetic infection must be suspected foremost in any knee that is painful after a total knee arthroplasty. Since its presentation may be quite indolent, it behooves the surgeon to pursue all avenues of diagnosis. Therefore, although it is reassuring to have a sedimentation rate and white blood cell count which are normal, it must be remembered that this is not inconsistent with a deep infection. In any postoperative painful knee, unless an obvious cause of pain is apparent (e.g. fracture) aspiration must be performed as part of the diagnostic process. Indeed, multiple negative aspirations may be necessary before one can definitely remove infection as a primary cause of pain. If suspicion still lingers, a synovial biopsy may be recommended.

Plain radiographs of the infected knee may demonstrate progressive radiolucency at the bone–cement interface, but this is not diagnostic. Gallium and indium scanning may help corroborate a clinical impression, but recovery of the infecting organism is the most definitive method of diagnosis.

Mechanical Failure (Loosening)

Once infection has been safely eliminated as the source of pain, mechanical causes of pain may be suspected. When the term mechanical is used, a myriad of painful failure modes may be defined. Additionally, most of the causes of a mechanical failure are secondary to technical factors at the time of the initial procedure. Although the end result is loosening of the implant, the cause of this failure of fixation is almost always the result of a technical error. The most common technical problems leading to pain and mechanical failure after total knee arthroplasty are malalignment of the implant, knee joint instability, suboptimal cement technique and patellofemoral instability. It is important to consider that these technical imperfections are avoidable. The need for careful pre-operative planning and attention to the primary concepts of surgical detail will often completely eliminate these potential mechanical problems.

Malalignment

A common cause of implant failure is insertion of the prosthetic components without restoration of the mechanical axis of weightbearing. This, along with implanting the components on a sloped surface will result in asymmetrical loading across the joint surface and promote loosening. Tension forces are significant on the less loaded side of the implant and will produce lift-off of the prosthesis. On the more severely loaded side compression forces will be excessive and may lead to collapse of bone and settling of the component. Radiographic evaluation of the knee will demonstrate this failure mode if the knee had not been implanted in the correct alignment.

Instability

Postoperative knee joint instability after joint replacement results from a failure to balance the ligaments at the time of surgery. This instability is compounded if the bone cuts are placed incorrectly. Such instability can be determined by stressing the knee into varus and valgus as well as evaluating weight-bearing radiographs of the knee. The instability causes tension in the collateral tissues on the concave side of the deformity and this is often painful. Pain can often occur in those cases in which the instability is so severe that the implants sublux from each other. In some patients, anteroposterior instability is present in flexion. This may be due to excessive tibial or posterior femoral condylar bone resection. Patients with this type of instability often complain of locking of the knee in flexion with severe posterior and anterior pain. Finally there are some patients in whom implants of insufficient thickness have been inserted. This leads to a recurvatum deformity when the patient bears weight and posterior popliteal pain.

Suboptimal Cement Technique

In addition to mechanical failure from technical errors producing malalignment and instability, poor cement technique can lead to deficiency in implant fixation and pain. The elements of proper cement technique include proper preparation of the bone, pressurization of the cement into the trabecular bone, and the avoidance of large columns of unsupported methylmethacrylate. The underlying bone must be well lavaged to remove debris and to allow penetration of cement into the bony interstices. Sclerotic bone must be drilled or fenestrated in some fashion to allow subchondral intrusion of cement. Methylmethyacrylate should not be used to fill defects greater than 5 mm in depth. Radiographic evidence of progressing radiolucency in a painful knee, often accompanied with evidence of implant shift, may indicate impending implant failure. Malalignment or instability may accentuate the problem as well.

Patellofemoral Dysfunction

Most investigators report that problems related to the patellofemoral joint are the major long term causes of pain after total knee arthroplasty (Scott et al. 1988; Aglietti and Buzzi 1988). There are several etiologies of patellofemoral pain and all must be considered in the evaluation of the painful total knee patient. These etiologies include patellofemoral subluxation or dislocation, patellar fracture, and peripatellar fibrosis.

Tracking problems can be identified easily on physical examination. The patient will usually complain of pain when arising from a seated position and while walking stairs. In cases of severe patellar instability the patient will walk with a stiff knee and will often be unable to extend the knee from the fully flexed position until the patella is manually replaced in the trochlear groove. Hozack et al. (1989) has coined the term "patellar clunk syndrome" for patients with anterior knee pain after total knee arthroplasty in whom crepitus is quite marked and pain occurs as there is a sudden shift in patellar position as it descends into the femoral groove during knee flexion.

Fractures of the patella appear to be diminishing in incidence, probably related to better surgical technique. Excessive resection of the patella and use of an oversized patellar implant may cause this problem. The source of the pain is easily identified by lateral and patellar radiographs.

Severe anterior knee pain can occur in those cases where the posterior cruciate ligament has been left excessively tight. It may also occur in cases where the posterior femoral rollback is excessive. Proper ligament balancing and filling of the flexion and extension spaces should obviate these problems.

Knee pain after total joint replacement may be due to inflammatory problems in the soft tissue about the joint. These inflammatory processes include tendonitis and bursitis. Pes anserine bursitis may also occur and produce disabling medial knee pain in some patients. Infrapatellar tendonitis is also seen in patients and can cause localized severe pain. These diagnoses are easily made on physical examination.

More diffuse knee pain can be encountered in patients in whom there is a limited postoperative range of motion. The knee can remain quite swollen and stiff. These patients can develop a clinical picture similar to reflex sympathetic dystrophy.

Soft tissue impingement along the surface of the prosthesis may produce pain (Hirsch 1989). This may occur in the area of the hamstring tendons and lead to popliteal pain. Retained fragments of meniscus and in some cases the popliteus tendon itself may prolapse into the articulating surface of the joint and become painful. The diagnosis may be difficult to confirm without arthroscopy.

Distant Sources of Pain

There exists a subset of patients who develop pain after total knee replacement and in whom no source of this pain can be identified. The diagnostic parameters described above may be followed without leading to a causative agent. These patients are among the most difficult and challenging in a surgeon's practice. There are a series of possible etiologies which must be considered in patients in whom no reasonable cause for pain can be discerned.

Arthritis arising in other areas with referred pain to the knee should be considered first. One of the more common causes of knee pain arising from a distant site is arthritic involvement in the spine with radicular symptoms from a degenerative disc or from spinal stenosis. Although pain from these etiologies tends to be more posterior they can cause anterior knee pain as well. A careful history, physical examination, and radiographic evaluation, often associated with CAT and MRI scans can help identify this source of pain. An epidural injection of corticosteroids may prove helpful in differentiating if the knee pain is spinal in origin.

In addition to spinal disease, knee pain may occur in patients with hip disease. The surgeon should do a careful hip examination and if necessary obtain radiographs of the hip if there is a suspicion that the hip joint is playing a role in the patient's pain. If after these evaluations there is still doubt, an intraarticular injection of a local anesthetic may be administered into the hip joint to see if this will alleviate the knee pain.

Knee pain can occur from a reflex sympathetic dystrophy. Normally these patients have a brawny swelling about the knee and a shiny atrophic appearance to the remaining soft tissues of the leg. These patients have pain both at rest and at night, and X-rays which demonstrate periprosthetic osteopenia. Sympathetic block has been helpful in some of these patients but no clear explanation exists as to the underlying nature of the dystrophy. Physical therapy, anti-inflammatory drugs and non-narcotic analgesics can be used. Antidepressants have been tried as well in those patients who are chronically disabled.

Claudication symptoms from arterial insufficiency may lead to limb pain extending from the knee to the calf. This pain can usually be identified by the nature of the symptoms, the diminution or absence of peripheral pulses, and the salutary response from vascular treatment.

After all of these disease processes are excluded there remain some patients with pain that may be psychological in origin. It may be related to an ongoing disability claim, or some other material or emotional secondary gain that is being achieved by the persistence of pain in the operated knee. Unfortunately a poor surgical result is often attributed to this cause rather than to the true technical or mechanical reason for failure.

References

Agliette P, Buzzi R (1988) Posteriorly stabilized total condylar knee replacement. J Bone Joint Surg (Br) 70: 211–216
Bourne M, Rand J, Ilstrup D (1988) Posterior cruciate condylar total knee arthroplasty. Clin Orthop 234: 129–136
Donaldson W, Sculco T, Insall J, Ranawat C (1988) Total condylar III knee prosthesis. Clin Orthop 226: 21–28
Ecker M, Lotke P, Windsor R, Cella J (1987) Long term results after total condylar knee arthroplasty. Clin Orthop 216: 151–158
Goldberg V, Figgie M, Figgie H, Heiple K, Sobel M (1988) Use of a total condylar knee prosthesis for the treatment of osteoarthritis and rheumatoid arthritis. J Bone Joint Surg (Am) 70: 802–811
Hirsch D (1989) Pain after total knee arthroplasty caused by soft tissue impingement. J Bone Joint Surg (Br) 71: 591–592
Hozack W, Rothman R, Booth R, Balderson R (1989) The patellar clunk syndrome. Clin Orthop 241: 203–208
Insall J, Lachiewicz P, Burstein A (1982) The posterior stabilized condylar prosthesis. A modification of the total condylar design. J Bone Joint Surg (Am) 64: 1317–1324
Scott W, Rubinstein M, Scuderi G (1988) Results after knee replacement with a posterior cruciate substituting prosthesis. J Bone Joint Surg (Am) 70: 1163–1173

Chapter 13

The Patella in Total Knee Arthroplasty

Hugh U. Cameron

Introduction

The patella has always been a problem area in total knee replacement (Aglietti et al. 1988). In the initial designs, the patella was simply ignored (Fig. 13.1). Later, a trochlear flange was added to the femoral component and the patella allowed to articulate with it. Finally, the patella itself was resurfaced, initially with all plastic buttons, and later with metal-backed plastic components. There remain, however, numerous questions about the patella and how it should be managed at the time of total knee replacement. This chapter will address some of those questions. I will describe my experience over the past fifteen years and give my rationale for prevention and treatment of patellar problems. As you will quickly see, there are no "right" and no "wrong" answers but rather many approaches to similar problems.

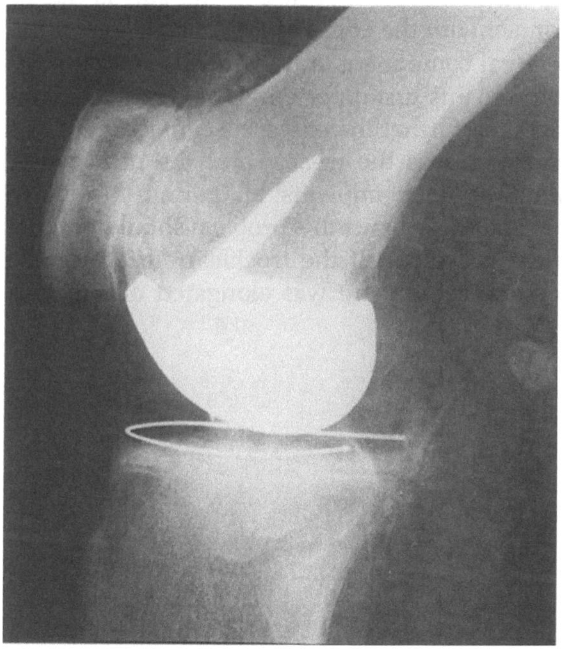

Fig. 13.1 In this early total knee, the patellofemoral joint was simply ignored.

Patellar Problems

Is It Necessary to Resurface the Patella?

Several investigators (Levai et al. 1983; Soudry et al. 1986) have suggested that if the patella is not resurfaced, there will be a high incidence of residual postoperative knee pain. Most of these studies, however, have drawn conclusions using different types of implants some of which have resurfaced the patella and some of which did not.

I have recently completed a study comparing the results of total knee replacement using the Tricon-P prosthesis with and without concomitant patellar resurfacing. The follow-up of these patients has been from 2 to 7 years. Sixty-eight knee replacements were performed with patellar resurfacing and 43 without. Using the Hospital for Special Surgery Rating System, the overall results appeared to be comparable. Fifty-eight per cent of the nonresurfaced knees were rated excellent while another 35% were rated as good. For the resurfaced group the corresponding percentages were 60% and 40%. However, when the data were scrutinized and the individual categories studied, it was found that there was anterior knee pain in 16.2% in the nonresurfaced group and 7.5% in the resurfaced group. Five of the knees in the nonreplaced group required revision for anterior knee pain. Stair climbing ability was similarly affected. For the nonresurfaced group only 21% could lead with the affected leg using no support. For the resurfaced group, 62% could climb stairs in this manner. There were two patellar fractures in the replaced group and none in the nonreplaced group. This study would appear to demonstrate that the benefits for patellar replacement far outweigh the potential complications.

What is the Best Design for a Patellar Component?

The loads across the normal patella are the results of muscular contraction and body weight, and normally are very high. The resurfaced patella has only half the contact area of a normal patella so that these loads are carried by a small area. It has been calculated that the load across the surface of a plastic patellar implant when the knee is flexed 30° are such that the yield strength of the polyethylene is exceeded, and the plastic will undergo cold flow.

In a clinical study of patellar wear patterns noted at the time of revision surgery, we have noted three patterns:

1. No wear was seen in cases where there was no contact between the patella and the femoral component. This occurs in severe patella alta or baja, or in cases of gross infection with a florid synovitis. In addition, low demand situations, such as in reflex sympathetic dystrophy, also demonstrated no wear of the polyethylene.

2. Mild single facet wear was the commonest pattern. The wear was usually centrally located. Occasionally in knees with patellar tilting, mild single facet wear was also seen. Severe single facet wear occurred in cases of frank patellar dislocation as the patella slid over the lateral femoral condyle during flexion (Figs. 13.2 and

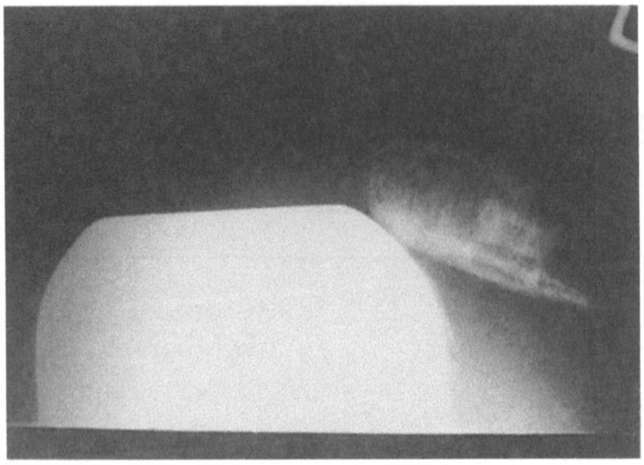

Fig. 13.2 This patella has dislocated and articulates with the lateral edge of the femoral component to produce severe single facet wear.

13.3). In every case of single facet wear the patellar component was surrounded by a dense meniscus of fibrous tissue with just a small area of patella showing through (Cameron and Cameron 1987). This finding was not a cause for concern since the presence of this patellar meniscus increased the congruity of the patella with the trochlea.

3. Double facet wear was seen in those knees which had obtained flexion beyond 100° (Fig. 13.4). At that level of flexion the patella makes contact with the edges of the cruciate gap of the femoral component only, while its central portion remains unsupported. This very small contact area further increases the contact pressures and increases the wear. Since the new generation of knee implants all permit flexion to beyond these limits this problem should become more prevalent. If the trochlear surface of the femoral component was elongated distally this

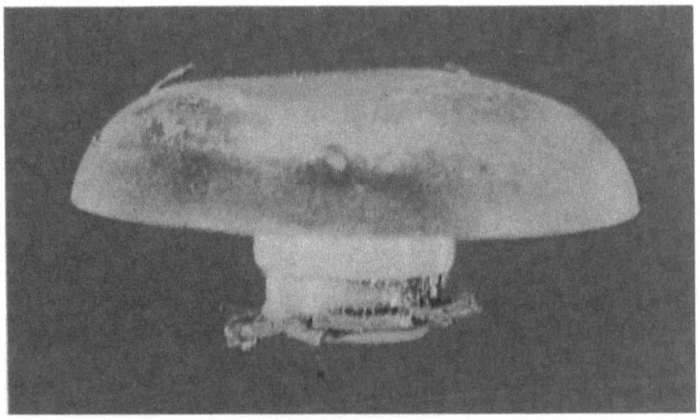

Fig. 13.3 This patella was removed and shows the common mild central single facet wear.

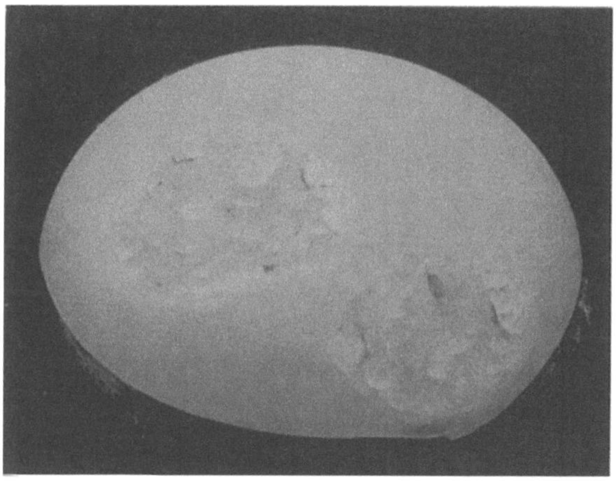

Fig. 13.4 This patella was removed and shows severe double facet wear. This occurred as the patella left the trochlear groove in flexion and articulated with the edges of the femoral condyles in the cruciate gap.

problem might be obviated. To do this however would require a radical redesign of the tibial component eliminating most of the intercondylar eminence. Another solution might be to utilize a high density polyethylene with a significantly higher yield point.

Since all patellae undergo some cold flow the question as to whether or not they should originally have facets may be moot. If allowed to articulate long enough, all patellar implants will develop a shape to match the corresponding femoral trochlear surface. Similarly, redesigning the patella so as to place the surface on a mobile bearing seems to have very little value. Bearing freeze occurs due to the development of the patellar meniscus and in any case, having a mobile bearing does nothing to obviate the problem of wear during flexion.

Should the Patellar Component be Metal-Backed?

Patellar metal-backing was introduced following the poor experience using the original unicompartmental knees (Laskin 1988). It had been noted that if the polyethylene used for tibial bearing surfaces was thinner than 6–8 mm, localized high loads would be transmitted to the cement bed resulting in its fragmentation. Placing a metal backing on the tibial component obviated this problem. These data were then extrapolated to patellar components and metal-backed components were fabricated.

There is a problem, however, when a metal-backed patellar component is onset on the bony patella. Bayley et al. (1988) and Lombardi et al. (1988) have both described metal on metal wear as the polyethylene on a metal-backed patellar component was worn through. The component that they used had a metallic endoskeleton as well as a metal base plate, and as a result, the amount of polyethylene in the implant was very small. This wear through of the polyethylene resulted in scratching of the trochlear groove leading to further patellar destruction and the generation of plastic and metal wear debris. At revision it was not possible to revise only the patella since the trochlear groove was also damaged. Therefore, if the patellar implant is inserted using the onset technique it should not be metal-backed, and especially should not be metal-backed with a metallic endoskeleton.

This problem can be avoided and metal-backed patellae used if the implant is inset rather than onset. A central hole is reamed in the patella exactly matching the shape of the patellar component. When the component is snapped in place, the metal base plate lies below the edges of the surrounding bone (Laskin 1988) (Fig. 13.5 a–c). This technique is beneficial in three ways. First, the shear loads on the patellar component are absorbed by the surrounding walls of the bony patella and not by the fixation pegs or studs. Second, by retaining the original patellar subchondral bone around the rim, the patella is not rendered as flexible as it would be if the entire articular surface was resected. It is just such flexibility which had led to fracture of some of the onset patellar metal base plates. Finally, if polyethylene wear occurs, the metal base plate is "shielded" from exposure to the trochlear surface.

The one drawback of insetting the patella is that the implant cannot cover the entire patellar surface. Some load must be transmitted through the patellar meniscus to the patient's own subchondral bone. This may potentially be a source of pain. In fact, as the Tricon-P study has shown, the incidence of this anterior knee pain is about 7.5%.

A further evaluation of pain in these patients demonstrated a relationship to the size of the implant. Only one size patellar component was

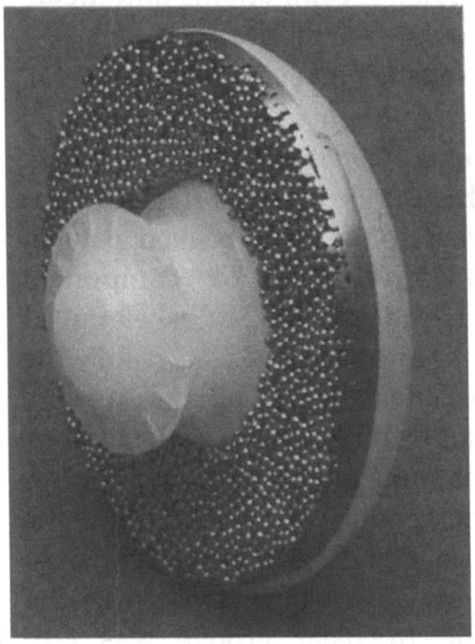

a

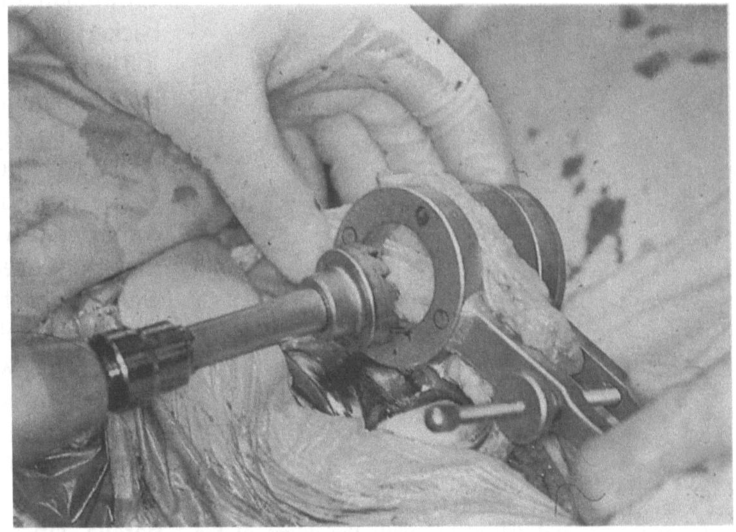

b

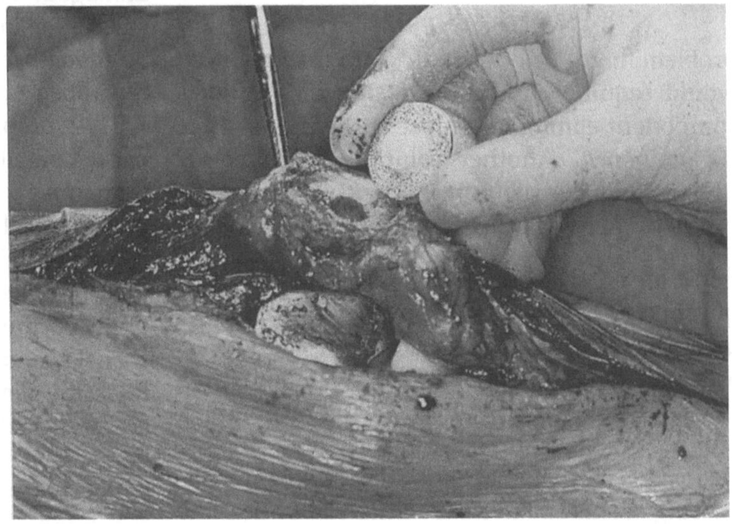

c

Fig. 13.5 a–c. The Tricon-M inset patella. **a** The porous metal surface of this implant will be inserted below the level of the surrounding patellar bone. **b** The patella is grasped with a clamp and a central hole is created to match exactly the shape of the patellar implant. **c** The patellar implant will be press fitted into the recess in the patellar bone.

available and in some patients with very large patellae, a large amount of rim contact occurred. Rim contact also occurred when there was patellar tilting greater than 7.5°. Tilting often occurred when a lateral parapatellar approach was used and the lateral retinaculum was left open at the close of the case (Fig. 13.6).

Two methods have been explored to decrease this residual patellofemoral pain. One was the use of a "winged patella." The same central inset component was used but the plastic surface was drawn out to give large wings, similar to the Charnley acetabular cement restricting cup. After reaming the central hole, the surrounding high spots on the patella were planed down and the component snapped in place. Three sizes were available. Since the patella is asymmetrical, the plastic would overhang in some areas. The overhang was trimmed off to allow concentric coverage of the bone. This solved the problem of rim bone contact and patellar tilting and eliminated patellofemoral pain.

There were, however, two drawbacks with this design. The wing portion of the implant was onset and most likely would wear through in time. The second drawback was that the surgeon was required to customize the implant.

Because of these two problems the technique was modified so as to leave the same central button but to recess the wings into the patella.

Fig. 13.6. The right patella is tilted and this has caused contact with the metal of the femoral component. Even if metal on bone contact occurs, less than 20% are painful.

With three sizes available, this does not give complete coverage, but it increases the coverage to the point where tilt is no longer a problem.

From a theoretical point of view, the patellar components should not increase in thickness as they increase in diameter. An increase in thickness could lead to an increase in retinacular tension (Dorr and Boiardo 1986). Furthermore an increase in thickness would require an increase in quadriceps tension to achieve the same degree of flexion (Wendt and Johnson 1985).

Although there are both cemented and uncement patellae presently available, I have virtually no experience with the cemented types. I see little need for cemented patellae since loosening of the noncemented implants has not be a clinical problem.

The majority of the noncemented patellae are metal-backed with a porous undersurface which may act as a substrate for tissue ingrowth. Mechanical problems related to metal–plastic dissociation and fracture of the base plate have been related to their design and are relatively easy to solve.

There are several press fit plastic patellae available. These are held in place initially by a ridged plastic peg, but the main retaining structure is the tight fit of the implant into a predrilled hole (Fig. 13.7). These patella have done remarkably well with virtually no reports of subsidence or loosening (Fig. 13.8).

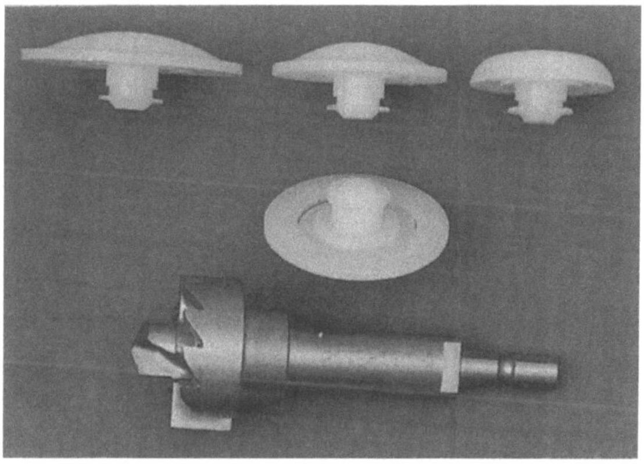

Fig. 13.7. This all plastic patellar implant is press fitted into a pre-drilled hole. The load is then taken on the walls of the implant rather than on the peg.

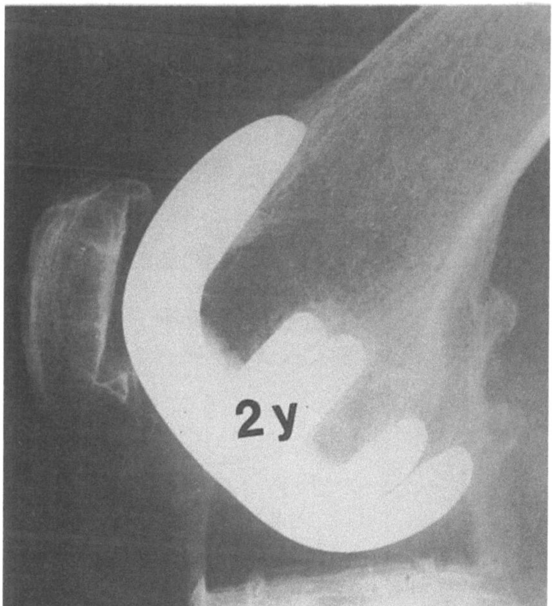

Fig. 13.8. The outlines of the press fit plastic button can clearly be seen. The walls of the button are recessed below the level of the surrounding patellar bone.

What Does One Do if the Patella is Absent?

When a prior patellectomy has been carried out, the results of total knee replacement with a

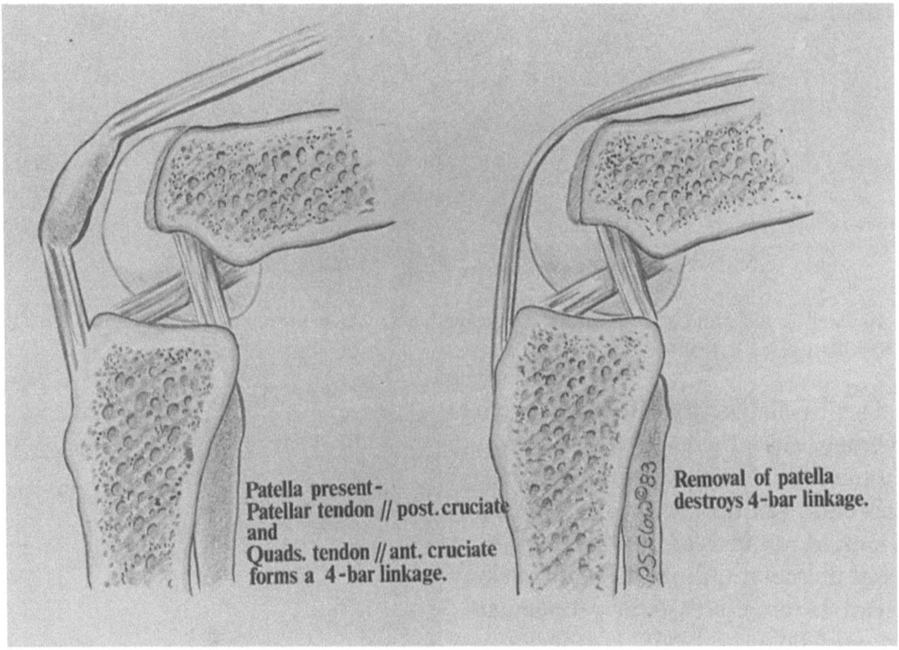

Fig. 13.9. A patellectomy alters the alignment of the extensor mechanism.

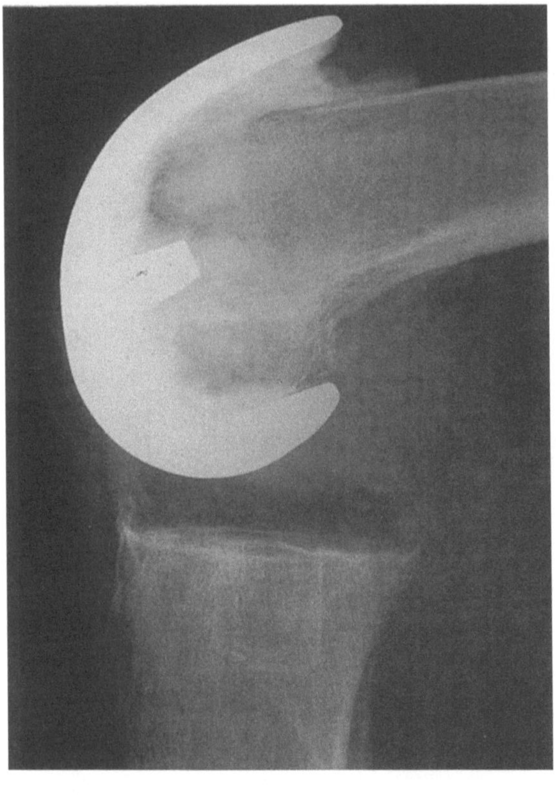

Fig. 13.10. Functional anteroposterior instability is present in 90° of flexion in this case in which both cruciates and the patella have been removed.

condylar posterior cruciate retaining prosthesis have not been good (Bayne and Cameron 1984; (Lennox et al. 1987). The reason for the poor results was anteroposterior instability.

With the patella in situ at 90° of flexion the patellar tendon is roughly parallel to the posterior cruciate ligament, and the quadriceps tendon is parallel to the anterior cruciate ligament. This forms a 4-bar linkage (Fig. 13.9). One or the other of these linkages may be resected without any deleterious anteroposterior instability (Cameron 1984). If both are resected, however, functional instability can occur (Fig. 13.10). Functional instability means that the knee may seem only mildly unstable on passive examination, but when the patient rises from a chair, marked anteroposterior shift does occur and this is usually painful. This will occur with most of the posterior cruciate retaining prostheses. This is not the case, however, in knees with a very deep or very constrained trochlear groove.

The author has tried two approaches to solve this problem. The first entailed using two individual unicompartmental components leaving both cruciate ligaments intact (Fig. 13.11 a,b). The results in a small study were reasonable – 3

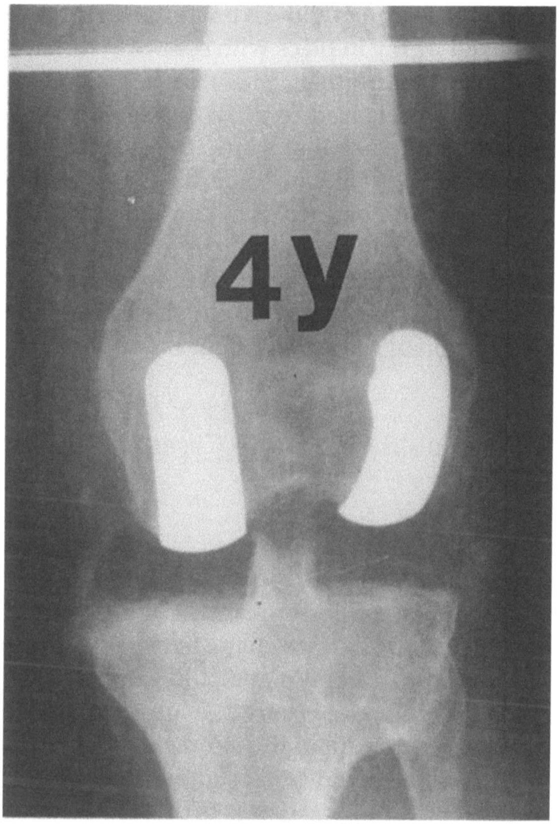

a

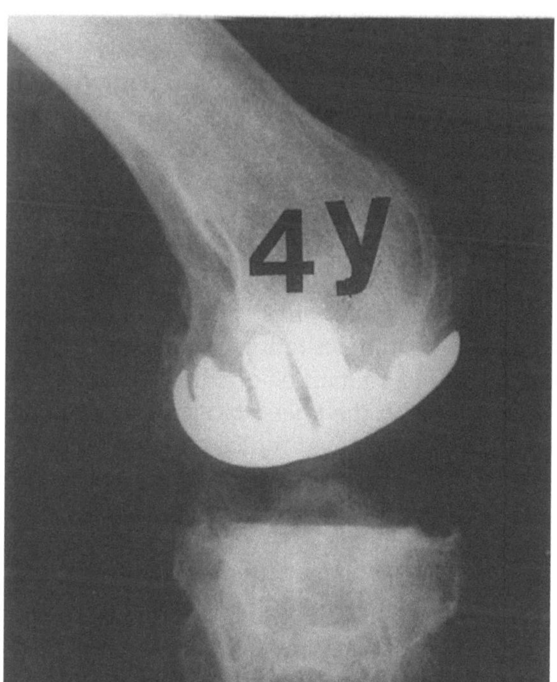

b

Fig. 13.11 a, b. Management of a patient requiring a total knee who had a prior patellectomy. A bicompartmental replacement has been performed retaining both cruciate ligaments. **a** P/A X-ray. **b** Lateral X-ray.

out of 5 patients were able to use the replaced knee as the lead leg on stairs. Unfortunately the technique of insertion of two unicompartmental components is very difficult and small discrepancies in position can severely compromise the results. A simpler solution appeared to be the use of a Posterior Stabilized knee. The early results in this study were even better than with the two unicondylar components – 5 out of 6 patients were able to use the replaced knee as the lead leg on stairs. Some patients, however, continued to have pain from rubbing of the patellar tendon on the metal.

In order to eliminate this anterior knee pain I have, on a very limited basis, attempted to replace the bony patella. In some very elderly patients with limited functional demands, I have simply drilled multiple holes about the edge of a large plastic patella and sutured it to the posterior aspect of the patellar tendon with non-absorbable sutures. In the short term, this seemed to work well. Hopefully, if plastic technology continues to improve, we can expect to obtain a polyethylene mesh that should be used to hold a patellar component in place by fibrous tissue ingrowth.

One final possible method to correct for an absent patella would be to place an iliac wing autograft in a pocket in the patellar tendon. It would appear that this procedure must be combined with a microvascular anastomosis in order to prevent avascular necrosis of the graft itself.

What Should One Do In Cases of Patella Baja?

Patella baja is rarely encountered in a knee that has not undergone prior surgery. Following a high tibial osteotomy, however, the patellar tendon may shorten and this may lower the level of the patella. Likewise, a Hauser type reconstruction with both distal as well as medial translation of the tibial tubercle may give rise to a patella baja and severe patellofemoral osteoarthritis (Blazina et al. 1979).

Patella baja may also be seen after a total knee replacement in which the prosthetic joint line was abnormally elevated. As most surgeons become aware that they must resect the same amount of distal femoral bone as the thickness of

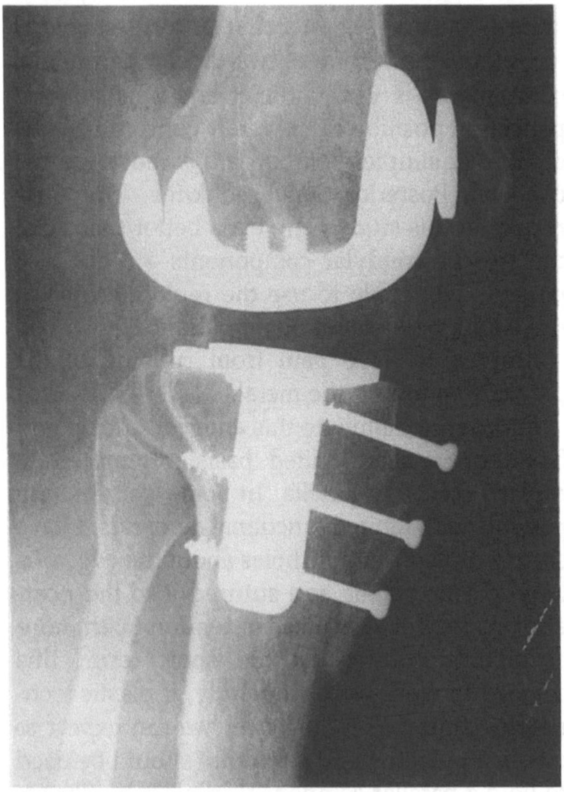

Fig. 13.12. Tibial tubercle osteotomy performed to correct a patella baja. The osteotomy is held in place with three screws.

the femoral component, this abnormality is decreasing in incidence. However, in cases where a large ligament release is required for soft tissue balancing, it is still possible unknowingly functionally to shift the joint line proximally. Likewise, when using a thin femoral component in a deformed knee with femoral bone loss, some elevation of the joint line may be required to seat the component on a flat surface.

The problem with a patella baja is that the implant may not make contact at all with the femoral component. This may result in a significant loss of flexion as well as catching as the patella abuts on the cruciate gap of the femoral implant.

When patella baja is present, entering the knee and dislocating the patella may be extremely difficult (Scott 1988). Even a V–Y quadriceps tendon division, as described by Coones and Adams, may not allow dislocation (Wendt and Johnson 1985). My preferred approach in these cases is a tibial tubercle osteotomy (Cameron and Jung 1988).

The tibial bone to be elevated should be a strip at least 8 cm long to allow it be shifted proximally and fixed firmly in place with screws at the close of the procedure (Fig. 13.12). A lateral release will also be required to allow proximal shift of the patella. Removal of a strip of bone from the anterior tibia results in some tibial weakening. Therefore, if a stemmed tibial component is to be used, some consideration might be given to spanning the inferior part of the gap with several transverse screws to strength the tibia before preparation of the central stem hole.

What Should One Do In Cases of Patella Alta?

Patella alta is usually not a problem for patients undergoing total knee replacement. If, however, it is noted that after implanting the prosthesis the patella articulates with the femur proximal to the anterior flange, it may "bump up" onto the implant as the knee is flexed. In order to prevent this the periosteum in the supracondylar region of the femur should be closed over the anterior surface of the femoral flange to present a smooth slope. In cases of very severe patella alta, the tibial tubercle can be moved distally.

Patella alta may occur postoperatively as a result of rupture of the patellar tendon. This, fortunately, is an uncommon occurrence. Most cases of rupture of the patellar tendon are noted within the first three months after surgery. A variant of patellar tendon rupture, avulsion of the tendon from the tibial tubercle, may be the iatrogenic result of over exuberant traction on the tendon at surgery in an attempt to expose the knee. This is a devastating complication in that the patient has a marked quadriceps lag and can walk only with the knee braced straight. Repair is therefore always indicated, but often is extremely difficult to obtain.

In order to hold the patella down to the correct level, wires have to be passed above the patella and looped through drill holes in the tibial tubercle (Fig. 13.13 a,b). If the knee is immobilized stiffness may result. Consequently the wires that are used should be very strong to allow early motion. Preferably, the wires should be multiphasic so as to work harden rather than weaken with use. It may be possible to reattach the patellar tendon remnant into the tibia by

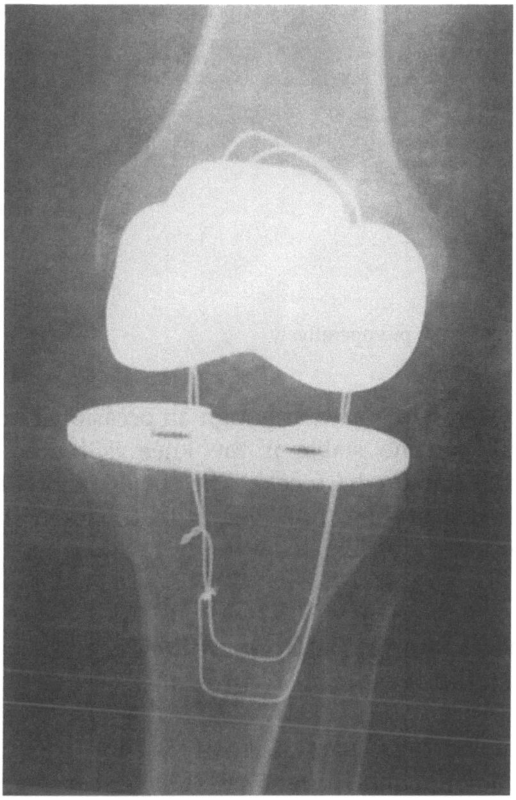

a

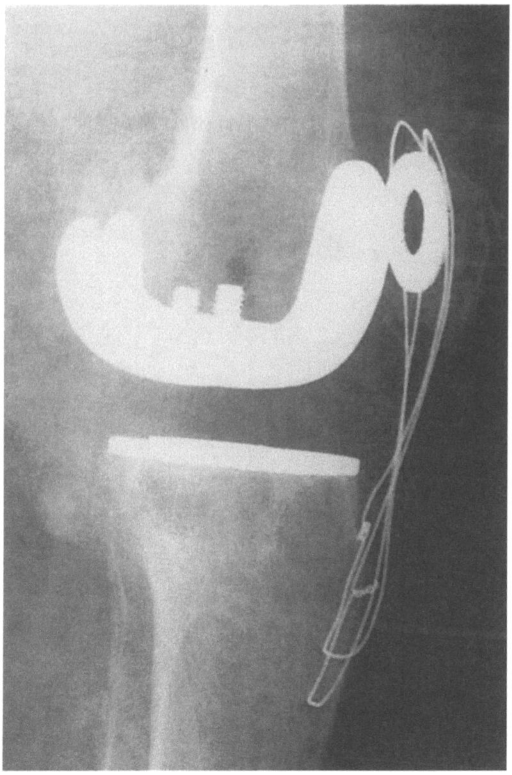

b

Fig. 13.13 a, b. Attempt at repair of an avulsion of the patellar tendon with a wire loop. **a** P/A X-ray. **b** Lateral X-ray.

means of a screw with a soft tissue washer. The tendon however may be so frayed and fragmented that a fascia lata graft is necessary. This is threaded in boot-lace fashion through a drill hole in the tibia and through the remnants of the patellar tendon.

How Should One Manage Patellar Subluxation?

There are several potential causes for patellar subluxation or dislocation. Using too thick a patellar component or cross faceting of a faceted patella can both force the implant out of the trochlear groove. Remove the patellar implant and replace it in the proper orientation, and, if necessary, thin the remaining patellar bone stock slightly to "thin-out" the bone-component dimension. Most of these situations will be evident at the time of surgery and should then be corrected.

The two commonest causes are tibial external rotation (that is placing the tibial component in relative internal rotation to the tibia) and a preoperative patellar subluxation. The treatment in these two situations is easy.

If the tibial component is placed in internal rotation with respect to the tibia the patella will sublux laterally. This can occur if the surgeon has inadequate exposure of the knee and cannot place the component in proper position, i.e. with its anterior midline aligned with the most medial quarter of the tibial tubercle. Adequate exposure will obviously correct this potential problem. Should severe patellar subluxation or dislocation occur and it is noted that the tibial component is internally rotated, it should be removed and replaced in proper position. In some patients with severe fixed valgus and flexion deformities, there can be a severe lateral patellar subluxation. The lateral trochlear ridge wears down and the patella drops over the edge (Fig. 13.14). In such knees the lateral tissues may be so contracted that even after properly placing the implants the patella will continue to track laterally. For some of these knees, a lateral release (sparing the lateral superior genicular artery) coupled with a vastus medialis advancement may be all that is necessary. For more severe cases, a proximal V–Y advancement medially, or a Roux procedure distally is indi-

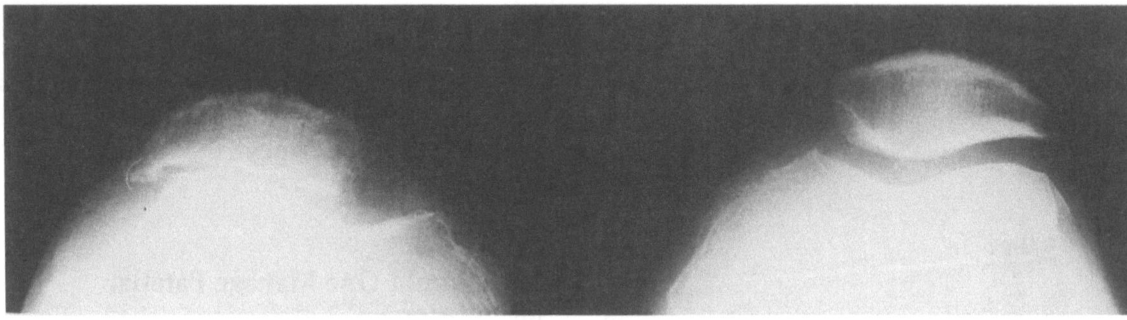

Fig. 13.14. Lateral patellar subluxation seen pre-operatively.

cated. In very severe cases it may be necessary to transfer the tibial tubercle.

When the surgeon anticipates a wide lateral release for a subluxing patella, it may be advantageous to perform a lateral parapatellar exposure of the knee. This spares the medial genicular vessels to the patella while allowing the subluxed patella to slide medially. The combination of the standard medial exposure and lateral release with tension or transection of the lateral superior genicular vessel may ultimately lead to avascular necrosis of the patella. When a lateral exposure is performed, patellar dislocation and exposure at surgery may be somewhat more difficult especially in the muscular patient. To facilitate this it may be necessary to split the patellar ligament longitudinally releasing the upper attachment from the patella and leaving it attached distally to the tibial tubercle. The assistant is then instructed not to pull the patella medially, which would apply tension to the ligament, but rather to pull distally to relieve tension on the ligament while still exposing the joint.

Initially I used to leave the lateral retinaculum open. It became apparent, however, that a very tight medial retinaculum with an open lateral retinaculum tended to tilt the patella. Consequently, a lateral retinacular closure is now routinely carried out. Curiously enough, patellar subluxation does not ocur after closure of the lateral retinaculum.

Patellar subluxation occurring after surgery in a knee in which there was good component tracking at surgery is a rare occurrence. One cause, however, can be disruption of the medial capsular repair. In such cases, the knee becomes unstable both anteroposteriorly and well as in rotation. In almost all cases some surgical correction is required although an occasional knee will become stable if the knee is braced in extension for 4–6 weeks. The obvious drawback of such bracing, however, is that marked stiffness can ensue.

What Should Be Done in the Face of Patellar Avascular Necrosis?

Patellar avascular necrosis is not common (Cameron and Huffer 1985). I have seen several

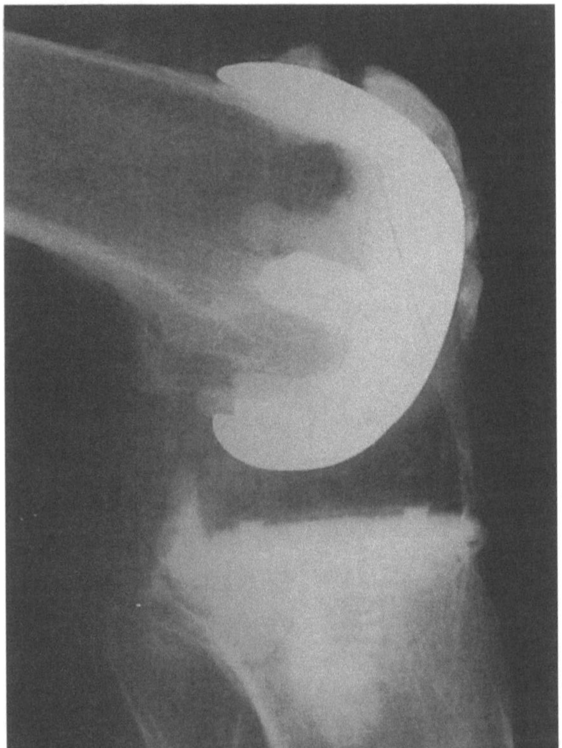

Fig. 13.15. Patellar avascular necrosis.

cases, however in which the surgery was performed through a medial parapatellar approach coupled with a lateral release of the retinacular tissues (Fig. 13.15). Since adopting a lateral parapatellar approach in those patients who obviously need a lateral release, this problem has all but disappeared. For those patients in whom a medial parapatellar approach was used and in whom at the end of surgery the patella is noted to sublux laterally, I perform the lateral release as far lateral as possible in order to spare the lateral superior genicular vessels.

Although avascular necrosis is a radiographic finding it rarely is a functional problem. In only two cases have I found it necessary to remove the avascular fragments. For most patients, the mild anterior knee discomfort that is seen after radiographic changes occur, disappears after a few months. A quadriceps lag is uncommon and, if it does develop, it can usually be controlled by simple bracing for 6 weeks.

Avascular necrosis is of significance only when patellar fracture occurs. Fracture of an avascular patella following total knee replacement will seldom heal by bone, in contrast to the normal fractured patella which virtually always heals. If minimal separation is present it is preferable simply to brace the patient for 6 weeks with the knee straight to allow healing by fibrous tissue. If wide separation has occurred with significant quadriceps lag, the patellar component should be removed and the remaining bone wired together. Union is unlikely to occur, but a fibrous non-union seems to function well (Fig. 13.16a,b).

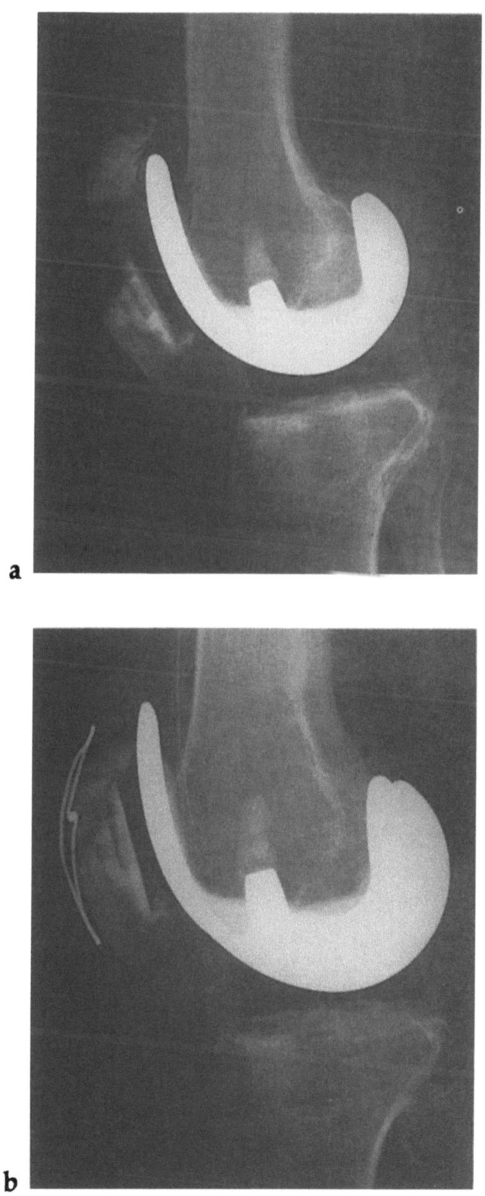

Fig. 13.16 a, b. Fracture of the patella. **a** The fragments are widely separated and there is an extensor lag. **b** Fixation with a wire loop tension band.

References

Aglietti P, Buzzi P, Gaudenzi A (1988) Patello-femoral functional results and complications with the posterior total condylar knee. J Arthroplasty 3: 17–25

Bayley JC, Scott RC, Edward FC, Holmes GB (1988) Failure of metal backed patellar components after total knee replacement. J Bone Joint Surg (Am) 70: 668–675

Bayne O, Cameron HU (1984) Total knee arthroplasty following patellectomy. Clin Orthop 186: 112–117

Blazina ME, Fox IM, DelPizzo W (1979) Patello femoral replacement. Clin Orthop 144: 98–101

Cameron HU (1984) Antero-posterior instability in total knee replacement. Acta Orthop Belg 50: 476–480

Cameron HU, Cameron GM (1987) The patellar meniscus in total knee replacement. Orthop Rev 3: 75–77

Cameron HU, Huffer B (1985) Avascular necrosis of the patella following total knee replacement. Acta Orthop Belg 51: 805–810

Cameron HU, Jung YB (1988) Patella baja complicating total knee arthroplasty – a report of two cases. J Arthroplasty 3: 177–181

Dorr LD, Boiardo RA (1986) Technical considerations in total knee arthroplasty. Clin Orthop 205: 5–22

Laskin RS (1988) Tricon-M uncemented total knee arthroplasty. J Arthroplasty 3: 27–38

Lennox DW, Hungerford DS, Krakow KA (1987) Total knee arthroplasty following patellectomy. Clin Orthop 233: 220–224

Levai JP, McLeod HU, Freeman MAR (1983) Why not resurface the patella? J Bone Joint Surg (Br) 65: 448–452

Lombardi AV, Engh GA, Volz RG, Albrigo H (1988) Fracture dislocation of the polyethylene in metal backed patellar

components in total knee arthroplasty. J Bone Joint Surg (Am) 70: 675–680
Scott RD (1988) Revision total knee arthroplasty. Clin Orthop 226: 166–175
Soudry M, Mestriner LA, Binazzi A, Insall JN (1986) Total knee arthroplasty without patellar resurfacing. Clin Orthop 205: 166–170
Wendt PP, Johnson RP (1985) A study of quadriceps excursion, torque and the effects of patellectomy on the cadaver knee. J Bone Joint Surg (Am) 67: 726–780

Chapter 14

Subsidence

Leif Ryd

Introduction

Loosening is generally recognized as one major complication in arthroplasty of the knee (Cameron and Hunter 1982; Thornhill et al. 1982; Goldberg et al. 1988; Rand and Coventry 1988). From an incidence of up to 10% in the 1970s (Skolnick et al. 1976; Freeman et al. 1978; Lacey 1978) the incidence has decreased significantly in more recent reports (Insall et al. 1983; Insall and Kelly 1986). During the last decade, a subgroup of loosening, i.e. subsidence of the tibial component, has emerged as a major cause of failure of knee replacements.

This chapter will deal with subsidence. By definition and also for empirical reasons, the tibial component is the one in focus; mechanical complications of the femoral component being much more infrequent. The chapter will deal with the causes of subsidence and possible ways to avoid it. It will not deal with the consequences. Revision arthroplasty because of subsidence is, in most cases, not different from revision for other reasons and will be dealt with in other sections of this book.

Definition

The Random House dictionary defines subsidence as "to sink to a lower level". Cameron and McNeice (1981) and Cameron and Hunter (1982), in a study on cases scheduled for revision, defined five different failure modes among which were "tilt and sink" as well as "compression mode". While "compression mode", i.e. sinkage of the entire prosthesis, may be the best equivalent to subsidence properly speaking, the "tilt and sink mode" is more common and it is certainly included in what is termed subsidence in the literature.

In this chapter, subsidence of the entire prosthesis or any part of it will be considered. When a distinction is needed, "sinkage" will be used to denote total subsidence while "tilt" will be used to denote subsidence of only a part of the prosthesis.

Review of the Literature

Subsidence or other terms indicating sinking of the prosthesis, or part of it, into the tibia, was mentioned already during the 1970s although the problem was quantitatively small. It also seems to have occurred in some specific types of prostheses. In the study by Cameron and McNeice (1981) subsidence occurred most commonly in unicompartmental components; Gunstons and Marmors. In other reports on unicompartmental arthroplasty the incidence of subsidence ranges from 0 to 16% (Table 14.1). Marmor (1985) reviewed his first 138 cases with

Table 14.1. Frequency of subsidence and revisions in reported series of knee arthroplasty

Author	% subsidence	Percentage revisions of those subsided
Unicompartment knees		
Laskin 1976	6	20
Cracchiolo et al. 1979	0	–
Jónsson 1981	16	25
Marmor 1985	4	100
Larsson et al. 1988	11	0
Total knees, cemented		
Ducheyne et al. 1977	4	100
Freeman et al. 1978	12.5	100
Insall et al. 1983	1	100
Townley 1985	0	–
Laskin 1988	4	0
Uncemented		
Hungerford and Krackow 1985	0	–
Audell and Cracchiolo 1987	8	100
Rand et al. 1987	34	0
Samuelson 1987	3	100
Albrektsson and Herberts 1988	11	80
Laskin 1988	45	5

an average follow-up of 6 years and found five cases of "depressed tibial components". Laskin (1976) reported settling in 5 cases out of 89 and Jónsson (1981) found settling in 16 out of 102 Marmor tibial components. Cracchiolo et al. (1979) reported five "loose" tibial components in 105 Polycentric arthroplasties but subsidence was not particularly mentioned. Finally Larsson et al. (1988), using the St. George "sledge prosthesis" reported 9 cases of subsidence out of 81.

For hinged prostheses, subsidence was not of any particular concern and the term was not mentioned despite a 15% incidence of loosening after 2 years for the Guepar prosthesis (Deburge et al. 1979). Kaufer and Matthews (1979) reported 10 cases of loosening defined as "a measurable shift in position of the prosthesis . . . with time or by stress films" in 134 cases of Spherocentric knee arthroplasty without specifically mentioning subsidence. Shindell et al. (1986) reported "subsidence" in all but one of 18 cases where the Noiles hinged prosthesis was used. Interestingly this subsidence occurred exclusively for the femoral components which had a very small cross-section area.

For bicompartmental prostheses, studies on the first generation types report subsidence from 0 to 12.5%. Cracchiolo et al. (1979) reported no problems of this type with the Geometric prosthesis. In a review of 632 Anatomic Total Knees, Townley (1985) reported a low incidence of loosening and no specific subsidence. Insall et al. (1983) reported on 125 Total Condylar knees and found two cases of loosening, one of which showed "progressive subsidence" on serial radiographs. Ducheyne et al. (1978), however, reported collapse and fragmentation of the trabecular bone in four cases out of 100 and Freeman reported a 12.5% incidence of sinkage in 200 consecutive ICLH prostheses (Freeman et al. 1978).

During the 1980s prostheses necessitating less bone resection, often in combination with noncement fixation, were introduced. In a minimum 2 year report on 96 Tricon-M arthroplasties, Laskin (1988) reported subsidence of at least 1 mm in 43 cases, of which two had subsided more than 2 mm. In that report the incidence of subsidence of cemented RMC tibial components was 2 out of 46 cases. Samuelson (1987) reported six cases of anteriomedial subsidence in 187 cases of uncemented Freeman-Samuelson arthroplasty and he stated that "the main problem with total knee component fixation is tibial subsidence". Using the same prosthesis, Audell and Cracchiolo (1987) reported subsidence in 4 cases out of 50 which occurred in an average of 21 months after surgery. Albrektsson and Herberts (1988) reported 12 cases of tilt in a series of 108 cases of uncemented ICLH arthroplasty. In a comparative study between cemented and uncemented PCA prostheses, Rand et al. (1987) found no significant changes in the component position between 2 month and 2 year evaluations in the cemented group (n=50). In the uncemented group (n=41), however, 14 cases with comparable serial radiographs showed anteriomedial sinkage. Hungerford and Krackow (1985), using the same uncemented prosthesis reported no problem with subsidence.

When reviewing the literature, it thus appears that although the problem of subsidence was recognized before 1980, it did not become a major one until the introduction of "modern" prostheses suitable also for uncemented insertion. The prostheses showing consistent subsidence, i.e. unicompartmental and "modern" (uncemented) total knees also seem to share a common design feature; they often lack central fixation posts and are more or less "lying" on the cancellous bone.

Incidence of Revision Due to Subsidence

The clinical consequences of subsidence per se are difficult to elucidate. It has been stated that a "change of position of prosthetic components", i.e. sinkage or tilt, is a definite sign of loosening (Kaufer and Matthews 1981; Schneider et al. 1982; Boegård et al. 1984; Harris 1984). Such loosening is, however, not always symptomatic and terms like "asymptomatic loosening (Rand and Bryan 1982; Schneider et al. 1982), "stable loosening" (Convery et al. 1980) and "biomechanical loosening" (Larsson and Ahlgren 1979) have been used. Kaufer et al. (1978) suggested four types of loosening: "Simple loosening", clinically satisfactory with or without demonstrable motion of the prosthesis with stress views or push-pull films, "symptomatic loosening" with some symptoms, "progressive loosening" mainly related to the formation of radiolucent zones, and "functional loosening" where, finally, a "progressive displacement of the implant" is included.

In the reported unicompartmental series the revision rate of the subsided prostheses range from 0 to 100%. In total knee arthroplasty the situation seems to be the same. Thus some authors have revised all of their subsided components, while others have revised none (Table 14.1).

The differences regarding the clinical consequences of subsidence reflect inevitable differences in attitudes and indications of the surgeons both regarding primary replacements as well as revisions. To some extent, also, the discrepancies can probably be explained by differences in interpretation of roentgenograms in combination with different radiographic techniques which are often not elucidated in a satisfactory way.

It seems quite clear, however, that subsidence today represents a clinical problem especially with noncemented tibial components.

Detection

Subsidence, i.e. true sinkage or tilt, is usually regarded as a sign of (impending) loosening (Schneider et al. 1982; Miller 1984). Such change in position is usually measured on standard radiographs, the technique of which is not always described. Angular tilt of the prosthesis is usually determined with reference to the long axis of the tibia in both planes, while sinkage is determined in relation to some point of reference in the tibia. Such a point of reference is sometimes the cut upper surface of the tibia which is left uncapped by the prosthesis at surgery (Laskin 1988; Whiteside and Pafford 1989). Schneider et al. (1982), however, pointed out that the latter is difficult to use as a landmark because on radiographs bony proliferations may develop around the prosthesis giving a false impression of subsidence. Also differences in projection between radiographs make the detection of bony landmarks difficult.

Some authors have tried to determine the accuracy of radiography in determining the change in the position of tibial components. Blaha et al. (1982) determined the observer error when measuring the same films twice and found that a tilt of 3° and sinkage of 2 mm was significant. This study did not include errors caused by radiographs in different projections. Albrektsson and Herberts (1988) reported a similar study and found an observer error of 1°. When adding the error introduced by differences in positions and projections during the radiographic examinations they did not accept angular changes less than 4° as significant.

A study using roentgen stereophotogrammetric analysis (RSA) as reference (Ryd et al. 1983), found the accuracy of conventional radiography regarding tilt, using a standardized technique, to be 3.6° at the 95% confidence limit.

In a recent study, measurements of apparent subsidence as indicated by the position of the prosthesis with reference to the cut upper surface of the tibia were made (Ryd, unpublished data). "Subsidence" of up to 15 mm was often accounted for by bony proliferations around the prosthesis despite little true change of position of the prostheses. This was especially true in uncemented cases. These bony proliferations

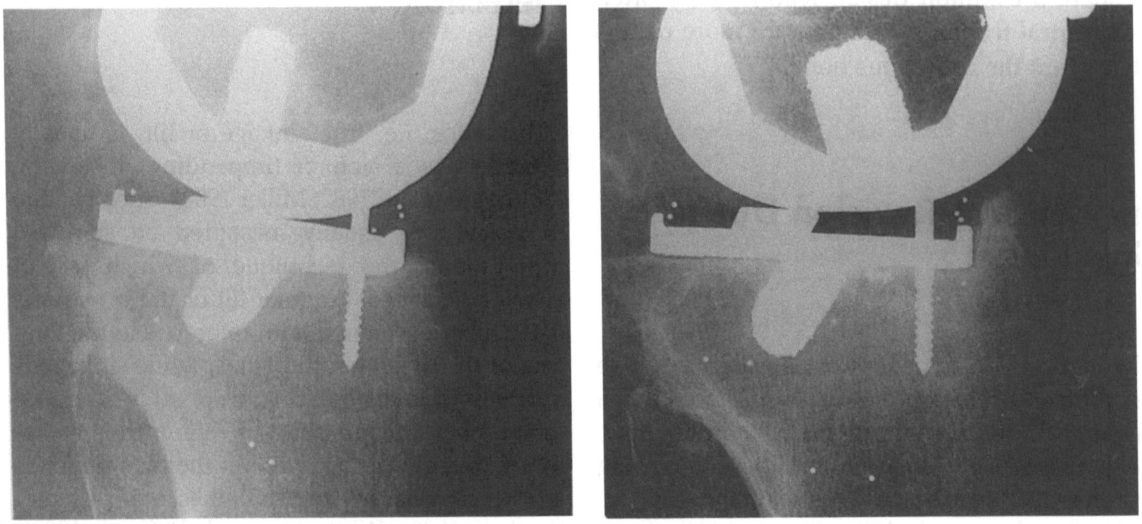

a b

Fig. 14.1 a.b. Radiograms of an uncemented PCA tibial component postoperatively (a) and after 4 years (b). As measured by RSA, this prosthesis had tilted 2.6° anteriorly, corresponding to a subsidence of 2.7 mm at the anterior margin. The remaining "subsidence" is accounted for by bony proliferation.

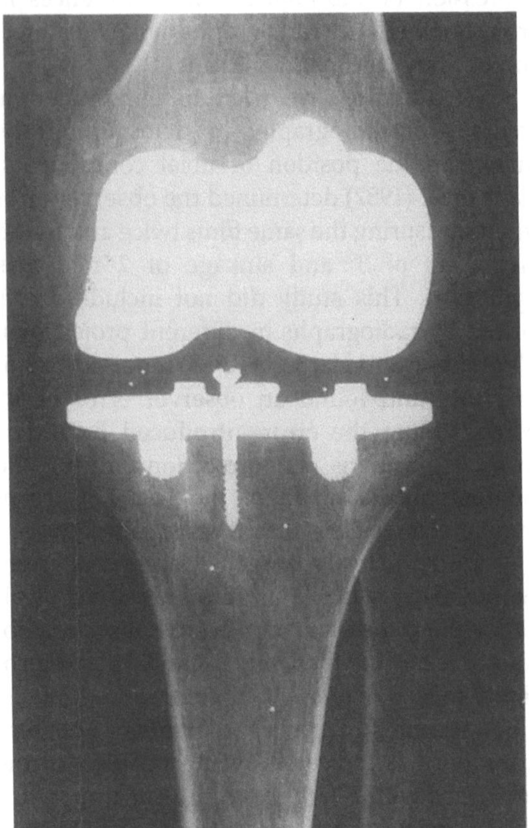

Fig. 14.2. Example of a knee arthroplasty marked by tantalum balls. Distinct marker images were achieved despite rather bad bone image quality, due to exposure characteristics set to keep the irradiation burden at a minimum (less than 1/10 of a routine knee examination: Ryd 1986).

developed during the first, and to some extent second, year (Fig. 14.1).

It thus appears that plain radiographs must be judged with the utmost caution in the context of subsidence, and changes in position of prostheses of less than 4° or 2–3 mm may not represent true subsidence.

RSA Studies

Among more precise radiographic methods to study prosthetic behavior are the "grid system" of Amstutz et al. (1986). Greene et al. (1983) used a system including calibration devices and marking of the objects of interest with metal balls. Perhaps the most comprehensive system to study skeletal kinematics, roentgen stereophotogrammetric analysis (RSA), was developed by Selvik (1974). RSA uses tantalum balls to mark the objects of interest. Tantalum has two advantages; it is inert in body fluids giving so-called osseointegration (Alberius 1983) and, due to the high atomic number (73), it gives very distinct images on radiographic films (Fig. 14.2). In this respect, marking also of metal objects, for example a hip prosthesis, can be done under certain conditions. By using proper exposure character-

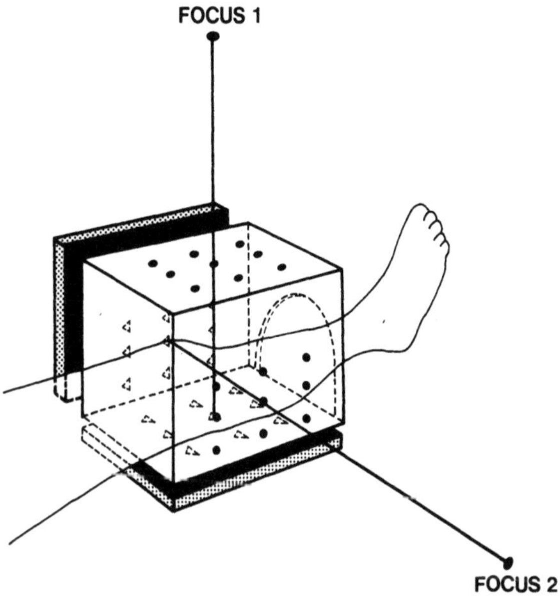

Fig. 14.3. Schematic view of the biplanar radiographic set-up during an RSA examination of a knee. Note two foci and a "calibration cage".

istics, the markers can be "seen" through the metal (Wykman et al. 1988). Radiograms, obtained in two planes under standardized conditions (Fig. 14.3), are measured using a precision digitizing table (Hasselblad, precision 10 μm). Data are obtained by using PC compatible micro computer programs (UNIKUM, Umeå University, Sweden). The KINEMA routine determines the motion between two objects while the GROWTH routine gives the growth pattern of a single object. The accuracy of RSA depends on the application, e.g. factors as number of markers, size of the marker configuration in each segment, etc. In knee arthroplasty the accuracy has been determined to 0.2 mm (Ryd 1986). RSA has found a number of applications including fracture healing, skeletal and tumor growth studies, studies of joint motion patterns and prosthetic fixation. Using RSA, or similar methods, a better understanding of the true micromotion of prostheses can be achieved both for the hip (Greene et al. 1983; Mjöberg 1986; Wykman et al. 1988) as well as for the knee (Greene et al. 1983; Ryd 1986; Ryd et al. 1983, 1986, 1987, 1988).

Since 1979 knee replacements of different designs have been entered into a RSA project now including approximately 400 cases. In this project micromotion of two types, migration and inducible displacement, have been studied (Ryd 1986):

1. *Migration*, i.e. motion over time, was studied by comparing the position of the prosthesis at an immediate postoperative examination, with the position after certain predetermined time intervals, usually 6 weeks, 6 months and yearly. The postoperative examination was always done before any weight was put on the knee, thus representing the position in which the prosthesis was inserted during the operation.
2. *Inducible displacement* was studied after a certain time interval after the operation, usually 1–2 years, when a stable prosthetic bed had been achieved. Here, the position of the prosthesis was determined while under the influence of external reproducible forces acting across the knee, and compared with the position at an initial supine exposure. After testing forces in every possible direction, e.g. valgus-varus and shear forces etc, rotatory forces, created by having the patient standing on a rotating plate with a 10 Nm force acting in both directions, were found to be the most yielding (Ryd 1986). 10 Nm rotation torque is within the physiological range (Bargren et al. 1978). These stress examinations were conceived of as simulating ordinary every-day life.

The direction of the migration or inducible displacement was presented as rotation and translation about or along each of the cardinal axes. The magnitude of these motions was given as the Maximum Total Point Motion (MTPM), the length of the three-dimensional space vector of the marker which moved the most. This value (=distance) does not have a direction and may represent motion in the downward direction (=subsidence) or in the plane of tibial bone resection (=rotation or translation).

Cemented Fixation

Migration has been shown to occur almost without exclusion. For cemented total tibial components without metal-backing of the Total Condylar design, migration of about 0.6 mm (MTPM) occurred in all 27 cases during the first

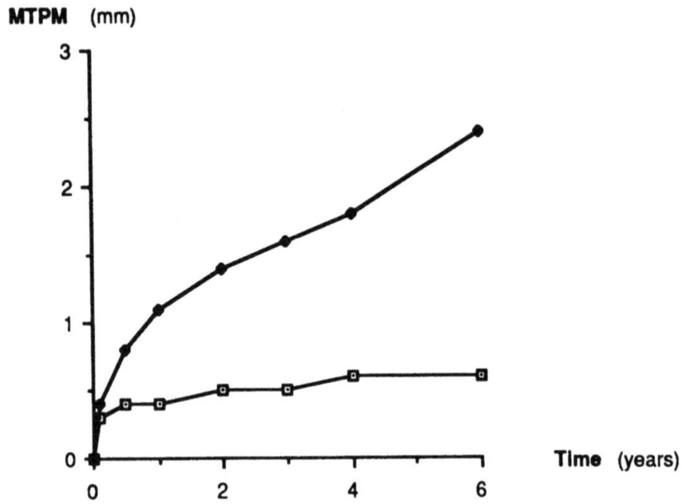

Fig. 14.4. Diagram of the migration of cemented polyethylene components of the Total Condylar (n=27) and Marmor (n=24) design. (*Black Squares*, continuous migration, n=17; *open squares*, initial migration, n=34).

year. After this time, a majority of prostheses stabilized and did not migrate any further, while a minority, eight cases, continued to migrate throughout the 4 year study period (Fig. 14.4). The maximum migration found in this group was 2.1 mm after 4 years. Inducible displacement was found in all these cases ranging between 0.2 and 1.0 mm (MTPM). In eight cases another stress examination was done about one year after the first one. Inducible displacement of the same magnitude was found in this second stress examination, indicating small further changes in the mechanical characteristics of the interface once a stable prosthetic bed has been reached (Ryd et al. 1987). Similar results regarding migration have been found for polyethylene components of the unicompartmental Marmor prostheses (Ryd 1986). Metal-backed cemented components have been tested, both total (bicompartmental) of the Kinematic (Ryd et al. 1986) and PCA (Ryd et al. 1988) designs as well as a unicompartmental prosthesis (Ryd 1986). Both migration as well as inducible displacement of the same magnitude as the polyethylene components were found, and metal-backing was thus not found to affect the mechanical properties of the interface as measured by RSA.

The direction of the migration of all these cemented prostheses was primarily in the plane of the tibial resection, i.e. subsidence was only an occasional finding.

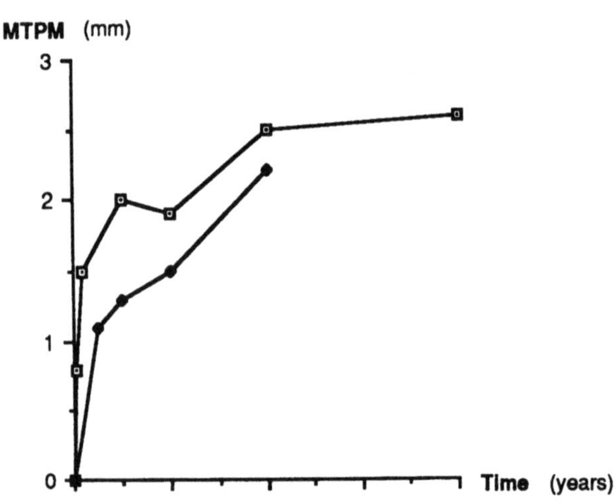

Fig. 14.5. Migration of uncemented PCA (*open squares*, n=13) and Freeman-Samuelson (*black squares*, n=5).

Noncemented fixation

Noncemented fixation has been studied both in a porous coated device as well as for a prosthesis of the intermediate interlocking concept ("magic peg", Freeman et al. 1981). The porous coated PCA total prosthesis showed considerable migration during the first postoperative year (Fig. 14.5). Already after 1 week approximately 1 mm of migration had occurred. This "first phase" migration was attributed to a harder impaction of the prostheses against the bone with weight-bearing and postoperative physiotherapy. During the remainder of the first year(s) additional "second phase" migration was found of a magnitude approximately similar to that found during the first year for cemented prostheses. After this point additional "third phase" migration occurred in only 3 out of 13 prostheses

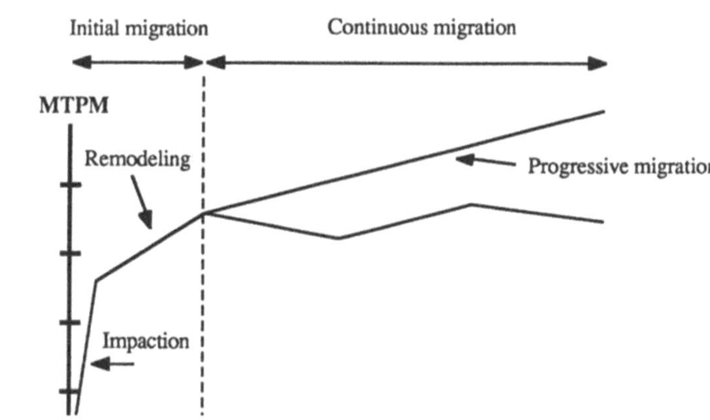

Fig. 14.6. Diagram of suggested three phases of migration for uncemented prostheses.

(Fig. 14.6). The direction of the migration was different than for the cemented cases and a subsidence of slightly more than 1 mm was a consistent finding after 1–2 years (Ryd et al. 1988). In individual cases subsidence exceeding 3 mm was recorded. Inducible displacement was found for all these noncemented PCA prostheses ranging from 0.4–1.3 mm, i.e. significantly larger than for the cemented prostheses (Fig. 14.7).

Noncemented prostheses of the Freeman-Samuelson design with magic peg fixation showed a migratory pattern similar to that of the PCA prostheses. Inducible displacement was, however, larger for these prostheses, with a mean of 1.9 mm (Fig. 14.7).

In conclusion, the RSA studies of tibial components have shown that:

1. Migration is a normal occurrence especially during the first year.
2. Subsidence is seldom found for cemented prostheses while it is a regular finding for noncemented prostheses. In clinically successful cases such subsidence may occasionally reach a magnitude of 3 mm.
3. Inducible displacement is found for all fixation concepts tested. It seems to be larger for noncemented prostheses.

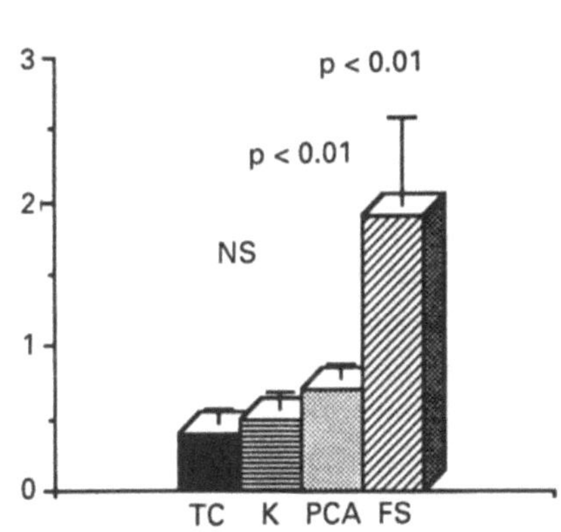

Fig. 14.7. Diagram of inducible displacement found by RSA for Total Condylar (TC, n=27), Kinematic (K, n=7), uncemented PCA (PCA, n=13), and Freeman-Samuelson (FS, n=6) prostheses.

It should be emphazised that, at the present stage, no particular pattern of micromotion can be connected to prosthetic failure by loosening or any other mode. The vast majority of these patients were clinically successful and none suffered from clinically obvious mechanical loosening.

Factors of Importance for Subsidence

Bone Strength

Perhaps the most immediate factor, and also one beyond the control of the surgeon, in considering subsidence is the bone strength. The cancellous bone of the tibial metaphysis is among the weakest in the body while the cancellous bone of the distal femoral metaphysis has been reported to be between 2 and 10 times stronger (Colley et al. 1978; Yusuki 1978). Furthermore, the strength of the cancellous bone decreases distally, both in the normal (Goldstein et al. 1983; Hvid and Jensen 1984) and in the diseased knee (Hvid 1988; Hvid and Hansen 1986).

In the normal knee, the medial condyle is stronger than the lateral one (Goldstein et al. 1983; Hvid and Jensen 1984), probably reflecting the larger proportion of weight carried by the medial condyle under dynamic conditions (Morrison 1970; Harrington 1976). In both condyles the strongest bone is found centrally, somewhat anteriorly in the medial condyle and posteriorly in the lateral condyle (Goldstein et al. 1983; Hvid et al. 1985). The strength decreases rather distinctly peripherally (Hvid et al. 1985).

In the diseased knee, malalignment in the varus or valgus direction distinctly influences the bone strength. In varus knees, the medial condyle is invariably the strongest one while the correlation is less distinct concerning the lateral condyle (Hvid 1988). Contrary to what one might think, the absolute strength of the cancellous bone, for example in the medial condyle, has been reported to be lower in an OA varus knee than in a normal knee. Also, the median value for bone strength in rheumatoid knees is only slightly less than in arthrotic knees although some rheumatoid knees have very weak bone (Hvid 1988).

Studies on the structural behavior of the tibial metaphysis together with prosthetic implants have been done both analytically and experimentally. Using a finite element model, Lewis et al. (1982) studied different configurations of tibial components under different kinds of load. In pure compression the stresses were generally less than 25% of the failure stress, but eccentric loading caused stresses ranging up to 91% of the failure stress. Considering the fact that a 2–3-fold margin of safety is needed to protect against fatigue failure, these results do not indicate any excessive strength of the cancellous bone. Similar tests were done experimentally by Bargren et al. (1978), who found the strength of the proximal tibia with a prosthesis to be considerably less than the normal knee using a number of different tibial components.

Walker et al. (1976) studied the fixation of a model unicompartmental tibial component experimentally on autopsy specimens, and found deflections, both in compression and tension, of up to 0.5 mm on "soft bone" using forces of a physiological magnitude. A keel reduced these deflections as did anchoring holes of cement. In a similar study, using a number of different tibial components resembling what is commercially available, deflections of 0.1 mm in pure compression and 0.2 mm for combined loads were found (Walker et al. 1981). Finally, Manley et al. (1987) reported considerable motion not only in the interface but within the cancellous bone itself underneath both cemented and uncemented tibial components in a dog study using "physiologic" forces.

In conclusion, available data on bone strength do not indicate a large margin of safety, and failure of the cancellous bone due to fatigue may well occur in a substantial proportion of the knee arthroplasties that are performed. The continuous migration found by RSA for a portion of the prostheses studied may represent such fatigue processes occurring continuously in the tibial metaphysis.

Cortical Bone Support

Cortical support of the tibial component has been advocated as an important means to achieve stronger fixation (Bargren et al. 1978; Freeman et al. 1978; Cameron and Hunter 1982). Other studies, however, have shown that the cortex at the level of resection is extremely thin, less then 0.5 mm, and should be regarded as an envelope of cancellous bone with small specific mechanical properties (Murray et al. 1984). In a mechanical study on the load transfer under the tibial component, Whiteside and Pafford (1989) concluded that load is transferred through the cancellous bone to the metaphyseal cortical bone "to a certain extent bypassing the proximal peripheral rim of the tibia". In the RSA studies coverage of the peripheral rim by the prosthesis did not correlate with the magnitude nor the direction of the migration (Ryd 1986) while Hvid et al. (1985) and Cheal et al. (1985) found that the inclusion of the periphery in the interface did not give a significantly stronger prosthetic support.

Given, however, the narrow margin of safety, every effort should be made to increase the strength of the tibial metaphysis. Larger prostheses cover more bone and thus increase the strength of the supporting bone corresponding to the area increase (Figgie et al. 1984). In clinical practice larger components have been reported to reduce the incidence of subsidence in an otherwise unaltered prosthetic design (Freeman et al. 1978) which, with small prostheses, was plagued by this complication. Thus, with only marginal safety regarding bone strength, undersizing of the tibial component should probably be avoided.

Prosthetic Macrodesign: Stem versus No Stem

Historically, modern knee prostheses evolved out of the hinges, pioneered by Walldius (Walldius 1957). Here the components, without cement, engaged the marrow cavities by long stems. When the importance of saving bone stock was realized, the intramedullary stems grew shorter and today, tibial components have either short stems, 3–5 cm long or short pegs. In pure compression, there does not seem to be any difference in the ability of these two designs to acommodate the loads that they are subjected to in the clinical situation (Bartel et al. 1982; Walker et al. 1981). However, tibial components are not always loaded in pure compression, but eccentric loading is also encountered during everyday life (Walker et al. 1981). With eccentric loading, considerably larger deflections, i.e. tilt, have been found between the bone and prostheses (Bartel et al. 1982; Walker et al. 1981). Experimentally, no differences in prosthetic behavior under eccentric loading were found between tibial components with one large central stem or with two small pegs (Walker et al. 1981) while Bartel et al. (1982) and Whiteside and Pafford (1989) found a more stable behavior for a single stem component than one with short pegs.

Using RSA, inducible displacement was most consistently found in eccentric loading when a 10 Nm rotatory torque was applied across the knee, while simple weight-bearing was less yielding. Perhaps the most consistent eccentric loading occurs when rising from a chair, especially for posterior cruciate retaining prostheses. With bending, there will be a posterior rollback of the femoral component in such designs. RSA studies have shown a consistent backward tilt (inducible displacement) of approximately 0.5°, corresponding to an anterior lift-off of 0.3 mm and posterior subsidence of 0.5 mm of PCA tibial components when weight-bearing in 60° of flexion (Ryd, unpublished data). An indication of such rocking of the prostheses in the sagittal plane is the tapered shape of the tibial component interface (Fig. 14.8), which has been reported (Ryd 1986).

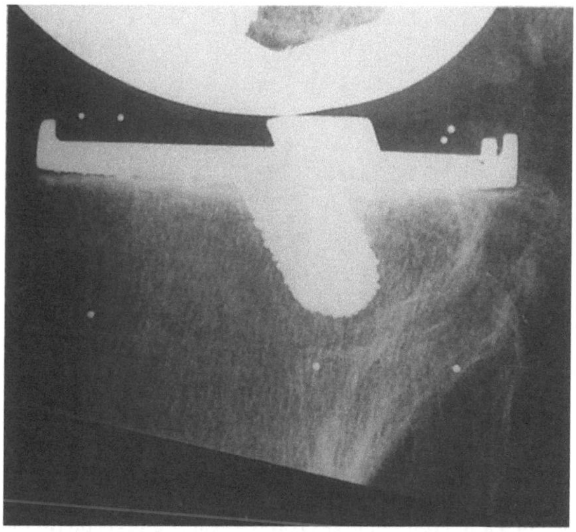

Fig. 14.8. Lateral radiogram of a PCA prosthesis showing tapered radiolucencies anteriorly and posteriorly suggesting rocking motion in the sagittal plane.

Furthermore, the addition of a long intramedullary stem, with a circular cross-section, to the Freeman-Samuelson tibial component has been shown to significantly control tilting migratory deflections as well as to decrease the inducible displacement as measured by RSA (Albrektsson et al. 1990).

The above-mentioned experimental and analytical studies consider bone of good quality. Clinically, prostheses are, however, often inserted in bone of poor quality, especially in rheumatoid patients. We have experienced two cases of catastrophic subsidence in rheumatoid patients (Lidgren, personal communication) with an anterior tilt of approximately 21° and 29° (as measured by RSA) necessitating revision (Fig. 14.9). It is possible that an intramedullary stem, resting on the posterior cortex would have prevented this complication.

Caution about intramedullary stems has been expressed because of the possible stress shielding effects of such stems (Bourne and Finlay 1986). In their study 15 cm long, heavy stems, being wedged into the medullary canal, gave a considerably reduced load on the entire metaphysis while 3.5 cm stems affected the load distribution in the proximal couple of cm only. Again, given the above-mentioned rather narrow margin of safety regarding cancellous

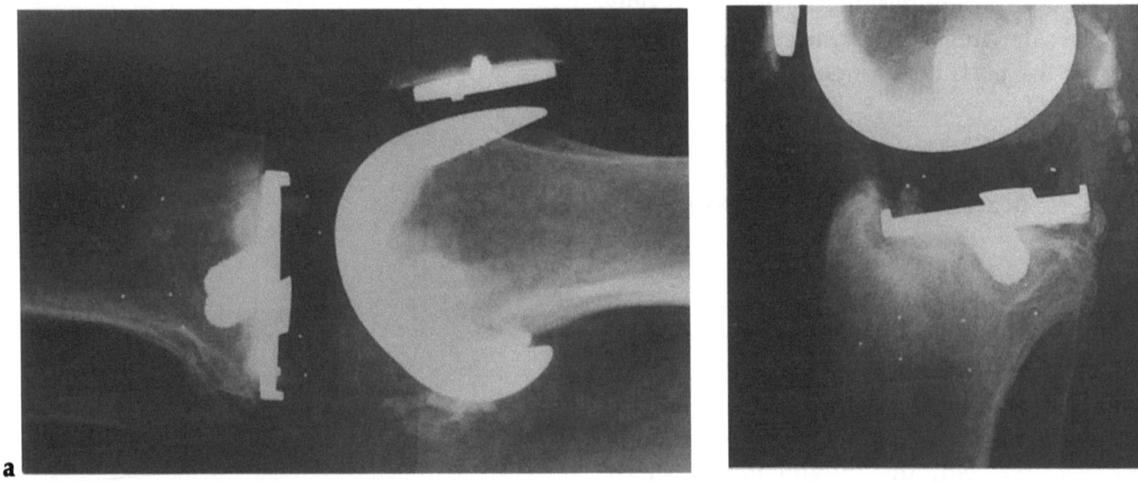

Fig. 14.9 a,b. Postoperative (**a**) and 4 year pre-revision (**b**) radiograms of a PCA prosthesis showing an anterior subsidence of 21° as measured by RSA.

bone strength, it is suggested that the problem in the upper tibia is one of overstressing rather than understressing the bone tissue. In conclusion therefore, a moderately long intramedullary stem may be feasible for the prevention of subsidence, especially in patients with cancellous bone of poor quality.

Articulating Geometry

In many contemporary knee prosthesis designs, stability is achieved solely by action of the surrounding ligaments. These tibial components usually have a rather flat articulating geometry giving unconstrained articulation between the femoral and tibial component (Kenna and Hungerford 1984). Such prostheses have been shown to give excellent motion patterns resembling the natural, for example in gait studies (Andriacchi et al. 1982). By definition, however, such designs allow for large excursions of the femoral component on the tibial one, with eccentric loading as a result. Such eccentric loading outside the central one third of the articulating surface gives tension in the interface and extremely eccentric loading can give catastrophic high compressive loads on the underlying cancellous bone (Bartel et al. 1982). On balance, therefore, a certain constraint of the prosthesis may be indicated in certain patient groups in order, again, to preserve the narrow margin of safety regarding bone strength.

Alignment

Proper alignment, i.e. a mechanical axis (Maquet et al. 1967) which passes through the center of the knee, is probably the single most important factor for the achievement of good long term results in knee arthroplasty (Lotke and Ecker 1977; Freeman et al. 1978; Coventry 1979; Rand and Bryan 1982; Bargren et al. 1983; Insall et al. 1983; Ecker et al. 1987). Specifically, subsidence has been correlated to malalignment (Insall et al. 1983; Albrektsson and Herberts 1988). Malpositioning of the tibial component, i.e. an angle deviating from the ideal one with reference to the long axis of the tibia, gives rise to considerable overload and shearing forces which jeopardize the fixation (Kagan 1977). Albrektsson and Herberts (1988) found that seven out of 11 ICLH arthroplasties which were malpositioned in this respect subsided.

In the RSA studies, neither alignment nor component position have been found to correlate with the magnitude of the overall migration (Ryd 1986). For noncemented PCA prostheses it has, however, been found that these factors correlate with progressive "third phase" migration. Thus malaligned knees or tibial components which deviated from the ideal position in the A–P projection resulted in significantly greater migration (MTPM) of the tibial components in the period after 2 years (Ryd et al. 1990). Although none of the arthroplasties in that report had failed after 4 years, the above mentioned implications of malalignment on long term results render such "third phase" migration ominous.

Proper alignment, therefore, is of the utmost importance to avoid subsidence, especially in uncemented cases.

Cement versus No Cement

Although susbsidence was reported for cemented prostheses, the literature suggests that it did not become an issue of concern until the introduction of uncemented prostheses. This may perhaps partly be explained by the fact that cement seems to "seal off" the proximal tibial cut and protects against bony overgrowth, which gives a false impression of subsidence on radiograms. Subsidence resulting in failure and revision has, however, been reported frequently in uncemented cases; the omission of cement then seems to make the arthroplasty particularly vulnerable to this type of complication. This stands to reason.

Cement serves to even out local irregularities and gives a smoother and more even stress transfer across the interface (Charnley 1960), i.e. the prosthesis is mechanically coupled to the bone. With the formation of soft tissue membranes (= "radiolucent zones"), these prostheses become "uncoupled" and may fail. Histological studies (Haddad et al. 1987; Cook et al. 1988; Hainau et al. 1989; Sumner et al. 1989) as well as the RSA studies suggest that the tibial component is not coupled to the bone in uncemented cases, i.e. sufficiently bony ingrowth does not consistently occur.

Why does not bony ingrowth consistently occur in humans despite the success in animal models (Bobyn et al. 1980; Hedley et al. 1982)? Ling (1986) has suggested a strain-stress diagram (Fig. 14.10) for prosthetic fixation where bony ingrowth is achieved only with minute strains. Such small strains can be obtained either with very secure initial fixation and/or with small initial loads. Available data suggest that this balance has not been struck (Manley et al. 1987) and that motion occurs in the interface during

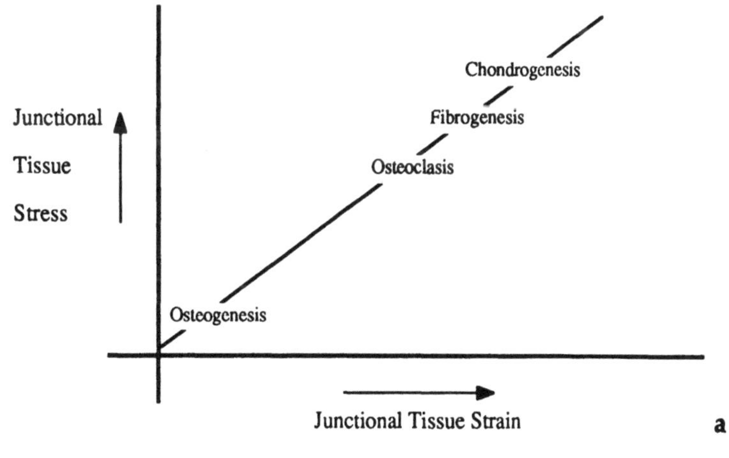

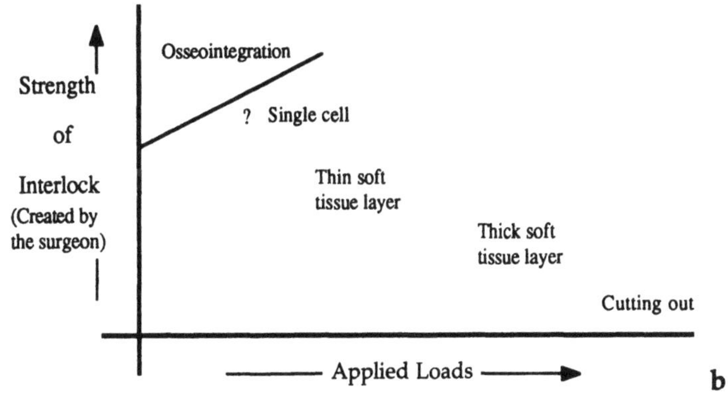

Fig. 14.10 a,b. Diagram of the connection between the mechanical properties of the interface region and the biological response in general terms (**a**) and specifically applied to knee arthroplasty (**b**) as suggested by Ling. (Reproduced by courtesy of the author and J.B. Lippincott.)

the postoperative period. Such motion prevents ingrowth (Cameron et al. 1973; Ducheyne et al. 1977; Hungerford and Kenna 1983).

How may micromotion between prostheses and bone be prevented? In a clinical study Whiteside and Pafford (1989) found a rather sturdy central stem to be a significant factor in protecting the soft cancellous bone and preventing anterolateral subsidence. Volz et al. (1988) studied the stability of various configurations of tibial components in an experimental model simulating everyday life and found subsidence and lift-off for a design with a central post and four cancellous bone screws only slightly greater than for a cemented component. Four screws or a central post resulted in larger micromotion, approximately 200–400 µm, while a design with two short pegs only resulted in large micromotion ranging up to 800 µm. Instantaneous inducible displacement for the PCA prosthesis of exactly the same magnitude was found by RSA. Further work on the design of the tibial components may thus be indicated.

Postoperative protected weight bearing is usually recommended after uncemented knee arthroplasty. There seems to be every reason for this recommendation. The loads across the knee can only be reduced to a certain extent, however, since postoperative motion exercises, giving considerable forces across the knee (Stulberg and Stulberg 1987), are a necessity. Possibly, CPM machines, which have otherwise been shown to be of little value in knee arthroplasty (Romness and Rand 1988), may have a particular place here as well as the use of shock absorbing insoles (Rööser et al. 1988). Together with principles known to be successful in achieving "bony ingrowth" in dental implants (osseointegration), such as atraumatic bone handling to avoid temperature trauma (Krause et al. 1982; Larsen and Ryd 1989) and close initial contact (Albrektsson and Albrektsson 1987), the concept of "bony ingrowth" may ultimately be successful.

Prevention in the Clinical Situation

Supported by the literature as well as by RSA data a plan of action in order to avoid subsidence can be envisaged. In the clinical situation a number of the factors here analyzed are beyond the control of the operating surgeon. Age, diagnosis, bone strength, of course, cannot be changed but these factors should be used as selection criteria. When inferior fixation can be anticipated because of poor bone quality, as in rheumatoid patients or when large osteoarthrotic bone cysts are present, a choice of procedure with the largest margin of safety should be considered. In such a case a large tibial component, resting on as much cancellous bone as possible, should be chosen. The component should have a central stem which abuts on the posterior cortex and cement should be used for optimum stress transfer.

When an uncemented procedure is considered, for example in young patients, minute attention to details in the operative technique is mandatory. One such important detail is alignment which must be within a couple of degrees from the optimum. The resection surfaces must be perfectly even and care should be taken to avoid improper damage to the bone tissue. In these cases every effort should be made to avoid postoperative micromotion of the prosthesis. Absolutely protected weight bearing is mandatory, and perhaps these patients should be trained preoperatively to use crutches consistently. CPM as well as thick rubber insoles can be considered.

References

Alberius P (1983) Bone reaction to tanatalum markers. A scanning electron microscopic study. Acta Anat 115: 310–318

Albrektsson T, Albrektsson B (1987) Osseointegration of bone implants. A review of an alternative mode of fixation. Acta Orthop Scand 58: 567–577

Albrektsson BEJ, Herberts P (1988) ICLH knee arthroplasty. A consecutive study of 108 knees with uncemented tibial component fixation. J Arthroplasty 3: 145–156

Albrektsson BEJ, Ryd L, Carlsson LV et al. (1990) The effect of a stem on the tibial component; A roentgen stereophotogrammetric analysis of stemmed and non-stemmed, uncemented tibial components in clinically successful Freeman-Samuelson knee arthroplasties. J Bone Joint Surg (Br) 72: 252–258

Amstutz HC, Ouzounian T, Grauer D, Flink C, Kirkpatrik J, Bassett L (1986) The grid radiograph. J Bone Joint Surg (Am) 68: 1052–1056

Andriacchi TP, Galante JO, Fermier RW (1982) The influence of total knee-replacement design on walking and stair climbing. J Bone Joint Surg (Am) 64: 1328–1335

Audell RA, Cracchiolo A (1987) The use of implants with

polyethylene peg fixation in total knee arthroplasty. In: Rand JA, Dorr LD (eds) Total arthroplasty of the knee. Proceedings of the Knee Society, 1985–1986. Aspen Publ. Inc., Rockville, Ma
Bargren JH, Day WH, Freeman MAR, Swanson SAV (1978) Mechanical tests on the tibial components of non hinged knee prostheses. J Bone Joint Surg (Br) 60: 256–261
Bargren JH, Blaha JD, Freeman MAR (1983) Alignment in total knee arthroplasty. Clin Orthop 173: 178–183
Bartel DL, Burstein AH, Santavicca EA, Insall JN (1982) Performance of the tibial component in total knee replacement. J Bone Joint Surg (Am) 64: 1026–1033
Blaha JD, Insler HP, Freeman MAR, Revell PA, Todd RC (1982) The fixation of proximal tibial polyethylene prosthesis without cement. J Bone Joint Surg (Br) 64: 326–335
Bobyn JD, Pilliar RM, Cameron HU, Weatherly GC (1980) The optimum pore size for the fixation of porous-surfaced metal implants by the ingrowth of bone. Clin Orthop 150: 263–270
Boegård T, Brattström H, Lidgren L (1984) Seventy-four Attenborough knee replacements for rheumatoid arthritis. Acta Orthop Scand 55: 166–171
Bourne RB, Finlay JB (1986) The influence of tibial component intramedullary stems and implant-cortex contact on the strain distribution of the proximal tibia following tibial knee arthroplasty. Clin Orthop 208: 95–99
Cameron HU, Hunter GA (1982) Failure in total knee arthoplasty. Clin Orthop 170: 141–145
Cameron HU, McNeice GM (1981) Mechanical failure modes in total knee replacements. Arch Orthop Traumat Surg 98: 135–138
Cameron HU, Pilliar RM, MacNab I (1973) The effect of movement on the bonding of porous metal to bone. J Biomed Mater Res 7: 301–311
Charnley J (1960) Anchorage of the femoral head prosthesis to the shaft of the femur. J Bone Joint Surg (Br) 42: 28–30
Cheal EJ, Hayes WC, Lee CH, Snyder BD, Miller J (1985) Stress analysis of a condylar knee tibial component: Influence of metaphyseal shell properties and cement injection depth. J Orthop Res 3: 424–434
Colley J, Cameron HU, Freeman MAR, Swanson SAV (1978) Loosening of the femoral component in surface replacement of the knee. Arch Orthop Trauma Surg 92: 31–34
Convery FR, Minteer-Convery M, Malcom LL (1980) The spherocentric knee: a re-evaluation and modification. J Bone Joint Surg (Am) 62: 320–327
Cook SD, Thomas KA, Haddad RJ (1988) Histologic analysis of retrieved human porous-coated total joint components. Clin Orthop 234: 90–101
Coventry M (1979) Two-part total knee arthroplasty. Evolution and present status. Clin Orthop 145: 29–36
Cracchiolo A, Benson M, Finerman GAM, Horacek K, Amstutz HC (1979) A prospective comparative clinical analysis of the first-generation knee replacements. Clin Orthop 145: 37–46
Derburge A, Aubriot JH, Genet JP and the GUEPAR group (1979) Current status of a hinged prosthesis (GUEPAR). Clin Orthop 145: 91–93
Ducheyne P, DeMeester P, Aernoudt E, Martens M, Mulier JC (1977) Influence of functional dynamic loading on bone ingrowth into surface pores of orthopedic implants. J Biomed Mater Res 11: 811–838
Ducheyne P, Kagan A, Lacey JA (1978) Failure of total knee arthroplasty due to loosening and deformation of the tibial component. J Bone Joint Surg (Am) 60: 384–391
Ecker ML, Lotke PA, Windsor RE, Cella JP (1987) Long-term results after Total Condylar knee arthroplasty. Clin Orthop 216: 151–158
Figgie HE, Davy DT, Heiple KG, Hart RT (1984) Load-bearing capacity of the tibial component of the Total Condylar prosthesis. Clin Orthop 183: 288–297
Freeman MAR, Todd RC, Bamert P, Day WH (1978) ICLH arthroplasty of the knee: 1968–1977. J Bone Joint Surg (Br) 60: 339–344
Freeman MAR, Blaha JD, Brown G et al. (1981) Cementless fixation of a tibial component for the knee. 27th Annual ORS, 157
Goldberg VM, Figgie MP, Figgie III HE, Heiple KG, Sobel M (1988) Use of a Total Condylar prosthesis for treatment of osteoarthritis and rheumatoid arthritis. J Bone Joint Surg (Am) 70: 802–811
Goldstein SA, Wilson DL, Sonstegard DA, Matthews LS (1983) The mechanical properties of human tibial trabecular bone as a function of metaphyseal location. J Biomech 16: 965–969
Greene DL, Bahniuk E, Liebelt RA, Fender E, Mirkov P (1983) Biplane radiographic measurements of reversible displacement (including clinical loosening) and migration of total joint replacements. J Bone Joint Surg (Am) 65: 1134–1143
Haddad RJ, Cook SD, Thomas KA (1987) Current concept review. Biological fixation of porous coated implants. J Bone Joint Surg (Am) 69: 1459
Hainau B, Reiman I, Dorph S et al. (1989) Porous-coated knee arthroplasty. A case report concerning bony ingrowth. Clin Orthop 239: 178–184
Harrington IJ (1976) A bioengineering analysis of force actions at the knee in normal and pathological gait. Biomed Eng 11: 167–172
Harris WH (1984) Advances in total hip arthroplasty. Clin Orthop 183: 4–11
Hedley AK, Clarke JC, Kozinn SC et al. (1982) Porous ingrowth fixation of the femoral component in a canine surface replacement of the hip. Clin Orthop 163: 300–311
Hungerford DS, Kenna RV (1983) Preliminary experience with a total knee prosthesis with porous coating used without cement. Clin Orthop 176: 95–107
Hungerford DS, Krackow KA (1985) Total joint arthroplasty of the knee. Clin Orthop 192: 23–33
Hvid I (1988) Trabecular bone strength at the knee. Clin Orthop 227: 210–222
Hvid I, Hansen SL (1986) Subchondral bone strength in arthrosis. Acta Orthop Scand 57: 47–51
Hvid I, Jensen J (1984) Cancellous bone strength at the proximal human tibia. Eng Med; 13: 21–25
Hvid I, Jensen J, Nielsen S (1985) Contribution of the cortex to the epiphyseal strength. Acta Orthop Scand 56: 256–259
Insall JN, Kelly M (1986) The Total Condylar knee prosthesis. Clin Orthop 205: 43–48
Insall JN, Hood RW, Flawn LB, Sullivan DJ (1983) The Total Condylar knee prosthesis in gonarthrosis. J Bone Joint Surg (Am) 65: 619–627
Jónsson G (1981) Compartmental arthroplasty for gonarthrosis. Acta Orthop Scand 52: Suppl 193
Kagan A (1977) Mechanical causes of loosening in knee joint replacements. J Biomech 10: 387–391
Kaufer H, Matthews LS (1979) Spherocentric knee arthroplasty. Clin Orthop 145: 110–116
Kaufer H, Matthews LS (1981) Spherocentric arthroplasty of the knee. J Bone Joint Surg (Am) 63: 545–559
Kaufer H, Matthews LS, Sonstegard DA (1978) Total knee loosening. Symposium on reconstructive surgery. CV Mosby, St. Louis
Kenna RV, Hungerford DS (1984) Design rationale for the Porous Coated Anatomic total knee system. In: Hungerford DS, Krackow KA, Kenna RV (eds) Total knee arthroplasty. A comprehensive approach. William & Wilkins, Baltimore, London

Krause WR, Bradburg DW, Kelly JE Lunceford EM (1982) Temperature elevation in orthopedic cutting operations. J Biomech 15(4): 267–275
Lacey JA (1978) A statistical review of 100 consecutive UCI low friction knee arthroplasties with analysis of results. Clin Orthop 132: 163–166
Larsen ST, Ryd L (1989) Heat elevation during knee arthroplasty. Acta Orthop Scand 60:439–442
Laskin RS (1976) Modular total knee-replacement arthroplasty. J Bone Joint Surg (Am) 58: 766–773
Laskin RS (1988) Tricon-M uncemented total knee arthroplasty. J Arthroplasty 3: 27–38
Larsson SE, Ahlgren O (1979) Reconstruction with endoprosthesis in gonarthrosis. Clin Orthop 145: 126–135
Larsson SE, Larsson S, Lundquist S (1988) Unicompartmental knee arthroplasty. A prospective consecutive series followed for 6 to 11 years. Clin Orthop 232: 174–181
Lewis JL, Askew MJ, Jaycox DP (1982) A comparative evaluation of tibial component design of total knee prostheses. J Bone Joint Surg (Am) 64: 129–135
Ling RSM (1986) Observations on the fixation of implants to the bony skeleton. Clin Orthop 210: 80
Lotke PA, Ecker ML (1977) Influence of positioning of prostheses in total knee replacement. J Bone Joint Surg (Am) 59: 77–79
Manley MT, Stulberg BN, Stern LS, Watson JT, Stulberg SD (1987) Direct observation of micromotion at the implant-bone interface with cemented and noncemented tibial components. 33rd Annual ORS: 436
Maquet P, Simonet J, De Marchin P (1967) Biomechanique du genou et gonarthrose. Revue Chir Orthop 53: 111–138
Marmor L (1985) Unicompartmental knee arthroplasty. Clin Orthop 192: 75–81
Miller J (1984) Fixation in total knee arthroplasty. In: Insall JN (ed) Surgery of the knee. Churchill Livingstone, New York
Mjöberg B (1986) Loosening of the cemented hip prosthesis. Acta Orthop Scand 57 [Suppl 221]
Morrison JB (1970) The mechanics of the knee in relation to normal walking. J Biomech 3: 51–61
Murray RP, Hayes WC, Edwards WT, Harry JD (1984) Mechanical properties of the subchondral plate and the metaphyseal shell. 30th Annual ORS, 9
Rand JA, Bryan RS (1982) Revision after total knee arthroplasty. Orthop Clin N Am 13(1): 201–212
Rand JA, Coventry MB (1988) Ten-year evaluation of Geometric total knee arthroplasty. Clin Orthop 232: 168–173
Rand JA, Bryan RS, Chao EYS, Ilstrup DM (1987) A comparison of cemented versus cementless Porous Coated Anatomic total knee arthroplasty. In: Rand JA, Dorr LD (eds) Total arthroplasty of the knee. Proceedings of the Knee Society, 1985–1986. Aspen Publ. Inc., Rockville, Ma.
Romness DW, Rand JA (1988) The role of continuous passive motion following total knee arthroplasty. Clin Orthop 226: 34–37
Rööser B, Ekbladh R, Lidgren L (1988) The shock-absorbing effect of soles and insoles. Int Orthop 12: 335.338
Ryd L (1986) Micromotion in knee arthroplasty. A roentgen stereophotogrammetric analysis of tibial component fixation. Acta Orthop Scand Suppl 220
Ryd L, Boegård T, Egund N, Thorngren KG (1983) Migration of the tibial component in successful unicompartmental knee arthroplasty. Acta Orthop Scand 54: 408–416
Ryd L, Lindstrand A, Rosenquist R, Selvik G (1986) Tibial component fixation in knee arthroplasty. Clin Orthop 213: 141–149
Ryd L, Lindstrand A, Rosenquist R, Selvik G (1987) Micromotion of conventionally cemented all-polyethylene tibial components in total knee replacements. Arch Orthop Trauma Surg 106: 82–88
Ryd L, Albrektsson BEJ, Herberts P, Lindstrand A, Selvik G (1988) Micromotion of noncemented Freeman-Samuelson prostheses for gonarthrosis. Clin Orthop 229: 205–212
Ryd L, Lindstrand A, Stenström A, Selvik G (1990) PCA tricompartmental tibial components; relation between prosthetic position and micromotion. Clin Orthop 251: 189–197
Samuelson KM (1987) Fixation in total knee arthroplasty: interference fit. In: Rand JA, Dorr LD (eds) Total arthroplasty of the knee. Proceedings of the Knee Society, 1985–1986. Aspen Publ. Inc., Rockville, Ma.
Schneider R, Freiberger RH, Ghelman B, Ranawat CS (1982) Radiologic evaluation of knee arthroplasty. Orthop Clin N Am 13(1): 225–244
Selvik G (1974) A roentgen stereophotogrammetric system for the study of the kinematics of the skeletal systems. Thesis, Universtity of Lund, Lund. Reprint in: Acta Orthop Scand 1989; 60 [Suppl. 232]
Shindell R, Neumann R, Conolly JF, Jardon M (1986) Evaluation of the Noiles hinged knee prosthesis. J Bone Joint Surg (Am) 68: 579–585
Skolnick MD, Coventry MB, Ilstrup DM (1976) Geometric total knee arthroplasty. J Bone Joint Surg (Am) 58: 749–753
Stulberg SD, Stulberg BN (1987) The biological response to uncemented total knee replacements. In: Rand JA, Dorr LD (eds) Total arthroplasty of the knee. Proceedings of the Knee Society 1985–1986. Aspen Publ. Inc., Rockville, Ma.
Sumner DR, Jacobs JJ, Turner TM, Urban RM, Galante JO (1989) The amount and distribution of bone ingrowth in tibial components retrieved from human patients. 35th Annual ORS: 375
Thornhill TS, Dalziel RW, Sledge CB (1982) Alternatives to arthrodesis for the failed total knee replacement. Clin Orthop 170: 131–140
Townley CO (1985) The Anatomic Total Knee resurfacing arthroplasty. Clin Orthop 192: 82–96
Volz RG, Nisbet JK, Lee RW, McMurty MG (1988) The mechanical stability of various noncemented tibial components. Clin Orthop 226: 38–42
Walker PS, Ranawat C, Insall J (1976) Fixation of the tibial components of condylar replacement knee prostheses. J Biomech 9: 269–275
Walker PS, Greene D, Reilly D et al. (1981) Fixation of tibial components of knee prostheses. J Bone Joint Surg (Am) 63: 258–267
Walldius B (1957) Arthroplasty of the knee joint using endoprosthesis. Acta Orthop Scand 27 [Suppl 19]
Whiteside LA, Pafford J (1989) Load transfer characteristics of a non-cemented total knee arthroplasty. Clin Orthop 239: 168–177
Wykman A, Selvik G, Goldie I (1988) Subsidence of the femoral component in the noncemented total hip: a roentgen stereophotogrammetric analysis. Acta Orthop Scand 59: 635–637
Yuzuki O (1978) Study on the mechanical strength and the inner structure of the knee. J Jpn Orthop Assoc 52: 537–549

Chapter 15

The Management of Bone Loss in Total Knee Replacement

Thomas P. Sculco, Hans W. Springorum, Ugo De Nicola, Walter J. Lowe and Richard S. Laskin

Bone Grafting in Total Knee Replacement

Thomas P. Sculco

Introduction

Over the past two decades, total knee arthroplasty has evolved into one of the most successful of orthopaedic procedures. The quality of the clinical result has become predictable and reproducible, pain is relieved, and function improved. These excellent results have been obtained in patients with and without severe angular deformities. This chapter, however, will concern itself with those more complicated knees with marked angular deformities in the varus/valgus, flexion/extension, or rotatory planes associated with bone defects.

Bone loss occurs most commonly on the tibial side of the joint. Most often it is localized posteriorly on the plateau due to the frequently associated flexion contracture. There may be associated fragmentation of the tibial plateau, but, as a rule, the tibial surface is flattened, extremely sclerotic and completely devoid of cartilage. Because there is frequently a subluxation of the femur on the tibia, there tends to be little, if any, preserved peripheral tibial rim. Consequently there is a steep descent from the middle of the tibial surface to the periphery.

Femoral bone loss on the concave side of an angular deformity occurs with much less frequency that does tibial bone loss. The sclerotic quality of the femoral subchondral bone and the ramshorn configuration of the distal femoral condyle favors the tibia collapsing rather than the femur. When femoral condylar collapse does occur there may be an element of osteonecrosis present which facilitates the destruction.

If marked degrees of bone loss are associated with fragmentation of bone, one must suspect an underlying neuropathic condition. Severe degrees of deformity with marked loss of joint stability are present and these are often out of proportion to the degree of pain. A careful history and neurological examination is paramount in these patients. The commonest cause of neuropathic joints in the United States is diabetes mellitus. Successful total knee replacement (or any other procedure) in the neuropathic knee is unlikely and therefore this pathologic entity should be viewed as a contraindication to total knee replacement.

The management of bone deficiency in total knee arthroplasty will vary depending upon the location and degree of the bone loss. Various methods have been employed with success including the use of methylmethacrylate alone (Lotke et al. 1985), methylmethacrylate reinforced with mesh or screws (Ritter 1986), bone grafting (Altchek et al. 1989; Dorr and Ranawat 1984; Dorr et al. 1986; Laskin et al. 1985; Ranawat

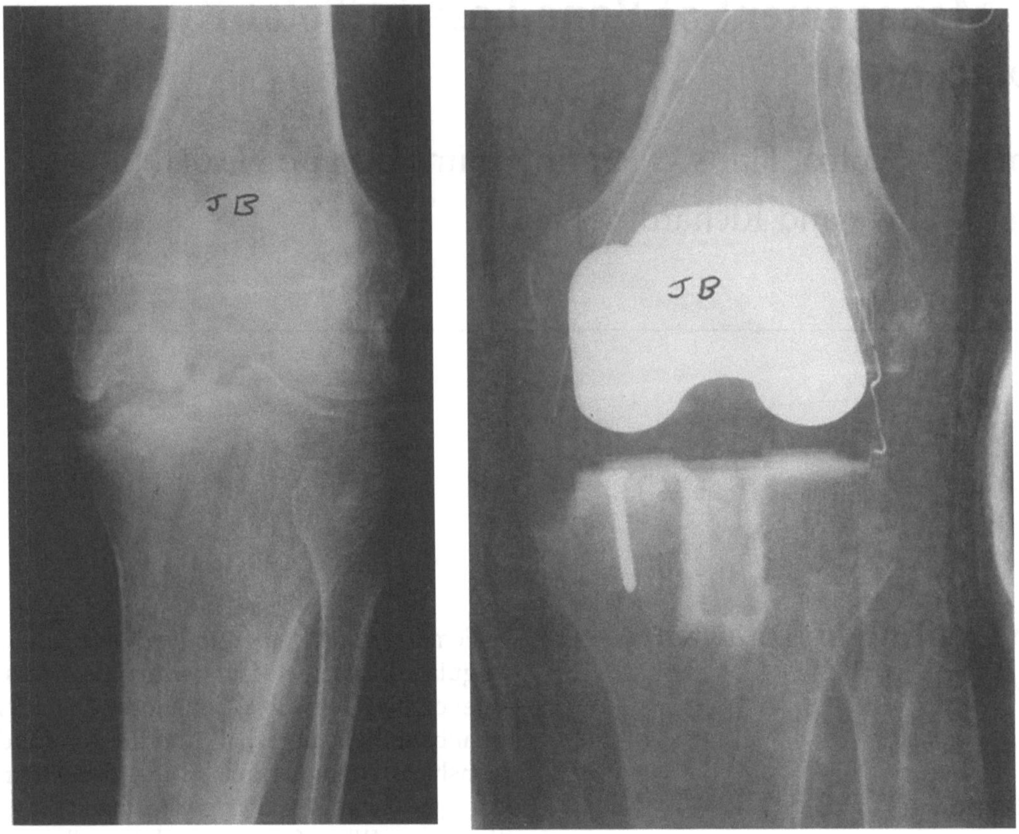

a b

Fig. 15.1 a,b. Treatment of small tibial defect. **a** Pre-operative X-ray. **b** Postoperative X-ray. The defect has been filled with methylmethacrylate supplemented by a cortical screw.

1985; Windsor et al. 1986) and the use of custom or augmented modular knee implants (Insall 1984).

Except in the mildest of bone defects (less than 8 mm) the tendency to resect additional bone from the tibia must be resisted. A series of problems arises when bone is resected too far distally, and these will further complicate the technique of the arthroplasty and any necessary subsequent revision surgery. If excess bone is removed the flexion gap is increased, requiring a thick implant for stability. This will alter the patellofemoral kinematics as the patella, tethered by the patellar tendon, will descend and may come into frank contact with the tibial implant itself. Furthermore the tibial component becomes seated on poor quality cancellous bone. Sizing problems will likewise occur because of the diminished cross-sectional area as one progresses down the tibia distally. Lowering the resection line on the tibia to deal with bone loss is an unsatisfactory method and should be utilized for only the smallest of defects.

Tibial Bone Loss

Defects 6–10 mm in Depth

There are several techniques to deal with bone loss on the tibial side of the joint which is less than 10 mm in depth and which encompasses less than one half of the tibial plateau surface.

Resection up to 8 mm can be performed. This may leave only a small defect remaining. In those cases, the remaining sclerotic bed is fenestrated with an 1/8 inch drill to allow penetration of bone cement into the subchondral bone. Up to 3 mm of remaining void can be filled with methylmethacrylate cement. Small amounts of unsupported methylmethacrylate have not been reported to fracture with time. Larger columns of methylmethacrylate, however, may fracture and initial support may be lost. This is especially true in the patient in which optimal alignment has not been achieved.

If after resecting the tibial plateau, a defect of 3–5 mm remains, screws can be used to reinforce the methylmethacrylate column. Two cortical screws are usually used placed in the area of the defect. The heads of the screws are placed so as to be just below the metallic tray of the tibial component. Acrylic cement is used surrounding the screws to fill the bone deficit. In order to avoid electrolytic problems, synergistic metals must be used for the screws and the metal base plate (Fig. 15.1 a,b).

Defects Greater than 12 mm in Depth

For defects greater than 12 mm in depth and in those encompassing more than 50% of the tibial surface an implant with a metallic wedge filler may be used (Insall 1984). Initially these implants had to be fabricated on a custom basis. At times, however, the implant in the operating room itself would not accurately fill the defect resulting in an unsupported column of acrylic between the wedge and the bone (Fig. 15.2). This column of acrylic could fragment causing loss of implant position. Furthermore, custom implants are costly and require considerable time for fabrication.

More recent advances in implant design have led to the evolution of modular component systems. These allow addition of metallic wedges of various thicknesses directly to the undersurface of the tibial component at surgery. The advantage of these devices lies in their flexibility and the ability essentially to build the component that is needed at the operating table.

In my experience, the best option available to the surgeon confronted with large tibial defects is the use of autogenous bone grafting procedures. The use of autogenous graft preserves bone stock. Furthermore it is theoretically attractive since the material used to support the implant is biologically active.

Autogenous bone is readily available at the time of primary total knee arthroplasty and can be harvested from a number of areas. Laskin et al. (1985) and Laskin (1989b) have reported on bone utilized from the posterior femoral condyle to use to fill tibial defects. This is a useful technique, however, at times this bone tends to be somewhat scant and not well suited since it is primarily subchondral and cortical with little cancellous substrate. The technique I will describe is the one that I have used for the past ten years and utilizes bone resected from the distal femur (Altchek et al. 1989; Windsor et al. 1986).

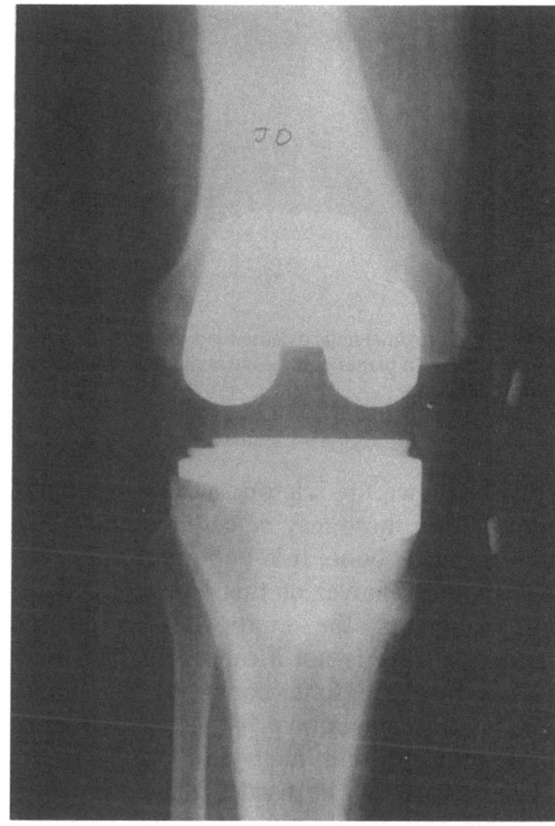

Fig. 15.2. A custom tibial prosthesis has been used. It is resting on an unsupported methylmethacrylate column due to an imprecise fit of the custom implant to the defect at the time of surgery.

The initial tibial proximal cut is made utilizing a standard tibial cutting guide. We are conservative in this proximal tibial cut, resecting at no time more than 8 mm of bone. An oscillating saw is then used to create an oblique osteotomy on the side of the tibial defect (Fig. 15.3). The concave surface of the defect should be resected. The deep surface of the bed should be 80%–90% cancellous in nature. There may be cystic areas

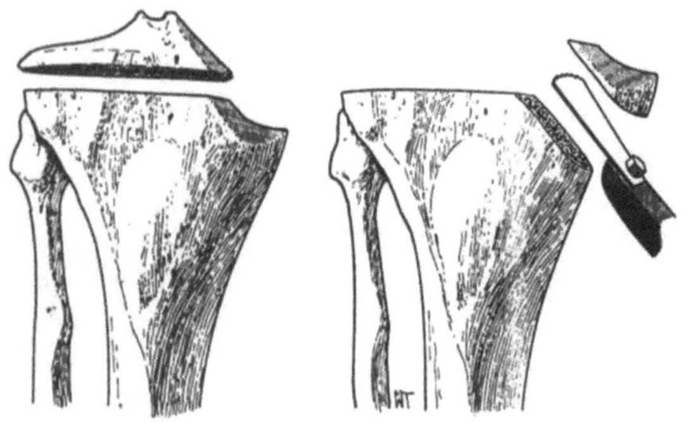

Fig. 15.3. The proximal tibial osteotomy is made in the usual manner and then a planar oblique cut is made to the base of the tibial deficiency.

in this bed once the sclerotic surface has been removed, and these may be curetted and filled with cancellous bone. It is important not to be timid in the removal of this sclerotic bed as consolidation of the graft will be greatly impeded if there is not a cancellous bed onto which to place the donor bone. The cut should be planar and smooth so that a flattened graft will fit intimately with the bed.

If the implant to be used has a central peg hole, this hole should now be made. This will assure that the fixation pins that are inserted can be placed so as to avoid the central stem hole. For implants with peripheral fixation peg holes this step is of less importance.

The next step is to remove the distal femoral bone. Generally, the resected distal medial femoral condyle is larger than the lateral condyle and therefore tends to be the better graft material. Having resected the distal femoral condyle, this segment of bone is rotated so that its cancellous surface faces against the cancellous surface of the recipient bed (Fig. 15.4). The defect should be filled by the bone. There will be an overhanging segment of bone which protrudes above the cut surface of the tibia. If there is any gaping between the bone and the recipient bed, the bed must be shaved. Once coaptation is precise, two K-wires may be used to stabilize the graft to the proximal tibia. The wires should be inserted from the periphery. After the graft is fixed in position, the overhanging bone should be removed using the tibial cut on the opposite tibial plateau as a guide. At this point the proximal tibia will be reconstituted. On observing the tibia from the top, the subchondral bone of the femoral condylar bone graft will act as the peripheral tibial bone of the upper tibia.

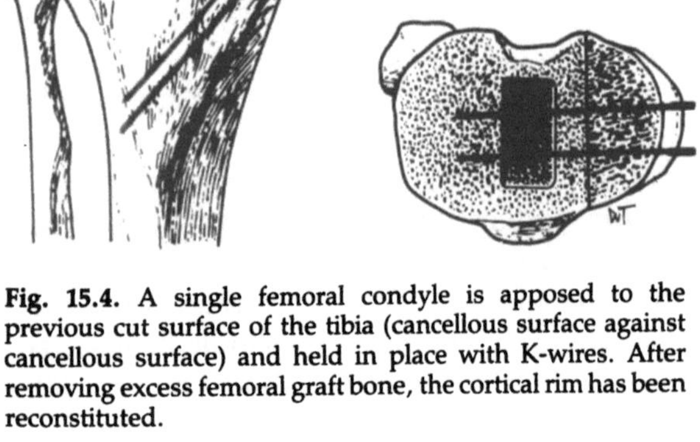

Fig. 15.4. A single femoral condyle is apposed to the previous cut surface of the tibia (cancellous surface against cancellous surface) and held in place with K-wires. After removing excess femoral graft bone, the cortical rim has been reconstituted.

The K-wires are then individually removed and replaced with screws. Cancellous malleolar screws may be used for fixation. As an alternative one can use cortical screws and overdrill peripherally so as to allow a lag effect. The peg hole should be examined when the holes are drilled. The screws should not violate or contact the peg of the tibial prosthesis, particularly if stainless steel screws are used.

It is of utmost importance that cement not be allowed to enter the interval between the graft and recipient bed. An excellent method of preventing this is to cement the femoral component first and use a small bit of doughy cement to caulk the upper surface of the tibia along the line of the graft and tibial host bone. This will harden so that when the lower viscosity tibial cement is inserted it will not penetrate into the graft interface. We devised this technique after our first case of bone grafting in which cement entered the graft-bed interface. The graft became sclerotic. We were fortunate, however, that there was some consolidation in the depth of the graft so that neither collapse nor prosthetic settling occurred (Fig. 15.5 a–c).

Postoperative rehabilitation for these patients is the same as for those patients without bone grafting. Because the tibial implant support is maintained on the more normal side of the tibia, and since the graft is securely fixed to the tibia, we have not felt that we must limit weight

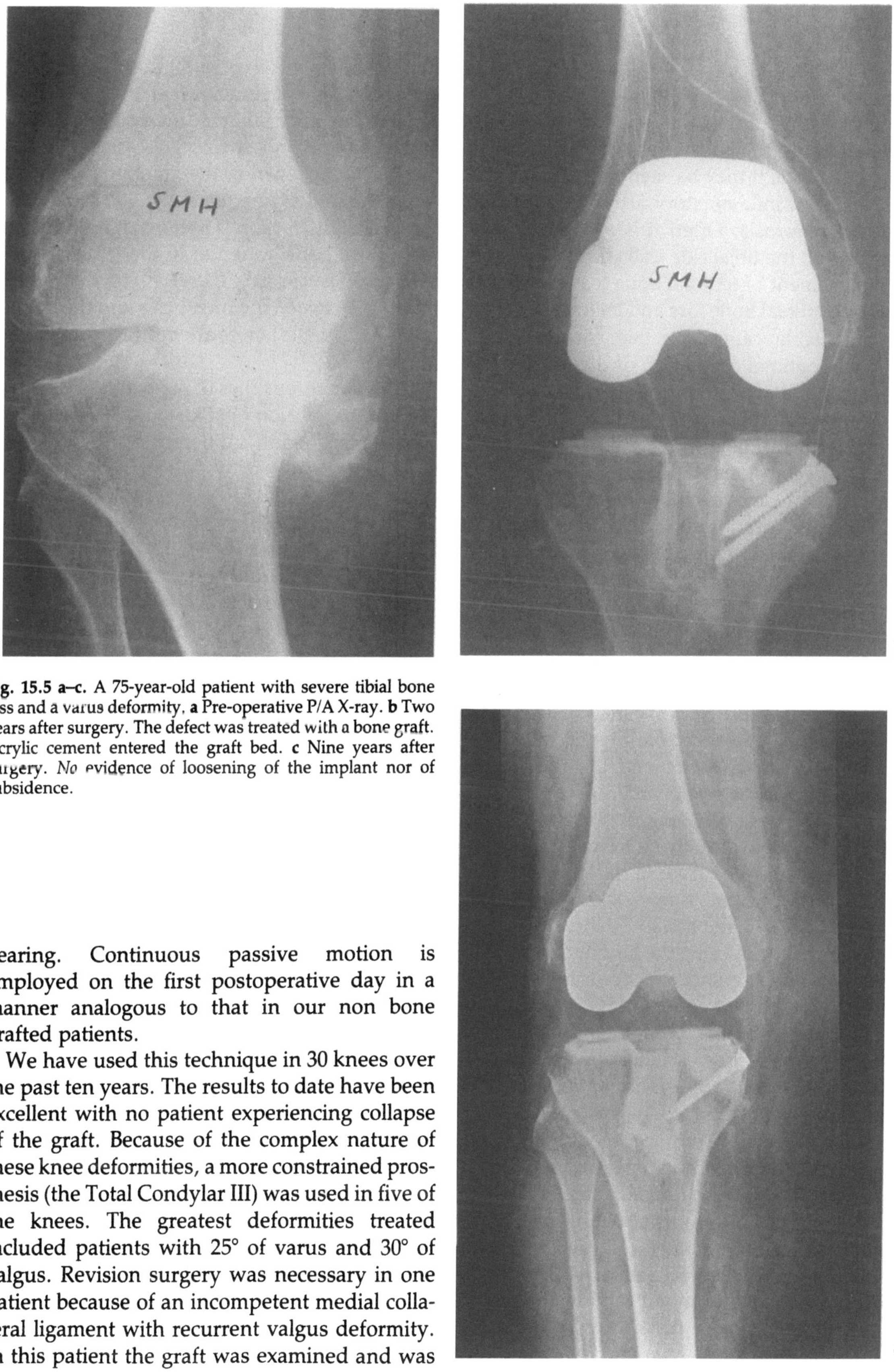

a b c

Fig. 15.5 a–c. A 75-year-old patient with severe tibial bone loss and a varus deformity. a Pre-operative P/A X-ray. b Two years after surgery. The defect was treated with a bone graft. Acrylic cement entered the graft bed. c Nine years after surgery. No evidence of loosening of the implant nor of subsidence.

bearing. Continuous passive motion is employed on the first postoperative day in a manner analogous to that in our non bone grafted patients.

We have used this technique in 30 knees over the past ten years. The results to date have been excellent with no patient experiencing collapse of the graft. Because of the complex nature of these knee deformities, a more constrained prosthesis (the Total Condylar III) was used in five of the knees. The greatest deformities treated included patients with 25° of varus and 30° of valgus. Revision surgery was necessary in one patient because of an incompetent medial collateral ligament with recurrent valgus deformity. In this patient the graft was examined and was found to be completely consolidated at the interface.

Femoral Bone Loss

Femoral bone loss occurs less commonly than tibial bone loss. It may be seen in posttraumatic arthritis or in inflammatory arthritis associated with osteonecrosis. Often it is associated with bone loss on the tibial side as well. The precepts of management of femoral bone loss are similar to those for tibial bone loss and include developing a suitable cancellous bed for the graft, achieving optimal coaptation of the graft to the bed, maintaining position of the graft with internal fixation devices, and re-establishing the joint line to its normal height.

The surgeon must adequately expose the distal femoral condyles in order to visualize the anterior and posterior margins of the bone. Any soft tissue at the interface between the collapsed and normal bone must be debrided from the bony surface of the femur to allow thorough evaluation of the defect. If the defect is primarily cystic without larger areas of segmental condylar loss, cancellous bone from the intercondylar area or from the tibial peg hole may be used to fill the defects. Bone can be compressed into these cavities with an impactor and the face of the femoral condylar osteotomy then shaped so as to accept the femoral component.

For extensive defects, bone from the intercondylar area may be used to fill the deficient condyle. The fixation screw(s) is inserted directly into the graft and advanced into the underlying femoral bone along the longitudinal axis of the femur. Since contact may occur between the femoral component and screw, compatible metals must be used. Care must be taken to insure that the recipient bed is primarily cancellous and that close apposition is present at the graft site. For small grafts in this area, K-wire fixation alone may be sufficient.

When determining the proper location for the joint line it should be remembered that the articular surface of the distal femur is approximately 17–20 mm from the most distal portion of the origins of the collateral ligaments. The articulating surface of the femoral component should be placed at this same distance from the collateral ligament origins.

Bone Grafting in Revision Total Knee Arthroplasty

Bone deficiency is a common finding in revision knee replacement surgery. It at times may be the cause of the knee failing, or it may be produced when the implants themselves are removed at the revision. Levering the component off may cause the underlying bone to collapse and fracture. Axial distraction is preferred, but even this may cause bone adhering to the component to avulse. It is crucial, therefore to disrupt the interface between the prosthesis and the bone as much as possible before attempting to extract the implant.

There are three types of bone defects found at the time of revision total knee replacement, and each is managed in a different manner.

Cystic Deficiencies

Cystic deficiencies are generally encountered on the surfaces of the tibia and femur after removal of the implants. They may be the result of acrylic which has penetrated into the subchondral bone and produced a punctate crater. They also may occur when the implant itself is removed from the bone and portions of the bone adhere to the implant. If the femoral component has condylar fixation pegs these may produce cystic areas of bone loss in the underlying bone. Usually these cystic areas are associated with larger plateau or condylar deficiencies and therefore combined techniques to handle both problems must be employed.

Cystic defects are easily filled with cancellous bone available locally at the time of revision. The base of the deficiency should be cleared of any adherent cement and soft tissue. The cancellous bone should be driven deep into the depression with an impactor. If sufficient bone is not available locally, iliac crest or allograft bone can be used. Normally we require bone from these other sources to augment larger deficiencies as well in the revision patient.

Central Medullary Deficiency

Central medullary bone deficiencies (Fig. 15.6 a,b) may be present on the femur or tibia during

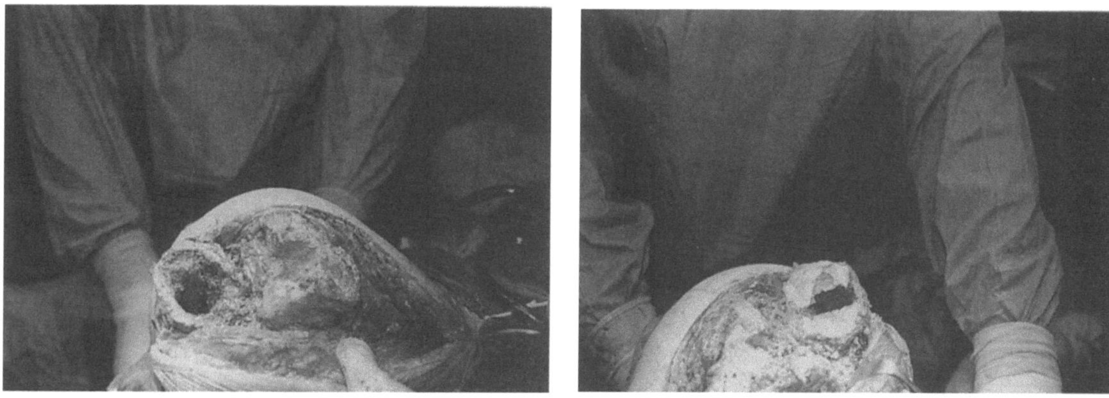

a b

Fig. 15.6 a,b. Large central medullary bone loss. a Large cavity noted in central tibia. b Treatment by autogenous bone grafting.

revision surgery. These most often occur if the primary implants used had central stems. This type of deficiency on the tibial side is usually funnel shaped. Often only the cortical rim is left without any cancellous plateau support on the medial or lateral side. If one is revising a hinged implant with a bulky femoral axle, there will also be a large amount of femoral bone loss. In some cases, the entire femoral condylar bone may be absent.

Because of the poor quality of supporting bone on the surface of the femur and tibia in these cases the surgeons must both add bone to the deficient areas, and then stress bypass the deficient bone by using long intramedullary stems. Usually autogenous bone is inadequate to deal with these larger defects even if the entire iliac crest is used. Femoral head allograft bone is often needed. It is shaped and placed so as to fill the defects and held in place by screws. There is some concern, however in using large fragments of allograft bone in that incorporation may remain incomplete and resorption of the graft may eventually occur.

To allow transfer of load away from the graft, stemmed components should be used. Now, with the availability of modular total knee systems, we are able to use large diameter fluted stems to bypass the previous stemmed area of the bone and obtain fixation in the more normal cortical bone. These stems are press fit in place, and cement is not inserted into the canals. Careful pre-operative planning is mandatory in these cases so that implants of the proper length and diameter are available.

Peripheral Tibial Plateau or Condylar Bone Loss

Peripheral rather than intramedullary loss can occur in those cases in which the previous implant had been malaligned. Bone collapse occurs on the overloaded side of the implant with tension forces on the opposite side causing lift off of the implant from the bone. The bone that is lost is wedge shaped either on the tibia or on the femur (Fig. 15.7). At times the entire plateau or condyle may collapse.

One must avoid the tendency to resect further bone to get below the base of the defect. We suggest using autogenous bone from the iliac crest or allograft to fill the defect. A large plate-like graft should be used. This graft should have a cortical component to it so as to prevent collapse once it is loaded. We have used the iliac crest with its cancellous surface against the cancellous surface of the tibial defect and its cortical surface apposed to the underside of the implant. Fenestrations should be made through the cortical surface, however, so as to allow interdigitation of the cement.

Although we prefer to use bone graft, modular wedge component may also be used for these large defects (Fig. 15.8). These are currently available and can be attached either with acrylic cement or screws to the undersurface of the tibial component. This method is useful in patients in whom bone is not available. Modular augments are also available to fill bone defects in the area of the distal and posterior femoral condyles. These metal fillers come in varying thicknesses and are

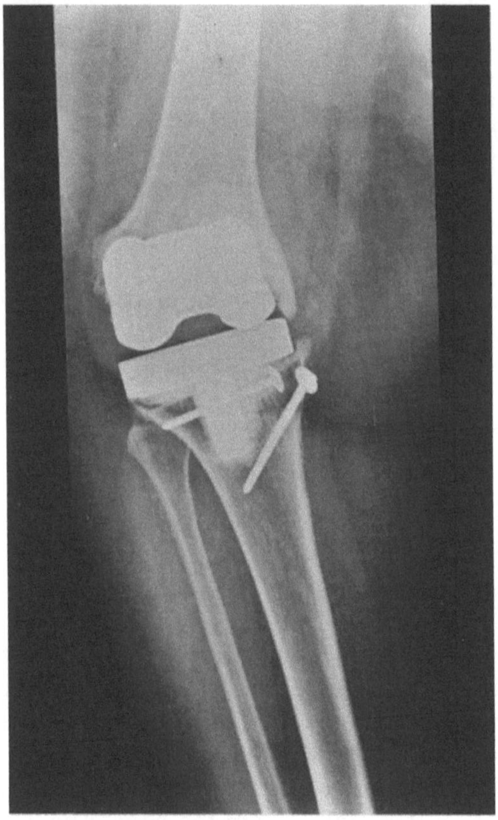

Fig. 15.7. Failed total knee replacement due to collapse of femoral condylar bone.

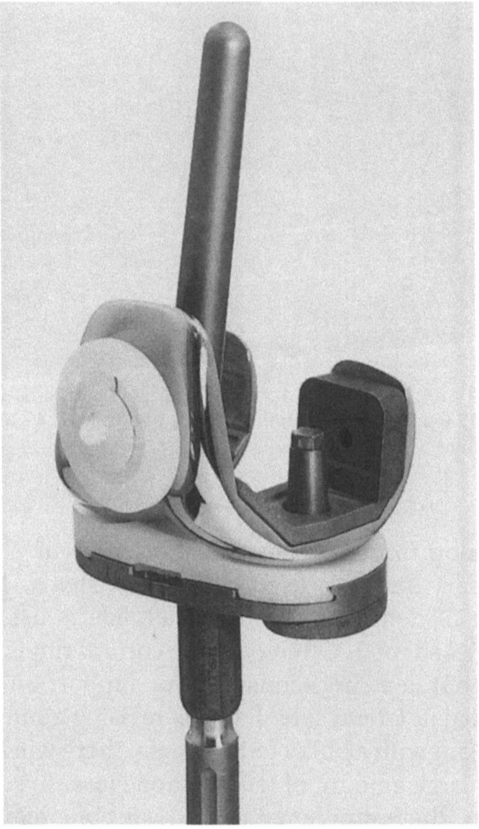

Fig. 15.8. Modular total knee system with wedge augment for filling plateau deficits in revision knee replacement.

attached to the femoral component by a locking device. Augments of different sizes must be required for each condyle.

In summary, bone grafting provides the surgeon with a biological approach to the management of bone deficiency either in the primary or revision total knee arthroplasty. Whenever possible, preservation of the underlying bone is vital to long term success of the replacement. In primary knee replacement with autogenous bone readily available, grafting should be employed rather than attempting to affix metal augments to the prosthesis. In the revision total knee replacement, the long term results of allografts are still unclear and recent. Recent experience with such allografts to correct for acetabular deficiencies raises questions as to the long term success in these grafts. Modular knee systems add yet another dimension, enabling the surgeon to customize the prosthesis and to supplement his use of bone grafts.

A New Technique of Defect-Filling in Cementless Total Knee Arthroplasty

H. W. Springorum, U. De Nicola, W. Lowe

Bone defects in the tibial plateau or femoral condyle are common in patients with severe gonarthrosis and anatomical axis deformities greater than 20° (Figs. 15.9, 15.10). In these situations many surgeons have recommended the used of fixed axis prostheses. This paper will describe a technique we have used at our center for correction of these bone defects. This technique enables us to avoid the use of fixed axis prostheses and instead insert a partially constrained uncemented prosthesis.

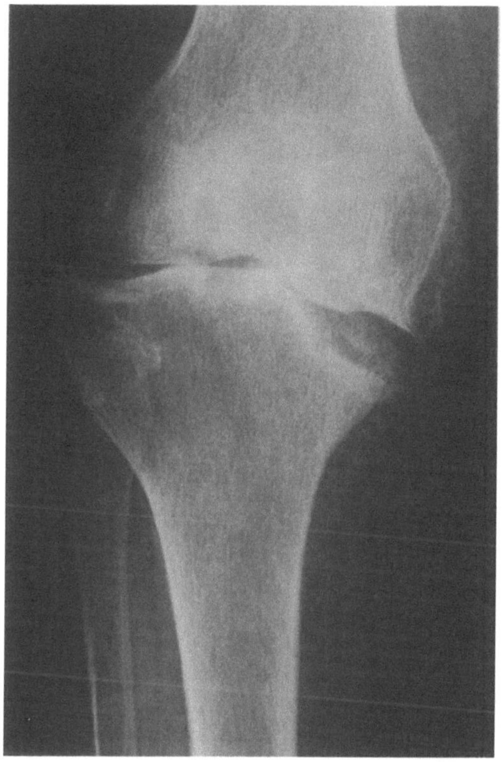

Fig. 15.9. Large medial bone loss from tibia with extensive osteophyte formation.

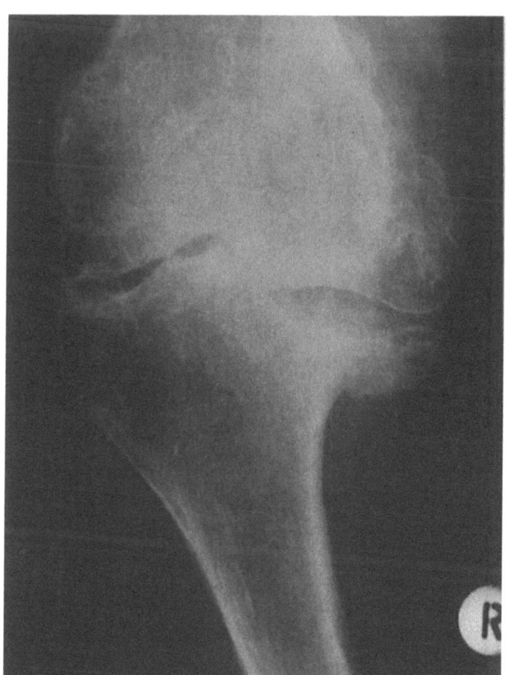

Fig. 15.10. Large medial bone loss associated with lateral subluxation of the tibia on the femur.

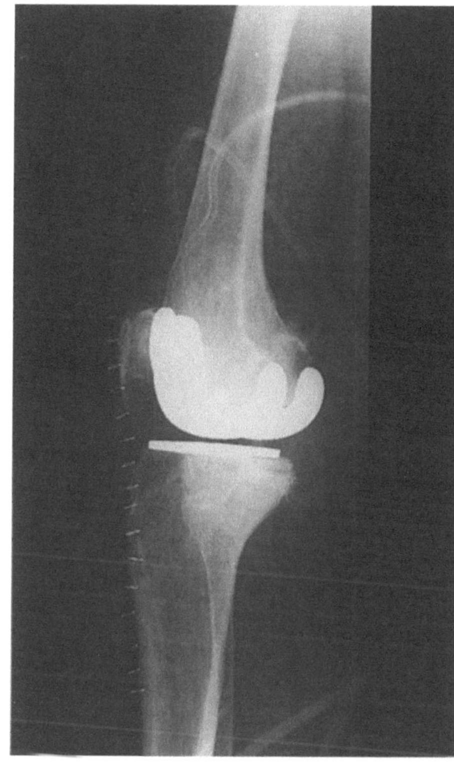

Fig. 15.11. Large corticocancellous bone chips used to fill a large posterior tibial cystic defect.

Small localized bone defects normally do not pose a problem. We usually fill these small cysts with cancellous bone taken from the bone resected from the distal femur. Fig. 15.11 shows a large posterior cystic defect which, after careful cleansing of all soft tissue, was filled with corticocancellous bone. Internal fixation was not necessary; the graft was held in place by the surrounding bone and the tibial component.

For larger defects supplemental fixation is usually required. One technique that we use consists of filling the defect with corticocancellous bone and fixing the bone to the tibial bed with wire pins or screws (Fig. 15.12 a,b). Normally we allow full weight bearing after a total knee replacement, cemented or cementless. For patients who have undergone this type of bone grafting and internal fixation, however, we routinely use a plastic leg brace for support and allow the patient to bear only partial weight on the leg for at least four weeks.

A second technique that we have used is called a basketplasty. We use the standard metal

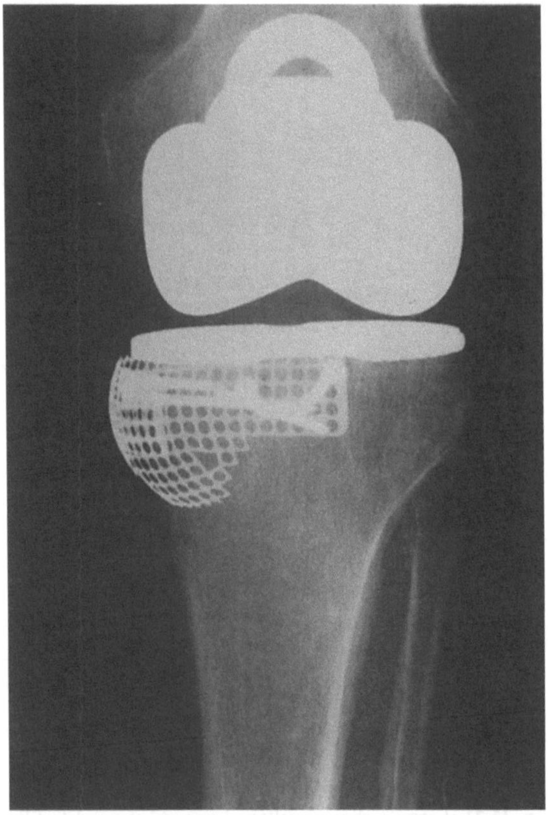

a

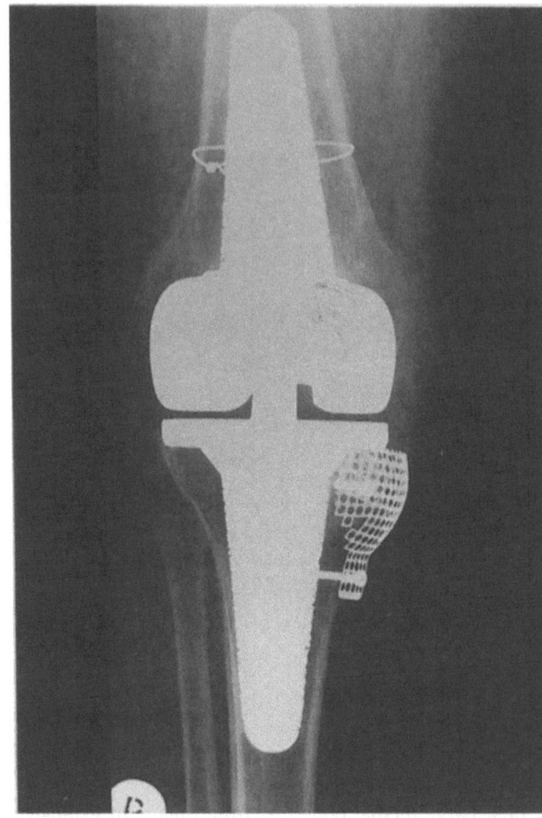

c

Fig. 15.12. The basketplasty technique. **a** Technique used to reconstruct medial tibial plateau with an uncemented Tricon-M prosthesis. **b** Technique used to reconstruct the medial tibial plateau with an uncemented Miller Galante Knee. **c,d** Technique used in a revision total knee replacement using a fixed axis prosthesis.

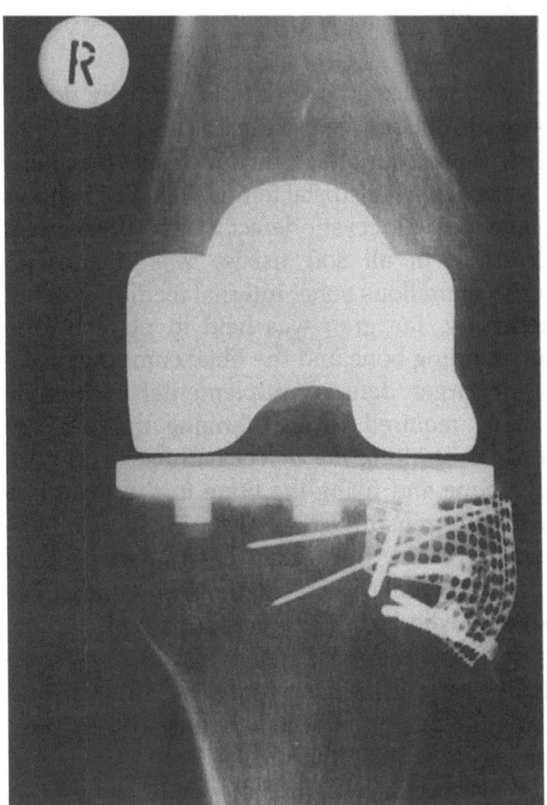

b

mesh that we use in total hip arthroplasty and cut and shape it so as to conform to the shape of the periphery of the proximal tibia. We then affix the metal basket with wire or screws to the tibia. The empty basket is filled with corticocancellous bone fragments (Fig. 15.12 a–d). Patients undergoing this type of reconstruction are also kept on a limited weight bearing and range of motion program similar to that described above.

In follow-up X-rays 4, 8, and 12 weeks after surgery we have found that the enclosed bone incorporates and amalgamates to the tibia in all cases. Longer follow-up three years after surgery has revealed no collapse of the bone nor migration of the implant.

Total Knee Replacement in the Presence of Large Bony Defects of the Tibia and Marked Knee Instability

Richard S. Laskin

Asymmetrical bone loss from the tibia is a common finding in the patient with advanced arthritis undergoing a total knee replacement arthroplasty. This bone loss leads clinically to an angular deformity and knee joint instability. Both of these problems must be corrected at the time of arthroplasty if optimum function of the reconstructed knee is to be expected. This chapter will discuss our results in performing total knee replacement arthroplasty in this group of patients with large bony defects and such marked instability. This includes a preliminary ligament balancing and equalization of the flexion and extension spaces. We subsequently will discuss the results with autologous bone graft to fill the defects and, the technique that we presently prefer, namely, filling of the defect with metallic wedges.

Table 15.1. Demographic data

Etiology of arthritis	
Osteoarthritis	11
Rheumatoid arthritis	11
Pigmented villonodular synovitis	2
Charcot arthropathy	2
Follow-up: 3.0 to 9.5 years	
mean 5.2 years	
Every knee had 20° varus/valgus instability in extension	
Source of bone for graft	
Local bone	22
Iliac crest	4
Prostheses used	
Posterior cruciate retaining	8
Posterior Stabilized	16
Insall-Burstein III	2

Materials and Methods

Out of our database of over 1800 total knee patients, we identified 26 patients who had severe pre-operative bone loss from the tibia and secondary varus/valgus instability of greater than 20°. The etiology of the patient's arthritis is noted in Table 15.1. The two patients with a neuroarthropathy both had severe adult onset diabetes mellitus. The diagnosis of pigmented villonodular synovitis was made by pathological interpretation of the synovial tissue combined with a history of prior recurrent episodic synovitis with hemorrhagic effusions. All the patients have been followed for at least 3 years with a mean of 5.2 years.

At surgery, the standard femoral, tibial, and patellar resections were made at the appropriate levels (Laskin 1989b). On the tibial side the resection line was approximately 4–6 mm below the surface on the normal side. In all but 4 knees, local bone was used for the graft. The bone that had been removed during the posterior femoral resection was often most appropriate. Cartilage was denuded, the subchondral surface scarified, and the entire fragment affixed to the tibia either with cancellous screws or Kirschner wires. In order to prevent fragmentation of the graft, the entire block of bone was affixed and the metallic pin or screw countersunk. The graft was then trimmed level with the previously cut surface of the normal tibial plateau. Ligament balancing and proper filling of the flexion and extension spaces was performed in a standard manner. We used capsular releases for any fixed deformities but did not perform any capsular reefings nor advancements in an attempt to "tighten up" the ligamentous structures on the convex side of the knee deformity. Although we routinely use acrylic in a low viscous state when we elect to cement in the prosthesis, we used a more doughy cement in these cases in an attempt to minimize interposition of the cement down between the graft and the tibial bed.

The types of implants that were used are documented on Table 15.1. The choice of implant was not based upon any basic preference of one type. Indeed both posterior cruciate sparing and Posterior Stabilized prostheses were used on an essentially randomized basis. No articulated implants were employed. All but two of the tibial components had a central stem and in all the arthroplasties, all three components were fixed with acrylic cement.

Postoperatively, the knee was placed in a Jones dressing for two days, and then in a fabric knee splint. The splint was used until the patient had regained sufficient quadriceps tone to lift leg unsupported from the examining couch. Range of motion exercises were begun on the third to fifth postoperative day. The patients used bimanual support for 6 weeks, and unilateral support for a subsequent 6 weeks.

The clinical data were summarized both pre- and postoperatively using the Hospital for Special Surgery Rating System. X-rays were routinely obtained at 3 months, 12 months and then at yearly intervals after surgery.

Results

The mean Hospital for Special Surgery Rating Score pre-operatively was 68. This was not statistically different from that seen in patients who were undergoing total knee replacement without having asymmetrical bony defects in their tibia. There was likewise no statistical difference between this group and the total knee group as a whole as related to age, diagnosis, or body weight. The mean Hospital for Special Surgery Rating Scores at three years after surgery was 82; that in the overall total knee group was 84. The difference was not statistically significant ($P<0.1$). There likewise was no statistical difference at the 3 month, 1 and 2 year scores.

At the three month evaluation, 19 of the 26 knees had no varus/valgus instability in extension. Three knees had less than 5°, 2 had between 5 and 10°, and 3 had >10°. One knee was markedly unstable at 3 months. This patient had a neuropathic arthropathy secondary to diabetes mellitus.

There was one case of massive bone graft dissolution within the first year after surgery. The implant had been placed in varus, referable to the tibial shaft and the overall tibiofemoral alignment had not been corrected. The patient's knee was markedly unstable but she declined the use of an external brace or any further surgery. The pre-operative diagnosis had been osteoarthritis.

Three further knees demonstrated evidence of graft dissolution with asymmetrical angular subsidence within the first year, all less than 3 mm. The subsidence did not progress after the first year, and none of these patients required bracing or further surgery. None of these knees has been revised. An additional three knees had bone grafts that demonstrated complete radiolucencies between the graft and the tibia. None of these implants showed any subsidence nor did the grafts appear to dissolve.

There was one case of a patellar ligament avulsion which occurred within the first two weeks after surgery. This occurred in a patient with marked intra-articular scarring who required extensive soft tissue elevation in order to dislocate the patella from the trochlear groove at surgery. An attempted repair using a tendon graft failed and the patient remained with a 20° extensor lag.

The patients who underwent surgery with the use of a Posterior Stabilized prosthesis were compared to those in whom a posterior cruciate retaining implant was used. There was no statistical difference in range of motion, pain, stability, or eventual rating scores between the two groups. One patient developed a supracondylar fracture of the femur at surgery when the intercondylar box was being fashioned to accommodate the Insall-Burstein Constrained III prosthesis. This was treated by screw fixation with excellent stability on the operating table. Within the first 3 weeks after surgery there was some displacement of the distal fragment, which then healed in approximately 30° of flexion.

A needle biopsy was performed in nine knees, one year after the arthroplasty. Positioning of the needle in the graft was assured by use of the image intensifier. In four of the grafts we could identify viable osteocytes; in the other five the lacunae were empty. None of these knees had demonstrated radiographic evidence of fragmentation of the graft or of subsidence.

Discussion

Tibial bone loss in the patient with advanced arthritis may have many etiologies including fractures (such as of the tibial plateau), erosive disease (as in rheumatoid arthritis of pigmented villonodular synovitis), and avascular conditions (such as osteonecrosis). In osteoarthritis, bone collapse can occur secondary to overload on the concave side of an angular deformity with areas of microcollapse coalescing into a large asymmetrical defect.

The instability occurs as the femoral condyle is displaced into the defect. The instability is almost always a flexible one, that is it is almost always correctable passively.

There have been numerous suggestions as to how to correct the bone loss. Among these have been: (1) filling the defect with acrylic cement, or cement "reinforced" with screws or mesh, (2) planing the tibial resection line inferiorly enough so as to be below the defect, (3) using shims or wedges to fill the defect (Brooks et al. 1984), and (4) using bone graft to fill the defect (Dorr and Ranawat 1984; Dorr et al. 1986; Windsor et al. 1986).

Filling the defect with cement can work for small circumscribed areas with an intact peripheral rim but is not applicable to those cases, such as occur in this series, where the bone loss is peripheral. Cement placed against such an oblique area of bone loss cannot obtain proper purchase and will easily loosen. Lowering the resection line will work for small areas of bone loss but not for large ones. As one progresses distally, important ligamentous attachments are sacrificed and the cross-sectional area of tibial bone available to support the implant is markedly decreased (Dorr and Boirdo 1986; Sneppen et al. 1981). Even more important is that the quality of the remaining bone is poor. A bony resection greater than 12 mm below the joint line sacrifices over 80% of the cancellous bone from the proximal tibia and will seat the implant on a rim of cortical bone. In this series, had the resection line been placed below the defect in each case it would have been at the level of the tibial tubercle in 12 cases.

We have previously shown that for severe fixed angular deformity, sacrifice of the posterior cruciate ligament was beneficial in order to obtain ligament balancing and optimal flexion (Laskin et al. 1988). In this group with flexible deformities, however, that was not the case. We compared the results seen in those knees in which a posterior cruciate retaining prosthesis was used with those in which a Posterior Stabilized prosthesis was chosen. There was no statistical difference in range of motion, stability, or component or limb alignment. The routine use, therefore, of a Posterior Stabilized implant in these patients is not indicated. The removal of bone from the intercondylar area that is required to insert either a Posterior Stabilized or constrained total knee can predispose the distal femur to fracture, especially in the osteoporotic patient. Although this not the only cause of distal femoral fractures about total knee prostheses (Merkel and Johnson 1986), we feel that is what occurred in our one patient with the supracondylar fracture.

Flexion and extension space balancing is crucial in order to obtain stability. If the plateau resection is made at the normal level, 3–6 mm below the joint surface, the resultant flexion and extension spaces can easily be filled using standard implants without having to resort to extremely thick or custom prostheses. Over 78% of the knees required the thinnest two sizes of tibial component available for the implant used.

Of the grafts that were biopsied, over 50% were not biologically alive. This may have been beneficial since the potential deleterious structural effects of creeping substitution could not occur. This cannot be the complete answer, however. Two of the knees that demonstrated graft dissolution on X-ray were biopsied; in one, osteocytes in lacunae could be identified and in the other they could not. Harris has stated that although during the early years massive bone grafts about the hip tend to do well, as time progresses many tend to fragment and dissolve. This may occur in the knee as well as these patients are followed beyond the 7–8 year period.

There were only three knees which had complete radiolucencies between the graft and the tibia. None of these implants subsided nor fragmented, however it is obvious that this is a tenuous situation with the graft not structurally incorporated to the tibia.

If we eliminate the one knee with a Charcot arthropathy and the two knees that developed surgical complications unrelated to the bone grating procedure, we are left with 24 knees. In four the graft fragmented, and in four more the graft was not incorporated. The "success rate" therefore is 67% at 5 years.

In the past we felt that the use of shims and wedges was not a reasonable alternative because of the inventory that would be required and because of our early feeling that the overwhelming number of our bone grafts did well. This does not appear to be the case however. We feel now that we are depending upon a poorly understood biological phenomenon to stabilize our implants; at times it is effective, but in over 30% of the knees it is not. In view of this we re-

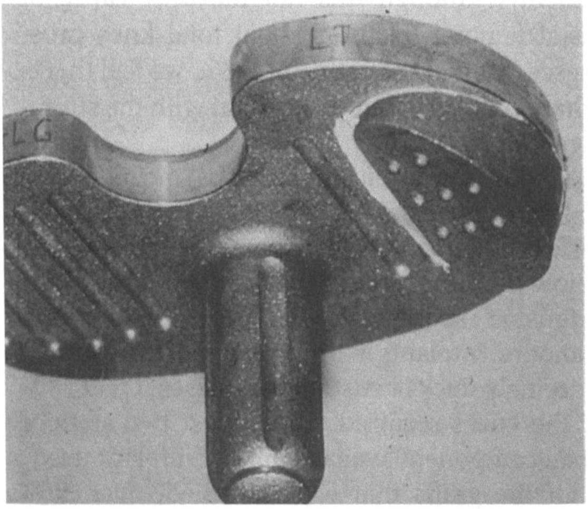

Fig. 15.13. Wedge affixed to tibial base plate by acrylic cement.

examined the wedges or shims as a possible alternative.

We presently have experience using two condylar prostheses that allow metal wedges to be directly affixed to the implants. In this manner, we are able to customize the implant at the time of surgery in a way that enables us to fill bone defects in the tibia or femur.

The Genesis total knee system has a system of wedges that can be affixed to the tibial component using acrylic cement (Fig. 15.13). The wedges come in a variety of sizes and shapes to accommodate for the shape of the bone defect (Fig. 15.14). Similar wedges are available for the distal and posterior portions of the femoral component. The Insall-Burstein II system likewise has a system of wedges. These wedges are affixed to the tibial component by small metallic screws. These wedges come in a more limited number of sizes that replace either one half or the entire tibial plateau surface (Fig. 15.4).

We have found both wedge systems to be effective and are presently evaluating this method to correct for bone loss, especially that occurring peripherally in the tibia. For small centralized areas of bone loss we continue to use autologous cancellous bone.

References

Altchek D, Sculco TP, Rawling B (1989) Autogenous bone grafting for severe angular deformity in total knee arthroplasty. J Arthroplasty 4: 151–156

Brooks PJ, Walker PS, Scott RD (1984) Tibial component fixation in deficient tibial bone stock. Clin Orthop 184: 302–308

Dorr LD, Boirdo RA (1986) Technical considerations in total knee arthroplasty. Clin Orthop 205: 5–11

Dorr LD, Ranawat CS (1984) Bone grafts for tibial deficits in total knee arthroplasty. In: Dorr LD (ed) Revision of total hip and knee. University Park Press, Baltimore, Md, p 143

Dorr LD, Ranawat DS, Sculco TP et al. (1986) Bone graft for tibial defects in total knee arthroplasty. Clin Orthop 205: 153–165

Insall JN (1984) Total knee replacement. In: Insall JN (ed) Surgery of the knee. Churchill Livingstone, New York

Laskin RS (1989a) The surgical technique for the performance of a total knee replacement arthroplasty. Orthop Clin N Am 20-3: 31–48

Laskin RS (1989b) Total knee replacement in the presence of large bony defects of the tibia and marked knee instability. Clin Orthop 248: 66–70

Laskin RS, Cameron H, Light R (1985) Correction of tibial bone loss during total knee replacement. A scientific

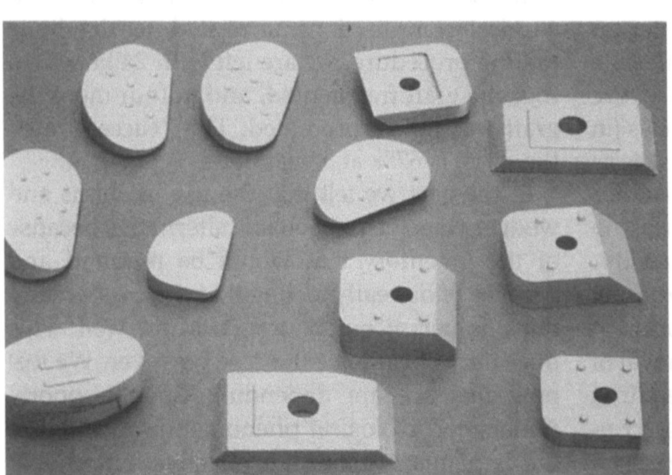

Fig. 15.14. Modular wedges for the femur and tibia – Genesis System (Smith and Newphew Richards Inc.).

exhibit presented at the 52nd annual meeting of the American Academy of Orthopaedic Surgeons, Las Vegas, Nevada
Laskin RS, Rieger M, Schob C, Turen C (1988) The posterior stabilized total knee prosthesis in the knee with a severe fixed deformity. Am J Knee Surg 1: 199–203
Lotke PA, Wong R, Ecker ML (1985) The management of large tibial defects in primary total knee replacement. A scientific presentation at the 52nd annual meeting of the American Academy of Orthopaedic Surgeons, Las Vegas, Nevada
Merkel KD, Johnson EW (1986) Supracondylar fracture of the femur after total knee arthroplasty. J Bone Joint Surg (Am) 68: 29–43
Ranawat CS (1985) How to compensate for bone loss. In: Ranawat CS (ed) Total condylar knee arthroplasty. Springer-Verlag, New York
Ritter MA (1986) Screw and cement fixation of large defects in total knee arthroplasty. J Arthroplasty 1: 125–130
Sneppen O, Christensen P, Larsen H, Vary PS (1981) Mechanical testing of trabecular bone in knee replacement. Int Orthop 5: 251
Vince KG, Dorr LD (1987) Surgical technique of total knee arthroplasty: principles and controversy. Techn Orthop 1: 69–82
Windsor RE, Insall JN, Sculco TP (1986) Bone grafting of tibial defects in primary and revision total knee arthroplasty. Clin Orthop 205: 153–165

Chapter 16

The Infected Total Knee Arthroplasty

Edward T. Habermann

Introduction

Sepsis following total knee arthroplasty is a catastrophic complication. Its management can be one of the most challenging and frustrating experiences in orthopaedic surgery. While infection is not the most frequent complication seen in total knee arthroplasty, it is probably the most dreaded. The incidence of deep infection following total knee arthroplasty has varied from less than 1% (Grogan et al. 1986; Insall 1986; Insall et al. 1983a; Poss et al. 1984) to greater than 20% (Jones et al. 1979) with the highest incidence being reported with early designs that used the hinged type of metal to metal bearing surface. With the more recently designed total knees, there has been a reduction in the incidence of deep infection to a level of from 1% to 5% (Insall 1986; Rand et al. 1986). Although this reduction is admirable, the incidence is still markedly higher than that seen following knee operations in which an implant is not utilized.

A variety of factors has probably played a significant role in reducing the infection rate in total knee arthroplasty. These have included: more recent design changes in the prosthesis, improved operative technique, better patient selection, better postoperative management and careful and judicious use of prophylactic antibiotic therapy. In addition, intra-operative contamination has further been decreased by better operative techniques, shorter operating times, and improved environmental conditions in the operation room including laminar flow systems, ultraviolet light, and exhaust suction systems for the surgeons. However, in spite of all of the advances in the environmental control, operative technique and design of prostheses, we have been unable completely to eliminate either early or late infection following total knee arthroplasty.

The treatment of the infected total knee arthroplasty has to be based on careful and critical assessment of a variety of factors and should include an orthopaedic surgeon and infectious disease consultant familiar with implant infections. The length of hospitalization, the long course of antibiotic therapy, the multiple procedures and the prolonged rehabilitation are often staggering in both monetary cost and emotional cost to the patient. The treatment plan must assess a variety of factors including:

1. Whether the infection is early or late.
2. The absolute diagnosis of the offending organism(s).
3. The radiographic appearance of the bone cement or prosthesis–bone interface.
4. The organism involved.
5. The patient's underlying disease including the presence or absence of immunocompetence.
6. The overall condition of the skin and soft tissues.
7. The type of prosthesis.
8. The patient's symptoms and physical findings.
9. The age and functional level of the patient and his future demands.

All of these factors, when carefully assessed, will lead the orthopaedic surgeon to an appropriate treatment plan for each individual patient.

Factors Associated with Increased Infection Rate

Underlying diseases such as rheumatoid arthritis have an increased rate of infection as compared to patients with osteoarthritis (Poss et al. 1984). Rheumatoid patients are more predisposed to late hematogenous infections and are more susceptible to bacteremia and soft tissue infection. This is due either to their immunosuppressed state or to impaired leukocyte phagocytosis. Rheumatoid patients have thinner skin and often have vasculitis in the small vessels of the skin and subcutaneous tissues. These problems may facilitate entrance of microorganisms into the joint. Other conditions such as systemic lupus erythematosus, psoriatic arthritis, or the seronegative spondyloarthropathies may also increase the risk of infection, although these have not been as clearly documented as those seen in rheumatoid arthritis. Conditions such as diabetes, chronic alcoholism, chronic renal failure and malignancy may likewise lead to an increased incidence of infection following total knee replacement. Any disease state that alters the host defense mechanism can potentially increase the infection risk.

Type of Prosthesis

The highest incidence of infection was reported with the early metal on metal prostheses, such as the Waldius and Guepar. This may have been due to the development of synovitis from wear debris caused by these fixed axis metal articulations. Often the patients requiring these types of prostheses were the most disabled, most immunocompromised, and most deformed. Prosthetic loosening, the amount of bone resection necessary and the poor vascularity of the peri-articular tissues may have provided a fertile site for bacterial invasion and subsequent infection. The wear particles from the articulation themselves may have directly caused macrophage impairment.

In recent years, there has been a major interest in the effects of biomaterials on host defense mechanisms and the role that these materials have played in the development of infection. Investigators have tried to predict the incidence of infection by studying the body's response to various metals. Rae (1975) in an in vitro study measured the levels of lactic dehydrogenase and gluco-6-phosphate dehydrogenase in macrophagic tissue near particles from metal implants. Elevations in the levels of those enzymes correlated well with the degree of cell damage and diminished activity. There has not, however, been any study to document a greater or lesser infection rate with one modern era alloy or metal as compared to another.

Investigators have tried to predict host response to materials by doing various types of skin patch tests and have been able to demonstrate positive skin patch tests for most biomaterials used in total knee arthroplasty, with the exception of methylmethacrylate (Deutman et al. 1977). Some investigators have been able to find a correlation between positive skin tests and local tissue responses, however others have been unable to duplicate these findings (Uchida et al. 1980). It has been shown that tissue responses are significantly lower around static implants than around articulating prostheses. In the latter group, there is less tissue response when metal articulates with polyethylene than when metal articulates with metal. The less the debris, the less the tissue response.

Gristina and others (1976, 1980, 1983) have focused their attention on the effect of biomaterials on macrophage activity. Adherence, which is concomitant with spreading and flattening of macrophages and polymorphonuclear leukocytes, is believed to be related to phagocytic capabilities (Rasp et al. 1979). Green's (1975) in vivo studies have shown that methylmethacrylate inhibits phagocytosis of *Candida albicans*. Leake and associates (1980) have shown that macrophages undergo various changes when they come in contact with different types of biomaterials. It has been postulated that if spreading is essential to the normal functioning ability of macrophages to fight infection, then the increased incidence of infection in the presence of methylmethacrylate or other biomaterials may be due to their affecting the shape of these cells. Gristina has shown that *Staphylococcus epidermidis* has the ability to adhere to the surface of a prosthesis and grow in a glycocalyx enclosed environment.

More attention is being paid to these areas of biomaterials and infection. It is too early to know whether the use of noncemented total knee prostheses will have a positive effect on infection by removing the negative effect of methylmethacrylate. Petty et al. (1985) have shown in a canine model that the use of methylmethacrylate made infection more likely in the experimental animal than that seen in controls with noncemented implants. This may have been the result of inhibition of leukocyte chemotaxis and phagocytosis that occur in the presence of methylmethacrylate (Rand et al 1984). Blomgren and Lindgren (1980) have suggested that the mere presence of a total joint prosthesis may impair local defense mechanisms and decrease the vitality of the surrounding soft tissues.

Wound Problems

Following any knee arthroplasty there is a hemarthrosis in the knee. With appropriate drainage systems that are usually employed for the first 24–48 hours this is kept to a minimum. Any remaining hemarthrosis or persistent bleeding into the joint may result in the formation of an ideal medium for bacterial growth. If the bleeding is excessive, capsular and even skin dehiscence may occur. Drainage from the Hemovac site may exist for a short period of time, but is worrisome if it exists much longer. One of the hardest decisions the orthopaedic surgeon faces in the early postoperative period is when to explore the knee when drainage persists. Any cultures that are taken must be obtained not from a skin swab, where they may be contaminated by skin flora, but rather by removal of fluid from the depths using a needle and syringe. Rest and temporary cessation of physical therapy may cause a resolution in erythema about the suture or staple line and clearly is a consideration when this is present.

Any skin slough or opening after a total knee arthroplasty is a dangerous situation. The skin slough may be related to the type of incision utilized and whether there had been previous surgery. It has been our usual policy to try to use previous skin incisions, if present, so as to avoid skin necrosis between the previous and new incisions. Problems with wound healing about the knee in primary operations are much less frequent than in revision operations.

The key to wound healing is maintenance of a good blood supply. The blood supply to the knee is both intrinsic and extrinsic. The intrinsic supply is derived primarily from the genicular branches of the popliteal artery whereas the extrinsic blood supply comes from the lateral circumflex femoral artery, the supreme, or descending genicular artery, and the recurrent branch of the anterior tibial artery. If prior incisions about the knee have been made, attention must be paid to these sources when deciding on the best approach for the new incision. If a previous lateral incision has interrupted the lateral blood supply, a medial incision which interrupts the superior medial genicular artery may lead to ischemia of the lateral flap. Wound healing may also be influenced by the general nutritional status of the patient, pre-existing vascular disease, the presence of rheumatoid arthritis or diabetes, a history of smoking, and whether the patient has had previous problems with wound healing.

Wound breakdown is a very significant and fearful complication after a total knee arthroplasty. If it is superficial in nature, it may be allowed to close secondarily by epithelialization and contraction. In some cases the ischemic area may be small enough that an appropriate debridement and secondary closure may suffice.

A more major problem occurs when a large area about the wound becomes ischemic and it is anticipated that there will be a full thickness loss of tissue. A decision must be made as to whether to excise this area surgically and then cover it with a graft of either skin, muscle or both. Timing is crucial in making this decision; we feel that earlier rather than late surgery is more appropriate. If too long a period of time is allowed to elapse after the wound compromise is noted, the patient will lose a significant range of motion. Infection of the joint with all its attendant complications may then occur.

In order to maximize the security of the suture line we close the capsule with interrupted sutures and then check the repair by flexing the knee prior to closing the more superficial tissues. The final skin and subcutaneous closure is done with the knee in some flexion rather than in full extension.

Antibiotics Usage

Perioperative antibiotics are now routinely used for all types of implant surgery including total knee arthroplasty. It has been clearly shown that antibiotics effectively reduce the incidence of deep wound infection following total hip arthroplasty (Carlsson et al. 1977; Hill et al. 1981; Norden 1983, 1985; Pollard et al. 1979). Cephalosporins and semisynthetic penicillins are generally utilized because of their activity against the most common pathogens seen in total knee replacement, namely staphylococci and streptococci. First generation cephalosporins should be used as the primary drug of choice. These drugs often have a short half life similar to the semisynthetic penicillins such as Nafcillin and Amoxicillin. Despite this short half-life they are very effective and one should not progress to a newer agent unless there is a specific reason to do so in a particular patient.

For patients allergic to penicillin or cephalosporin, we use Vancomycin. Vancomycin is an effective prophylactic drug especially against methicillin resistant staphylococci. Unfortunately, it has the potential disadvantages of causing skin rashes, nephrotoxicity or hypotension in occasional patients.

At the present time we give our peri-operative antibiotics 30 minutes prior to making the skin incision and continue them for 24–48 hours depending on when the closed suction drain is removed. Longer prophylactic antibiotic therapy should not be a routine but occasionally be used in special circumstances. At times there may be wound drainage, accompanied possibly by cellulitis or changes in the soft tisues about the wound. This is a very critical situation and all attempts should be made to clarify whether indeed an infection is present and what organism is present prior to beginning long term antibiotic therapy.

Prophylactic use of antibiotics is suggested for all patients with total knee replacements who are undergoing any surgical or manipulative procedure involving the genito-urinary tract, gastrointestinal tract, or the mouth and teeth. These procedures frequently produce a transient bacteremia and prophylaxis is recommended in an attempt to prevent subsequent seeding to the prosthetic joint. We use the oral antibiotic program that is recommended by the American Heart Association for prevention of bacterial endocarditis for prophylaxis in our total joint patients. Prompt attention should be paid to any local source of infection such as the skin, respiratory, intestinal or genitourinary tracts to prevent hematogenous spread from these areas. It should be noted that the rheumatoid patient is at a very high risk for such secondary bacteremic seeding.

Reduction of local contamination at the operative site is another important factor. Different operating rooms have a variety of techniques to control the environment including body exhaust suits, laminar air flow systems, and ultraviolet light. Surgical technique, length of the surgical procedure, frequency of air exchange, the operating room traffic and the surgical attire have all been shown to be potential sources of infection (Fitzgerald and Kelly 1979; Salvati et al. 1982).

The use of antibiotic impregnated cement in the prevention of infection in total knee arthroplasty appears attractive. It has been clearly shown that the local concentration of antibiotics in the bone and soft tissue following its release from the cement surface is many times higher than the concentrations obtained by intravenous antibiotic therapy (Elson 1985). In addition, the serum concentrations of antibiotics released from the cement are low, thereby reducing the risk of toxicity. Where there are scarred tissues, such as seen in a revision case, the devascularized tissues often cannot receive adequate doses of antibiotics via a parenteral route and antibiotics in the cement may be indicated.

The potential disadvantages of utilizing impregnated antibiotic cement include allergic reactions and potential weakening of the cement itself. This latter problem, however, represents only a mild one, as long as the antibiotic is inserted in powder, not liquid form (methylmethacrylate is extremely hydrophobic and will not uniformly mix with an aqueous preparation, leaving voids in the mass). The use of antibiotic impregnated cement in total hip replacement, for instance, has not been associated with an increase in mechanical failure rate as compared to standard nonantibiotic impregnated cement.

At the present time there does not appear to be any significant advantage of antibiotic impregnated cement as compared to intravenous prophylactic antibiotic therapy in the standard primary total knee replacement. Its value in septic revision cases is considerable. Its use following removal of infected total knee implants will be discussed later in this chapter.

The Diagnosis of Infection

Often it is difficult and perplexing to differentiate between superficial inflammation and deep infection, but the necessity to do this is quite obvious. Local inflammation about the suture site, which is not an uncommon finding, is usually representative of a superficial reaction. However, when persistent erythema, induration, and edema occur, this is more alarming. A high index of suspicion must be present in all patients, however, since with some infections there may be minimal swelling, no erythema and only scant drainage.

Classification of infection into acute, subacute and late stages is based on arbitrary time spans. The acute infection occurs within the first 3 months after the operation and probably represents contamination at the time of surgery. The subacute infection occurs between 3 months and 1 year and may represent the result of operative contamination with a low virulence organism or hematogenous spread from a distant focus. The late infection occurs after one year and almost always represents hematogenous spread.

Pain

The characteristics of the pain may at times be helpful in making the diagnosis of infection. Although pain secondary to mechanical loosening usually has a more sudden onset than does pain seen after infection, this is variable at times. Antibiotics may decrease the pain from infection, but again, not consistently. Insidious onset of pain may be due to infection, or a variety of other conditions.

Laboratory Findings

Acute phase reactants such as the sedimentation rate and C-reactive protein are usually elevated in a patient with an infected knee arthroplasty. Unfortunately, however, the sedimentation rate may be elevated for some period of time following any joint arthroplasty in the absence of infection. Therefore the sedimentation rate may be helpful only when it is normal in ruling out the presence of infection. The white blood count level is equally variable. The most important laboratory diagnostic tool is analysis of the synovial fluid. This evaluation included cell count, differential, gram staining, glucose and protein determination, and eventually culture and sensitivity. Bacteriological studies are especially important in planning a total knee arthroplasty if the patient has had previous surgical procedures in the joint. If the patient has been taking antibiotics, the laboratory should be alerted to look for L-forms. In every case, however, the culture should be evaluated for at least 5–7 days.

Reports by Gristina and others (1976, 1980, 1983, 1985) have identified that bacteria are surrounded by a polysaccharide membrane called the glycocalyx. Costerton et al. (1978) determined that this surface "slime" on some naturally occurring bacteria enabled them to colonize and adhere to smooth surfaces. The glycocalyx slime consisted of polysaccharide fibrils derived from a carbohydrate component in the bacterial cell wall. Its adhesive properties allowed both aerobic and anaerobic species to adhere tightly to each other as well as to other surfaces (such as metal implants) in symbiotic protective colonies called consortia. This adherence between biomaterials and their colonization by glycocalyx-producing bacteria explained the higher incidence of infection in operations where biomaterials were used. This also explained the resistance of those infections to macrophagic attack and antibiotic penetration. This concept also explained the difficulty with growing these bacteria on a culture medium. With routine culture techniques, samples of free-floating bacteria rather than samples of the tightly bound colonies are usually examined. Because the tightly bound adherent pathogenic species are inconsistently present in the floating debris, they are seldom identified. Since these adherent bacteria are not transferred to the culture medium, standard reports of bacterial concentrations and minimum inhibitory concentrations can give false impressions of the true problem and lead to improper antibiotics being given.

Pathological examination and culture of the tissues at the time of surgery is critical and is often the most reliable technique in diagnosing sepsis. Obtaining tissue from the bone cement or prosthesis-cement interface is crucial.

General Findings

Any patient presenting with chronic pain and swelling without a mechanical etiology such as loosening should be suspected of having sepsis. A persistently low grade fever that is unexplained is also suggestive of infection. Component loosening associated with chronic induration of the pericapsular tissues is most commonly associated with an infection with a low virulence microorganism. The knee presenting with a chronic draining sinus presents no problem for the diagnosis of infection. Unfortunately, a low grade infection due to *Staphylococcus epidermidis* or to anaerobic organisms usually presents with pain, and few, if any, local findings.

Organisms Encountered

Many organisms may be found in infected total knee replacements. In our experience, the usual organism, both in early and late hematogenous infections, is *Staphylococcus aureus*. Strangely enough, *Staphylococcus epidermidis*, which is not an uncommon organism in infected total hips, is less common in infected total knees (Table 16.1). Infections after seeding from urinary or gastrointestinal sepsis are usually gram negative. Infections following dental procedures frequently involve streptococci. Mixed infections are more common in cases of skin breakdown and direct extension (Thornhill and Maguire 1987). Enterococci are also common in those patients with skin breakdown as well as in those with seeding from infections in the urinary or gastrointestinal tracks. *Pseudomonas* and *Serratia* occur primarily where there have been open wounds and where various courses of antibiotics have been given previously.

Table 16.1. Frequency of infecting organisms (cases)

Staphylococcus aureus	18
Staphylococcus epidermidis	3
Streptococcus	2
E. coli	2
Proteus mirabilis	1
Pseudomonas	1
Serratia	1
Mixed	3

Collaboration with a member of the infectious disease staff with an interest in these problems is extremely important in formulating the most effective treatment plan. Dosage of synergistic combinations of drugs on the basis of bacteriocidal levels will determine the treatment regimen. The antibiotics that are chosen must maintain adequate bacteriocidal levels, and must be monitored for potential systemic toxic effects.

Imaging Techniques

Radiographs may not be helpful in diagnosing an infection. Prosthetic loosening may be present in long standing infections, but it is often difficult to differentiate septic from aseptic loosening. Periosteal new bone formation is highly suggestive of infection but is infrequently present. Radiographic changes, when present, may take many months to occur. When these changes are found it may indicate a more chronic situation rather than an acute one. Cortical scalloping, which is commonly seen with infection after total hip arthroplasty, is an uncommon finding after knee replacement. Arthrography hasn't been found to be useful in the diagnosis of infection.

Bone scanning may be helpful, although activity in the technetium scan is often found for many months after non infected knee arthroplasties. Furthermore the bone scan may be positive in cases of loosening, whether septic or aseptic. Associated differential gallium and technetium scans may be beneficial in distinguishing septic from aseptic loosening. If the uptake of a gallium scan is equal to or exceeds that on the technetium scan, infection is likely. Sinograms can certainly demonstrate the continuity into the deep tissues and the prosthesis, although when a sinus track and drainage is present, the diagnosis of infection is usually not difficult to establish.

Treatment Options and Results

The treatment of an infected total knee arthroplasty has to be based on careful assessment of a variety of factors. The time interval between the onset of infection and the initial surgery is important. This interval may determine what type of treatment may be necessary. Treatment may include soft tissue debridement and intravenous antibiotics, removal of the prosthesis, direct exchange, delayed exchange, arthrodesis, or resection arthroplasty. Factors to be considered include the time between diagnosis and treatment of the infection, the organism(s) involved, the patient's general health, the overlying soft tissues, the type of prosthesis in place, and the patient's needs and expectations.

Aspiration and Antibiotics

There are only certain indications for this treatment protocol and these criteria must be strictly met. The prosthetic components must be firmly fixed and the overlying skin and soft tissues must be intact. Any soft tissue changes such as draining sinuses and open wounds are contraindications to this form of treatment. In an extremely ill patient who is not toxic from the infection, the risks of major surgery may outweigh the attempts at a true cure and on occasion, this form of therapy may then be used. Johnson and Bannister (1986) found that long term antibiotic treatment was successful in eradicating symptoms of deep infection in only 2 of 25 cases. Bengtson and associates (1989) reported that only 2 of 32 patients had been successfully treated with antibiotics alone following deep infection after total knee arthroplasty. There have been isolated instances of successful outcomes by antibiotic therapy alone. One of the few organisms that may be controlled by this method of treatment is streptococcus.

Early Debridement and Antibiotics

Debridement carried out for chronic infection has not been demonstrated to be curative. For acute infection, however, surgical debridement done either open or through the arthroscope has had some success. Five of six patients reported upon by Freeman et al. (1985) were rendered free of infection following debridement and antibiotic therapy. Morrey and associates (1989) reported that this treatment yielded satisfactory results in 80% of their cases when patients were followed for more than 6 years after their infection. Their regimen included three weeks of intravenous antibiotics in hospital followed by a minimum of 3 months of oral antibiotics subsequently. Borden and Gearen (1987) related the success of debridement and antibiotic therapy to the acuteness of the infection. Their overall success rate was only 45%.

Debridement of the soft tissue with prosthetic retention and intravenous antibiotics should only be considered in acute perioperative and acute hematogenous infections in which the organisms are sensitive to antibiotics and the prosthesis is well fixed without interface changes.

Whether more adequate debridement will be able to be achieved in the future with the newer modular designs where the tibial component tray can be removed so as to facilitate exposure of the posterior aspect of the knee is still speculative. We have been gratified in several cases utilizing this approach in combination with a gastrocnemius flap in order to bring a better blood supply to the area.

Arthroscopic debridement is a viable alternative to open debridement in appropriate settings. The use of an implantable continuous effusion antibiotic pump for treatment has been described by Perry and associates (1988). This technique enables maximum local antibiotic levels to be achieved with minimal systemic levels, thereby decreasing the potential for general toxicity.

This technique should not be confused with the old "drip and suction" technique used to treat osteomyelitis. Continuous irrigation and drainage of antibiotic fluids into the knee joint has no place in the treatment of an infected total knee replacement. The incidence of secondary superinfection (especially with gram negative organisms) using this technique is unacceptably high.

One Stage Reimplantation

The advantages of this procedure are obvious. It requires just a single operation, a shorter hospitalization and potential in the decrease of soft tissue contractures. This procedure, however, is rarely indicated. It possibly might be used in an immunocompetent patient who is severely ill, who could not undergo multiple procedures, and in whom the organism is of low virulence. There should be no soft tissue or bone changes. Obviously the number of patients who will fulfill these criteria is very small. The results of one stage exchange have not been as satisfactory as those seen in two stage exchanges.

Delayed or Two Stage Reimplantation

This is the most common, and so far, the most successful form of treatment for an infected total knee arthroplasty. Success rates as high as 90% have been reported (Borden and Gearen 1987; Insall et al. 1983b; Wilde and Ruth 1988). Rand and Bryan (1983) reported on their experience with 14 total knee prostheses that were infected with re-implantation of a new prosthesis within two weeks of removal. Salvage was successful in 6 of 7 patients with low virulence organisms but only in 2 of 7 patients with a high virulence infection. Of the 8 patients for whom the result was a functioning prosthesis, two had significant restriction of motion and one had moderate pain. Eliminating these from the analysis, the overall success rate was only 35%. This low success rate was probably due to the short time used between removal and reimplantation.

The delayed exchange protocol includes:

1. Removal of all the components and methylmethacrylate.
2. Thorough debridement and synovectomy.
3. Obtaining appropriate deep cultures from the various tissues and interfaces.
4. Using antibiotic impregnated beads or spacers.
5. Primary closure.
6. Closed suction drainage.
7. Intravenous antibiotics.

Following an appropriate period of time, the wound is recultured, and if sterile, another prosthesis inserted. Attempts in all of these procedures should be made to preserve as much bone stock as possible.

The interval between removal and re-implantation varies between surgeons. If all the parameters for re-implantation are met, the re-implantation can usually be performed between 4 and 6 weeks after removal. Our usual protocol is that at 6 weeks we operate on the knee, take frozen sections and gram stains, and if no infection is found, do our re-implantation. We use antibiotic impregnated cement and continue the intravenous antibiotics for 48–72 hours or sometimes for several weeks.

The MIC levels that are eluded from antibiotic impregnated cement are many times higher than those that can be achieved by intravenous antibiotics alone. The highest levels adjacent to the cement will occur within the first 2–3 weeks and then diminish over the next 3–4 weeks. The two antibiotics that have been most widely used are Gentamicin and Tobramycin. Even though their primary indications are for gram negative organisms, the high levels that are obtained in the local area make them bacteriocidal for gram positive organisms as well. The usual dose level is 0.5 – 1 g of powdered antibiotic for each bag of methylmethacrylate powder. In no case should liquid antibiotics be used. Likewise since there is a potential risk of an allergic reaction to the antibiotics, the beta lactams should not be used in cement. Finally there has been evidence in Europe to suggest that the amount of antibiotic that is eluded from the cement is more even using Palacos rather than Simplex as a base.

Antibiotic impregnated cement beads or spacers are routinely used during the interval between removal and reimplantation. They have the dual effect of delivering high doses of antibiotics to the local area while reducing the dead space. The spacer blocks can be easily fashioned and modified to fill the intramedullary canals. They are somewhat easier to remove at the time of re-implantation than are the beads. The blocks will likewise maintain the collateral ligaments at length and help prevent contractions. Wrobleski has reported leaving the blocks in place permanently in patients in whom the risk of secondary re-implantation surgery was too great. The antibiotic dose for the beads or blocks is similar to that described previously.

At the time of reimplantation multiple frozen sections should be taken. If there is *any* doubt about the persistence of infection as demonstrated either on a gram stain or biopsy, the knee should be redebrided and closed. It is better to be conservative in the timing for reimplantation. Treating a reinfected reimplanted total knee prosthesis is often a disaster.

The use of allograft or autograft bone in cases where there is significant bone loss has been performed without untoward effect on the infection rate. Custom implants have also been utilized and these can be designed during the interval period between removal and reimplantation. It has been suggested that the surgeon make a cement mold at the time of the initial surgery to facilitate fabrication of a custom implant. Most recently, the availability of prostheses that can be customized at surgery by the addition of wedges or stems has diminished the need for pre-customized prostheses.

The gastrocnemius myo-cutaneous flap (McCraw et al. 1978; Salibian and Anzel 1983; Sanders and O'Neill 1981) has been useful in our hands in the salvage of infected total knees both in the two stage exchange as well as in attempting to salvage and retain an infected total knee arthroplasty. Sanders described the use of this flap in eight patients with preservation of the prosthesis in six of the eight cases. The joint and prosthesis were covered with this flap in order both to provide a fresh blood supply as well as to provide a reliable and stable skin cover. Selection of the flap that is used is governed by the position of the defect. In many cases, lateral defects can be closed by the use of a medial flap, the latter being longer, more robust and more mobile than a lateral flap. The gastrocnemius flap has offered us the opportunity to salvage five of six prostheses without having to proceed with the removal of the prosthesis. We have been using it earlier in our decision making process when there is a skin defect or when viability of the tissues seems impaired. At times the flap may be used at the time of prosthesis insertion hopefully to prevent the breakdown of the scarred soft tissues.

Multiple difficulties frequently are encountered with the soft tissues at the time of re-implantation. Quadriceps contractures may necessitate lengthening procedures such as described by Coonse and Adams (1943), Thompson (1944) and Scott and Saliski (1985). Tibial tubercle osteotomy is sometimes necessary, although the complications of this procedure that have been reported are very high (Wolff et al. 1989). I have not experienced that high complication rate with our tibial tubercle osteotomies.

Arthrodesis

Arthrodesis of the knee is sometimes required for a failed total knee replacement. Arthrodesis was the usual method of treatment to salvage the failed infected total knee prior to the era of reimplantation. Arthrodesis still may be indicated where there is poor skin coverage and inadequate soft tissues to provide a functional total knee arthroplasty. Arthrodesis will often give good pain relief whereas a revision arthroplasty alone may not completely eradicate the pain.

Successful arthrodesis depends upon the type of prosthetic component removed. Brodersen et al. (1979) reviewed 45 arthrodeses for failed total knee arthroplasty and reported an 81% success rate following removal of condylar type prostheses, whereas only a 56% arthrodesis rate following failure of a hinged implant. In a series of 85 arthrodeses, Knutson et al. (1985) reported a success rate of 50% when fusing after removal of a semiconstrained prosthesis, whereas the success rate was only 20% after removing hinged prostheses. Both Hagemann et al. (1978) Salvati and Insall (1980) reported two small series of attempted arthrodeses having only very limited successes, less than one third eventually achieving solid fusion. Even successful arthrodesis may have significant functional drawbacks such as shortening, increased energy expenditure when walking, and problems related to other joints in the lower extremities and back.

It is clear that arthrodesis after infected total knee replacement is more difficult to obtain when the arthroplasty and/or cement has sacrificed or damaged large volumes of cancellous bone. Cortical bone may be gone as well especially if there has been extensive osteolysis as is often seen after hinged implants are removed.

External fixation methods at this time seem to offer the best success rates for arthrodesis following failed infected total knee arthroplasties. The advantages of external fixation devices are that they allow for easy access and continued wound management, for compression at the arthrodesis site, and for control of stability. They allow for maintenance of whatever available bone vascularity is present by not requiring extensive stripping of the soft tissues. External fixation must be performed using pins in multiple planes. Anteriorposterior half pins are important to resist the pull of the quadriceps and hamstring muscles. Wade and Duhan (1984) reporting on the Portsmouth external fixator had a 100% success rate in a small series as compared to only a 39% success rate using the four pin Charnley method.

Arthrodesis can also be obtained using an intramedullary rod as described by Matthews (Falahee et al. 1987). Pre-operative planning is critical to determine the rod size as well as delineate the shape of the femur and tibia. Bone grafting may be used with any arthrodesis. Pulsed electromagnetic fields have been utilized as well to enhance the arthrodesis if there had been a delayed union (Bigliani et al. 1983).

Although reimplantation gives the best opportunity for a functional knee, arthrodesis still has a place in the orthopaedist's armamentarium. It remains especially beneficial where re-implantation has failed, where infection cannot be adequately controlled, or where there is extensive soft tissue loss.

Arthrodesis by a long intramedullary rod has served us by eradicating the infection as well as obtaining a fusion in selected cases.

Resection Arthroplasty

Resection arthroplasty as described by Falahee et al. (1987) is a salvage procedure for an infected total knee arthroplasty. They reported that systemic signs of infection were eradicated in all their 26 patients, while local signs of infection were eradicated in 89%. After resection arthroplasty, 15 of their patients could walk independently. Those patients who had a severe pre-op disability found their resection to be more satisfactory than those with lesser disability.

Resection arthroplasty leaves the patient with a functionally poor limb. It should be saved therefore for those patients in whom a life threatening infection cannot be controlled or those in whom a prior revision total knee replacement has failed. It also may be used in patients who are non-ambulatory or who have very limited functional demands.

Amputation

The indications for an above knee amputation include uncontrollable infection despite radical attempts to salvage the knee, unmanageable soft tissue defects where wound closure cannot be achieved, and life threatening sepsis. In these cases a standard above knee amputation should be performed.

Conclusions

Infection in total knee arthroplasty will not disappear. However, identifying the at-risk patient, careful pre-operative planning and intra-operative technique with environmental control and perioperative antibiotics will reduce the infection rate to very low levels.

Once infection is present, an early diagnosis and aggressive treatment will give the best opportunity for eradication and salvage of the infected knee. The critical factors involved in evaluating the best protocol for treatment include:

1. The time interval between surgery and infection.
2. The radiographic findings and whether the bone-cement and bone-prosthesis interface is involved as well as whether or not the prosthesis is loose.
3. The nature of the patient's symptoms.

4. The organisms and their response to antibiotics.
5. Whether reimplantation can be performed.
6. What type of prosthesis is present and how much bone loss may be present upon its removal.
7. The functional demands of the patient.

Taking all these considerations into account, one can usually arrive at a reasonable management plan with the appropriate treatment.

Early treatment and diagnosis of infection may lend itself to debridement, antibiotic therapy and retention of the prosthesis, especially when the organism virulence is low and the implants are not loose. When these criteria are not met, the prosthesis should be removed and after debridement and local augmented antibiotics, the implant reimplanted at a second stage. When the infection cannot be controlled or where the skin and soft tissues are irreparably involved and damaged, then arthrodesis may be the best approach. Resection arthroplasty and amputation are reserved for special circumstances where either reimplantation or arthrodesis are not possible.

References

Bengtson S, Knutson K, Lidgren L (1989) Treatment of infected knee arthroplasty. Clin Orthop 245: 173–180

Bigliani L, Rosenwasser M, Caulo N et al. (1983) The use of pulsing electromagnetic fields to achieve arthrodesis of the knee following total knee arthroplasty. J Bone Joint Surg (Am) 65: 480–485

Blomgren G, Lindgren U (1980) The susceptibility of total joint replacement to hematogenous infection in the early postoperative period: an experimental study in the rabbit. Clin Orthop 151: 308–320

Borden LS, Gearen TF (1987) Infected total knee arthroplasty: a protocol for management. J Arthroplasty 2: 27–32

Brodersen MP, Fitzgerald RH, Peterson LPA, Coventry MB, Bryan RS (1979) Arthrodesis of the knee following failed total knee arthroplasty. J Bone Joint Surg (Am) 61: 181–185

Carlsson AS, Lindren L, Lindberg I (1977) Prophylactic antibiotics against early and late deep infections after total hip replacements. Acta Orthop Scand 48: 405–410

Coonse K, Adams JD (1943) A new operative approach to the knee joint. Surg Gynecol Obstet 77: 344–347

Costerton JW, Geesey GG, Chenk KJ (1978) How bacteria stick. Sci Am 238: 86–95

Deutman K, Mulder THJ, Brian R, Nater JP (1977) Metal sensitivity before and after total hip arthroplasty. J Bone Joint Surg (Am) 59: 862–865

Elson RA (1985) Antibiotic loaded acrylic cement. In: Uthoff HG (ed) Current concepts of infections in orthopaedic surgery. Springer-Verlag, Berlin, pp 247–250

Falahee MH, Matthews LS, Kaufer H (1987) Resection arthroplasty as a salvage procedure for a knee with infection after total arthroplasty. J Bone Joint Surg (Am) 69: 1013–1019

Fitzgerald RH, Kelly PJ (1979) Total joint arthroplasty: biological causes of failure. Mayo Clin Proc 54: 590–595

Freeman M, Sudlow R, Casewell M, Radcliff S (1985) The management of infected total knee replacements. J Bone Joint Surg (Br) 67: 764–768

Green SA (1975) The effect of methylmethacrylate on phagocytosis. In: Proceedings of the Orthopaedic Research Society. J Bone Joint Surg (Am) 57: 583

Gristina A, Costerton J (1985) Bacterial adherence to biomaterials and tissue. J Bone Joint Surg (Am) 67: 264–273

Gristina AG, Kolkin J (1983) Total joint replacement and sepsis – current concepts review. J Bone Joint Surg (Am) 65: 128–138

Gristina AG, Rovedre GD, Shoji H, Nicastro JF (1976) An in vitro study of bacterial response to inert and reactive metals and to methylmethacrylate. J Biomed Mater Res 10: 273–281

Gristina AG, Costerton JW, Leake E, Kolkin J (1980) Bacterial colonization of biomaterials. Clinical and laboratory studies. Orthop Trans 4: 355

Grogan TJ, Dorey F, Rollins J, Amstutz HC (1986) Deep sepsis following total knee arthroplasty. J Bone Joint Surg (Am) 68: 226–232

Hagemann WF, Woods GW, Tullos HS (1978) Arthrodesis in failed total knee replacement. J Bone Joint Surg (Am) 60: 790–794

Hill C, Flamant R, Mazas F (1981) Prophylactic cefazolin versus placebo in total hip replacement. Report of a multicentre double blind randomized trial. Lancet i: 795–797

Insall JN (1986) Infection of total knee arthroplasty. In: Anderson LD (ed) AAOS instructional course lectures, vol 25. CV Mosby, St. Louis, p 319

Insall JN, Hood RW, Flawn LB, Sullivan DJ (1983a) The total condylar knee prosthesis in gonarthrosis. J Bone Joint Surg (Am) 65: 619–625

Insall J, Thompson F, Brause B (1983b) Two-stage reimplantation for the salvage of infected total knee arthroplasty. J Bone Joint Surg (Am) 65: 1087–1098

Johnson DP, Bannister GC (1986) The outcome of infected arthroplasty of the knee. J Bone Joint Surg (Br) 68: 289–291

Jones EC, Insall JN, Inghs AE, Ranawat CS (1979) GUEPAR knee arthroplasty results and late complications. Clin Orthop 140: 145–152

Knutson K, Hovelius L, Lindstrand A, Lindgren L (1985) Arthrodesis after failed knee arthroplasty. A nationwide multicenter investigation of 91 cases. Clin Orthop 191: 202–210

Leake ES, Wright MJ, Gristina AG, Earle CP (1980) Macrophage attachment and bacterial colonization of biomaterials. Presented as a poster session at the National Meeting of the Reticuloendothelial Society, Tampa, Florida

McCraw JB, Fishman JH, Sharzar LA (1978) The versatile gastrocnemius myocutaneous flap. Plast Reconst Surg 62: 15–23

Morrey BF, Westhold OPA, Schoifet S, Rand JA, Bryan RS (1989) Long term results of various treatment options for infected total knee arthroplasty. Clin Orthop 248: 120–130

Norden CW (1983) A critical review of antibiotic prophylaxis in orthopaedic surgery. Rev Infect Dis 5: 928–932

Norden CW (1985) Prevention of bone and joint infections. Am J Med 78 (Suppl 6B): 229–232

Perry C, Davenport K, Vossen M (1988) Local delivery of

antibiotics via an implantable pump in the treatment of osteomyelitis. Clin Orthop 226: 222–230
Petty W, Sapnier S, Schuyster J, Silverthorne C (1985) The influence of skeletal implants on incidence of infection. J Bone Joint Surg (Am) 67: 1236–1244
Pollard JP, Hughest SPF, Scott JE et al. (1979) Antibiotic prophylaxis in total hip replacement. Br Med J i: 707–709
Poss R, Thornhill TS, Ewald FC et al. (1984) Factors influencing the incidence and outcome of infection following total joint arthroplasty. Clin Orthop 182: 117–126
Rae T (1975) A study of the effects of particulate metals of orthopaedic interest on murine macrophages in vitro. J Bone Joint Surg (Br) 57: 444–450
Rand J, Bryan R (1983) Reimplantation for the salvage of an infected total knee arthroplasty. J Bone Joint Surg (Am) 65: 1081–1086
Rand J, Morrey B, Bryan R (1984) Management of the infected total joint arthroplasty. Orthop Clin N Am 15: 491–504
Rand JA, Peterson LFA, Bryan RS, Ilstrup DM (1986) Revision total knee arthroplasty. In: Anderson LD (ed) AAOS instructional course lectures, vol 25. CV Mosby, St. Louis, p 305
Rasp PL, Clawson CC, Hoidal JR, Repine JE (1979) Quantitation and scanning electron microscopic comparison of human alveolar macrophage and polymorphonuclear leukocyte adherence to nylon fibers in vitro. J Retic Soc 25: 101–109
Salibian AH, Anzel SH (1983) Salvage of an infected total knee prosthesis with medial and lateral gastrocnemius muscle flaps. J Bone Joint Surg (Am) 65: 681–684
Salvati EA, Insall JN (1980) The management of sepsis in total knee replacements. In: Savastano AA (ed) Total knee replacements. Appleton-Century Crofts, New York, pp 49–58
Salvati EA, Robinson RP, Zeno SM et al. (1982) Infection rates after 3175 total hip and total knee replacements performed with and without a horizontal unidirectional filtered airflow system. J Bone Joint Surg (Am) 64: 525–531
Sanders R, O'Neill T (1981) The gastrocnemius myocutaneous flap used as a cover for the exposed knee prosthesis. J Bone Joint Surg (Br) 63: 383–396
Scott RD, Saliski JM (1985) The use of a modified V–Y quadricepsplasty during total knee replacement to gain exposure and improve flexion in the akylosed knee. Orthopaedics 8: 45–48
Thompson TC (1944) Quadricepsplasty to improve knee function. J Bone Joint Surg (Am) 26: 366
Thornhill T, Maguire J (1987) Infected total knee arthroplasty. In: Scott WN (ed) Total knee revision arthroplasty, Grune and Stratton, Orlando, Fla,. pp 79–88
Uchida S, Yoshino S, Doi M, Kudo H (1980) Side-effects of prosthetic materials on the human body. Int Orthop 3: 258–291
Wade PJF, Duhan RA (1984) Arthrodesis of the knee after failed knee replacement. J Bone Joint Surg (Br) 66: 362–366
Wilde A, Ruth J (1988) Two stage reimplantation in total knee arthroplasty. Clin Orthop 236: 23–35
Wolff AM, Hungerford DS, Krackow KA, Jacobs MA (1989) Osteotomy of the tibial tubercle during total knee replacement. A report of twenty-six cases. J Bone Joint Surg (Am) 71: 848–852

Chapter 17

Special Considerations in Arthroplasty of the Rheumatoid Knee Joint

Anders Wigren

Introduction

The most striking factor in comparing the rheumatoid knee joint to the knee joint with primary osteoarthrosis, posttraumatic osteoarthrosis and osteochondritis is its environment – the rheumatoid person. Rheumatoid arthritis is often severe affecting many joints in both the upper extremities, lower extremities and cervical spine. Thus the rheumatoid knee joint is only a small part of a systemic problem. The knee joint must be looked upon and evaluated in light of the individual's total functional and social situation.

In the United States there are about 3.6 million people suffering from inflammatory joint disease (Brashear and Raney 1978). In Sweden about 200 000 (approximately 1.2% of the general population) are affected. About 15% of all of these patients have severe disease and require knee surgery. The knee joint is by far the prime causal factor when these patients become wheelchair bound (Brattström et al. 1977). The result of a successful arthroplasty on such a wheelchair dependent person may miraculously change the patient's functional classification (Wigren 1988).

The bone quality of the rheumatoid knee is often much worse than that in the osteoarthrotic knee because of severe osteoporosis. The surgical technique must therefore be varied and individualized. This differs from the surgery in the patient with osteoarthrosis where relatively uniform rules can usually be followed. Implants and solutions which cannot be used in osteoarthrosis are frequently the only solution in a severe rheumatoid knee (Fig. 17.1). This is especially true in revision surgery and in fractures close to an arthroplasty in a rheumatoid knee (Fig. 17.2).

The evaluation of results of arthroplasties in rheumatoid cases must be related to the type and severity of the disease as well as to the functional classification of the patient, otherwise there cannot be a fair comparison between different methods of treatment. Consequently, the various scoring systems used to evaluate the functional results after knee surgery in degenerative or traumatic osteoarthrosis cannot be applied to the rheumatoid patient. Likewise a suitable roentgenographic classification for rheumatoid joints has to be used in order to allow a comparison between different series. Most European rheumatologic surgeons prefer a roentgenographic classification such as that proposed by Larsen et al. (1977, 1979).

The Influence of Patient Related Factors on Knee Arthroplasty

The mental situation of the patient is important. There is often a depression and gloominess in rheumatoid patients that make them see surgery

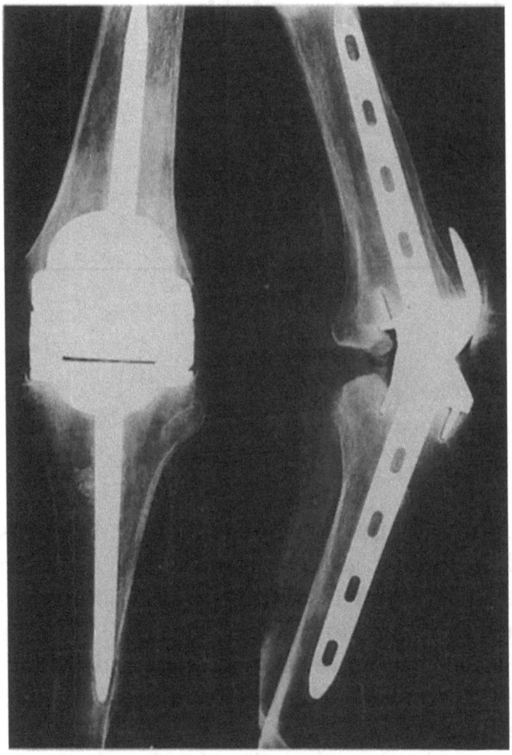

Fig. 17.1. A Walldius hinge prosthesis might be a solution in a knee with severe bone loss and osteoporosis in a wheelchair bound person with rheumatoid arthritis.

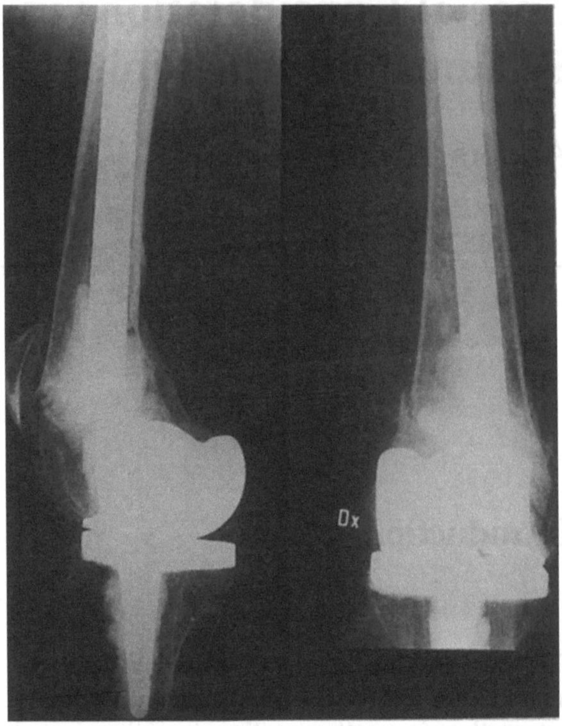

Fig. 17.2. This fracture close to an endoprosthesis was solved with a combination of a Spherocentric knee and a Küntscher nail.

as a "magical solution" which could cure an otherwise desperate life situation. The orthopaedic surgeon on the other hand must be aware of these unrealistic expectations on the part of a desperate patient. The patient must always be asked why he wants surgery and what he expects out of it (Brattström H 1976 personal communication). If the answers are unclear it is better not to perform an arthroplasty but rather to see the patient again after some time for a new discussion. If the surgeon works in concert with a rheumatologist, a physiotherapist and a social worker these psychological problems are often easy to recognize and solve. In the rheumatoid patients, an arthroplasty must not be performed merely on account of the X-ray appearance of destructive arthropathy. There must also be clear clinical indications and expected functional benefits.

The experience of a rheumatology team is often needed to evaluate how disabled the patient is and if there are realistic possibilities that a knee arthroplasty will change the functional situation. Even if the knee joint is the main reason for the patient needing a wheelchair there are always many other factors such as a decreased muscular strength, other diseased joints and it is especially important to evaluate the motivation of the patient. Knee arthroplasty possibly may give the patient a chance to get out of the wheelchair but to achieve this he or she must persist with an exercise and rehabilitation program.

The patient's housing and living conditions may influence not only the indication for a knee arthroplasty but also the choice of endoprosthesis itself. For instance, if the patient lives in the countryside with rough or hilly ground, and that situation cannot be changed, it may be wise to choose a semiconstrained implant which can give stability and security while walking. Walking downstairs and upstairs demands 110° of flexion ability and the endoprosthesis must be chosen according to this. We have found (Wigren 1988) that the ability to cope with stairs is improved by using a completely unconstrained surface to replace prosthesis, such as the Modular knee. (Richards Medical Company, Memphis, Tenn.)

After a total knee replacement, some restriction in the attitude to work and sports is advisable in people with osteoarthrosis. Fortunately this is rarely a problem in the rheumatoid patient. For many reasons their activities are already reduced. Although they still may participate in activities such as dancing, cycling, and crosscountry skiing, their general disease will usually preclude those activities which can lead to implant loosening: i.e. jogging and contact sports.

The Influence of Medical, Social and Surgical Resources

In a depressed health economy it is hard for chronic diseases like rheumatoid arthritis to compete with other more acute dramatic conditions like heart surgery (Calltorp 1989). Despite this, however, the deteriorating rheumatic knee joint must be taken care of without much delay if severe deformities and ensuing technical problems that attend them are to be avoided (Fig. 17.3). Waiting for surgery often means functional loss for the individual and eventually a more extensive type of treatment followed by a prolonged rehabilitation. Special units and resources for these patients give the best results with the greatest safety (Wigren 1987 a, b). A so-called waiting list for surgery which is common in the Scandinavian countries is dangerous and must be controlled very carefully so as to avoid delay in treatment of these patients.

We must remember that the knee joint is just a part of a general disease process. The cooperation of a rheumatologist who can take care of the drug treatment and the complications related to the disease is essential. The nursing of the severe cases is best taken care of in a rheumatological ward with opportunity for total rehabilitation. After surgery the social situation and the housing situation must be planned together with the social workers.

A surgical team experienced in rheumatological surgery is crucial. It is necessary that anesthesiologists and otolaryngologists experienced in nasotracheal anesthesia are part of this team because of the high incidence of temporomandibular and cervical spine disease. Regional and epidural anesthesia are often preferred. In the operating room, vacuum mattresses and positioning facilities must be available for these severely handicapped patients with multiple joint contractures. There must be a very high standard of sterility peri- and intra-operatively as these patients have a higher risk of infection.

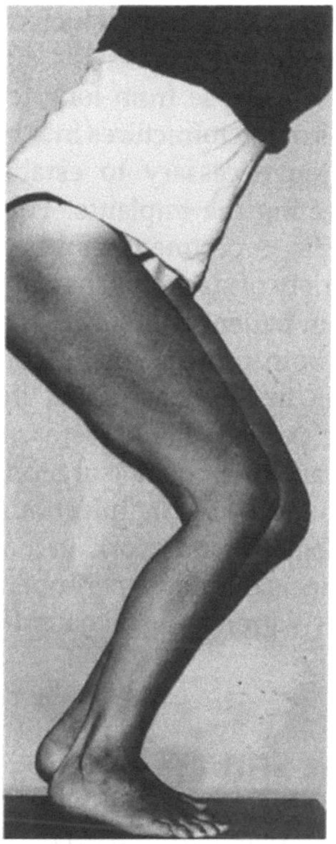

Fig. 17.3. This 25-year-old woman has fixed deformities of 90° in her hips, knee and ankle joints which are an extremely difficult surgical problem to solve.

Special problems such as blood incompatibility and bleeding diatheses are more prevalent in these patients. High demands are often put on the blood banking services of the hospital. These patients often have a very long lasting salicylate or other nonsteroid anti-inflammatory medication which severely impairs the function of their thrombocytes. Even if all laboratory tests are normal, significant bleeding can occur when the tourniquet is released at the end of the procedure. Hypotensive anesthesia may diminish intra-operative bleeding and the use of blood recovery machines is preferable.

There is also a need for a bone bank or an association with such a bank which offers good service. Rheumatoid patients often have advanced bone collapse from long term use of corticosteroids or microfractures into cysts. Bone grafts are often necessary to establish a flat surface for seating the implants. Furthermore, the orthopaedic department must stock prostheses in a variety of sizes and shapes to account for variances in patient anatomy.

Infections, both primary and secondary, are more common in the rheumatoid than in the osteoarthrotic patient. For this reason a team consisting of an orthopaedic surgeon, a plastic surgeon and specialists in infectious diseases and bacteriology should work in harmony to plan surgical incisions and a peri-operative antibiotic regime (Wigren and Hakelius 1986).

Symptoms and Objectives

Pain in the knee both with weight bearing and at rest is the most important surgical indication to perform an arthroplasty. If the knee arthroplasty does not produce a painless knee joint or one with only a minimal amount of episodic pain, the result is unsatisfactory. Most rheumatoid arthritis patients will accept some residual discomfort in the knee after an arthroplasty. The general pain level to which these people are accustomed makes them tolerant of some residual pain in a way not seen in the patient with osteoarthrosis. Walking ability and walking distance, which are the important goals for the osteoarthrotic patient, especially one with only a single joint problem, will often be of secondary interest for the rheumatoid patient. This is one reason why most score evaluation systems are not applicable to the rheumatoid knee (Barck 1988). At least one knee joint of the rheumatoid patient should be capable of flexing more than 100°, since this range of motion is necessary for standing up from a chair or the toilet.

A special indication for a total knee replacement in a patient with rheumatoid arthritis is rapid and progressive bone loss that can accompany collapse of granulomas and cysts. The result will often be a malposition of the joint with a severe valgus or varus deformity. Even if the pain situation is not severe, knee joint arthroplasty may be needed as part of a total rehabilitation program to enable the patient to walk.

Because of the frequent involvement of the shoulder, elbow and hands, it is often difficult for the rheumatoid arthritis patient to walk without bearing weight on the painful joint. Surgery, therefore, may be indicated at an early stage before the upper extremity disease has progressed to the point when rehabilitation becomes extremely difficult.

Timing of Surgery

The best time to perform an arthroplasty is when the symptoms have progressed to the point that they are significantly impairing the patient's ability to participate in the activities of daily living. The patient with rheumatoid arthritis, however, has a generalized disease which may fluctuate in activity. To perform surgery during an acute arthritic flareup may be unwise because the general medical condition is often poor. If, however, the knee joint is deteriorating rapidly, arthroplasty should be done even in the face of active synovitis elsewhere. The need for a total rheumatology team approach in these situations is even more crucial.

Unilateral involvement of the hip, knee and foot to such an extent that all joints need surgery makes surgical timing and planning even more important. We recommend performing foot surgery first followed by the hip and then the knee. Foot surgery in rheumatoid arthritis is often complicated by healing disturbances (Sahlberg 1987) and therefore it should be done before proximal arthroplasty surgery (Karlström and Wigren 1978; Kaufer et al. 1980; Lidgren et al. 1987). Otherwise, there may be a risk of hematogenous or lymphogenic spread of an infection from the foot to the artificial joint. Furthermore, the manipulation of the leg that accompanies hip surgery might otherwise overstress a knee arthroplasty. This is another reason that I feel that for most patients the hip should be operated upon before the knee.

The results of ipsilateral arthroplasty of the hip and the knee at the same time are often less successful than when the arthroplasties are done

one at a time. On the other hand bilateral knee arthroplasties may spare time for the patient and make rehabilitation faster and more easy than when the joints are operated on at separate sessions. Optimal resources must be available for bilateral arthroplasties. We prefer to have a new theater for each arthroplasty so as to minimize the risk of infection. The postoperative exercise program progresses slightly slower in the bilateral patient as compared to the patient who is having only one knee operated upon. Despite this, we feel that this delay is only a minor setback when compared to the benefit of having two pain free joints present during the rehabilitation period.

Contraindications for Knee Arthroplasty

Lack of cooperation is one of the most important contraindications for an arthroplasty of the knee. The patient's need of an arthroplasty must be assessed properly and their unspoken hopes for the outcome success of the surgery be ascertained. If the indications are not clear it is better to postpone the surgery.

A relative contraindication is the absence of appropriate facilities for the post-discharge rehabilitation. The home environment must be evaluated and at times modified in order that the patient can function and exercise with a minimum amount of encumbrance.

The age of the rheumatoid arthritis patient is seldom a contraindication. Even very young persons may have a knee arthroplasty since for many, their functional demands are limited.

An unstable cervical spine may be a relative contraindication and should best be stabilized before the arthroplasty. In any case,the arthroplasty should be performed with the patient wearing a cervical collar and probably using spinal or epidural anesthesia.

An almost invariable contraindication for knee arthroplasty is an ongoing active infection somewhere in the body. Such an infection must be treated before an arthroplasty is performed. Recurrent infections of the urinary tract, which are so common in women, should be treated before the arthroplasty.

Pathoanatomy and Pathophysiology and Their Relation to Knee Arthroplasty

Rheumatoid arthritis normally causes a decrease in the activity level of the patient. This results in osteopenia and a diminution in muscle strength. Weakness can also occur from inflammatory disease in the muscle itself. Synovitis is present in all patients at some stage of their disease. Over and above the swelling and the attendant loss of motion, the synovitis also affects the cartilage and ligaments.

The instability of the knee joint seen in the rheumatoid patient is caused by loss of cartilage and bone and not by damage to the collateral ligaments. The collateral ligaments themselves are completely normal (Coomes 1962). This is not the case, however for the anterior cruciate ligament. In our own study of 100 knee arthroplasties, we found that the anterior cruciate ligament was almost universally absent, while the posterior cruciate ligament usually remained intact. This is easily understandable when we realize that the anterior ligament is intra-articular and is enclosed in a synovial sheath while the posterior is not. Indeed, the posterior cruciate ligament is partially extra-articular.

The inflammatory tissue can invade the subchondral bone and cause granulomas in the metaphysis. A collapse of the articular surface over these granulomas can then lead to severe angular deformities and cause problems at surgery if they are not appreciated roentgenographically before surgery. Filling in such granulomas with bone cement can lead to fracture and loosening of the prosthesis (Fig. 17.4) (Wigren et al. 1980). Bone grafting of the granuloma with cancellous bone can obliterate the defect and result in a stable flat base for the implant (Fig. 17.5 a,b) (Rosendahl and Wigren 1987).

Flexion contractures or extension deficits of the knee joint were considered by Helfet (1974) to be caused by soft tissue contractures. Other authors found that bone impingement was the commonest cause of extension lag (Marmor 1973; Brattström 1977; Gschwend 1977; Smillie 1974; Kolstad et al. 1980; Laskin 1988). In order to get a full range of motion in such a knee joint the anterior impingement between tibia and femur must be removed (Fig. 17.6 a,b).

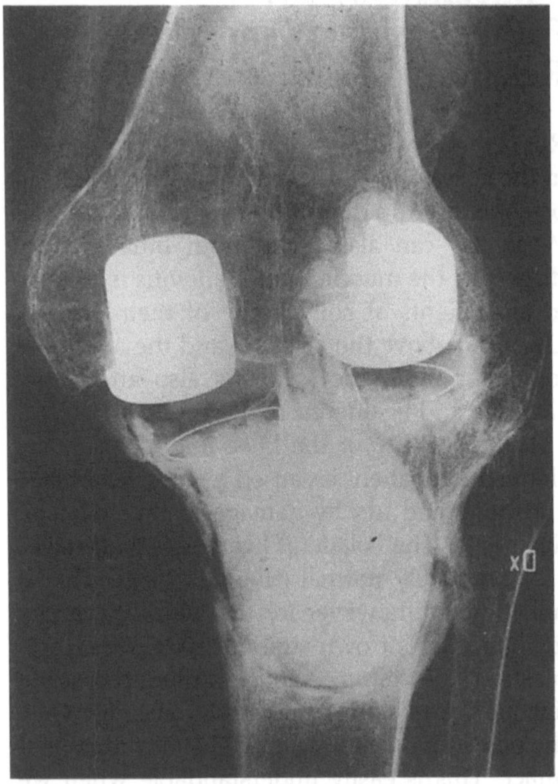

Fig. 17.4. This giant metaphyseal granuloma was filled with bone cement. The surgeon had not observed it on the X-ray. Fracture of the proximal tibia with loosening of the prosthesis was the natural outcome with severe revision problems. The histology of the cortical bone, three years after the cement filling revealed no living bone.

Patients with juvenile rheumatoid arthritis present special problems. The bones may be extremely small and gracile, requiring specially sized implants. Furthermore there is high incidence of fibrous ankylosis in these patients and this may modify the soft tissue releases that are required.

Most rheumatoid patients undergoing total knee replacement are younger than their osteoarthrotic counterparts. Therefore they are more likely to undergo one or more revisions as they get older. One must therefore attempt to get as good a functional result as possible with the first operation, while still using an implant that will spare as much bone as possible.

It would be beneficial if the original operation could be performed without cement since any revision would be technically easier and result in less bone ablation. Unfortunately, uncemented prostheses are often not suitable because of the poor bone stock in the patient with inflammatory arthritis. Since rheumatoid arthritis involves the entire joint, unicompartmental replacement is of little value. We have, however, performed bicompartmental replacement in some of these patients in order to maximize motion while minimizing bone loss (Wigren 1988). The procedure of bicompartmental replacement is exacting and requires meticulous attention to ligament balancing and cementing technique. Furthermore there must be good peripheral cortical support on the tibia in order to prevent subsidence (Fig. 17.7). Bicompart-

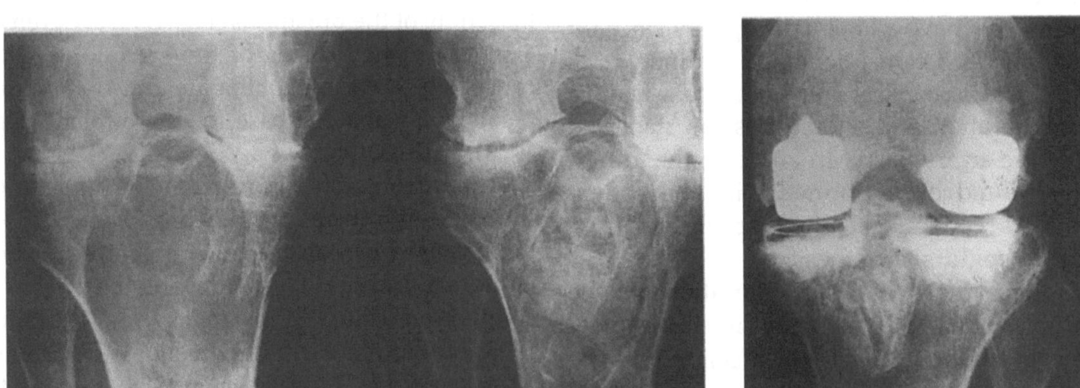

a b

Fig. 17.5. a A giant metaphyseal granuloma grafted with cancellous bone. **b** Four months after the surgery shown in **a**, bicompartmental unicondylar Marmor arthroplasty was performed. There was no loosening and good function, eight years postoperatively.

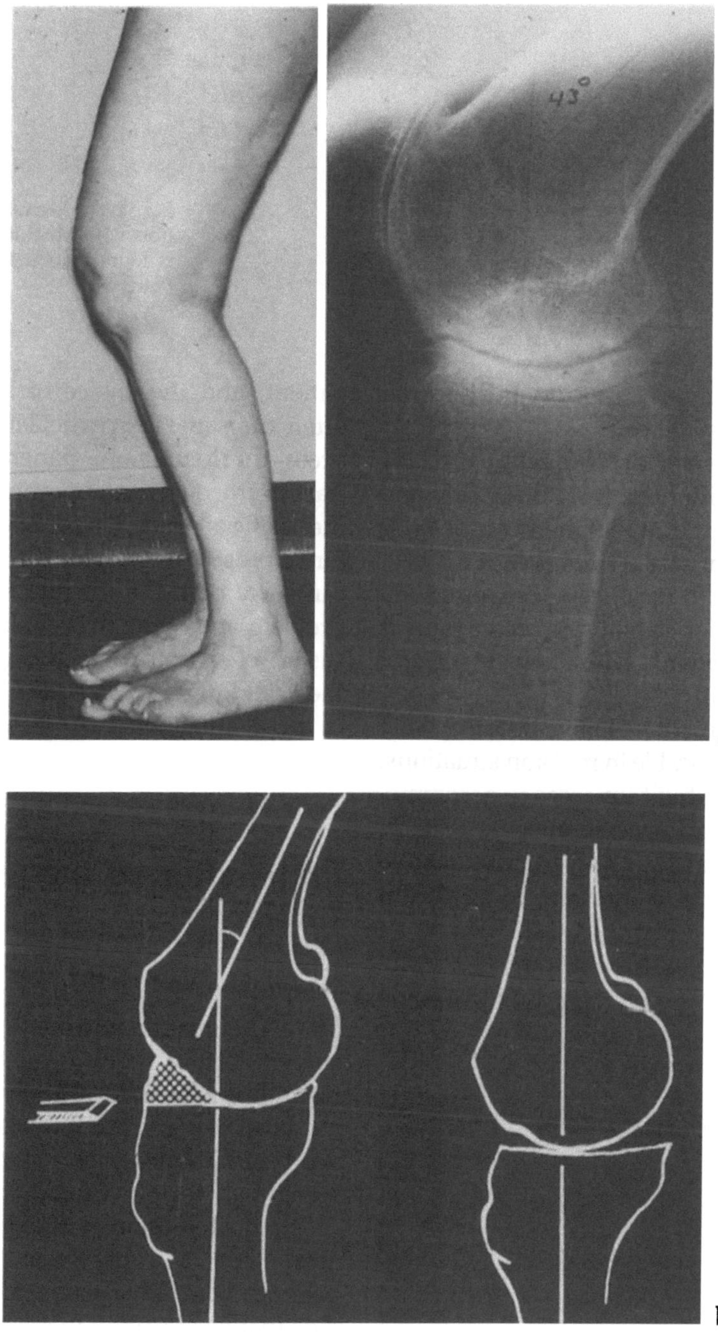

a

b

Fig. 17.6. a A fixed extension defect of 45° is shown. There is anterior impingement between the anterior part of the tibia and the femur. **b** After resection of the anterior part of the tibia, full extension was possible.

mental replacement should not be used in those patients with severe fixed soft tissue deformities. At present, the commonest arthroplasty performed in the rheumatoid knee is a variant of the total condylar system, which, when properly cemented in place, can give excellent results (Laskin 1988).

Regardless of which prosthesis is used it is advantageous to attempt to retain the posterior cruciate ligament. Retention of the ligament

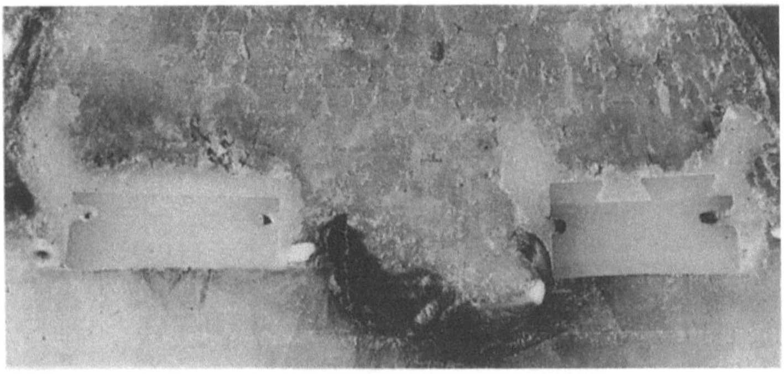

Fig. 17.7. A cross-section of the proximal tibia with Modular implants. Good contact is found between the cement and cortical bone.

lessens the risk of hyperextension and secondary ligamentous instability.

For severe combined deformities, especially those associated with bone loss, instability and poor muscular strength, the Spherocentric knee has given good ten year results (Wigren 1988). This cemented prosthesis does not require competent soft tissues for stability. Its main value is in the elderly patient with low functional demands (Fig. 17.8).

Most recently, prostheses have become available that will be applicable in revision situations. Many of these have built up areas to accommodate for bone loss in specific areas. The technique for a revision arthroplasty in a rheumatoid patient is the same as for an osteoarthrotic patient, and the choice of implant is likewise often the same. A particular problem that will occur in rheumatoid patients, however, is a fracture through osteoporotic bone adjacent to the artificial joint. Under such circumstances a hinge prosthesis with long intramedullary stems can solve both the fracture and endoprosthetic problem and make the rehabilitation somewhat easier. We have had good experience using both the Walldius as well as the GSB endoprosthesis in these situations.

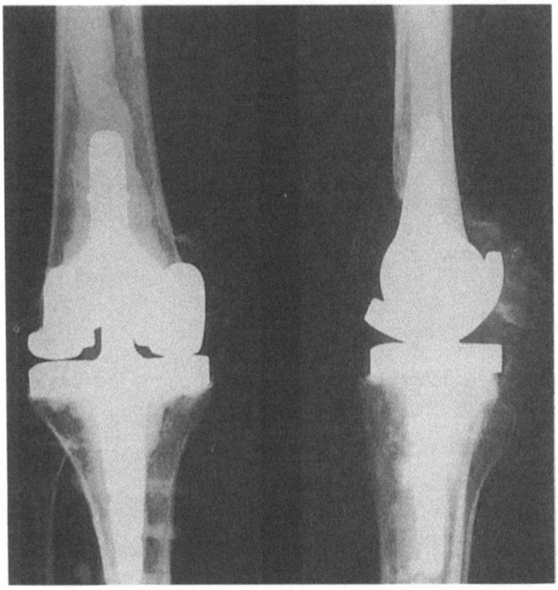

Fig. 17.8. The Spherocentric endoprosthesis has given good lasting results in a rheumatoid arthritis patient with severe pre-operative bone loss and severe knee instability.

Preparation of the Joint for the Implant

Many rheumatoid patients have had prior knee surgery before requiring a total knee replacement. It is wise, if technically possible, to follow old surgical scars. For knees in which there have not been any previous operations, we prefer a straight anterior incision.

Rheumatoid skin is friable and easily bruisable. This is a particular problem in those patients who have taken systemic corticosteroids that has resulted in dermal thinning associated with those medications. It is preferable to use moist closure over the wound edges and to avoid pressure from hard instruments. The assistants must be especially wary lest they damage the skin with their fingers or with retractors.

If there has been a good range of knee motion preoperatively, wide exposure of the knee can usually be easily obtained. This usually requires elevation of a small amount of periosteum and tendon from the tibial tubercle as well as separation of the vastus medialis muscle from the rectus femoris tendon high up in the thigh. When flexion is limited preoperatively, the surgical incision usually must include release of any scarring from the proximal and lateral recesses of the joint. Further exposure may be obtained, especially in very stiff knees by performing a modified proximal Coons-Adams release (Scott and Siliski 1985). Although osteotomy of the tibial tubercle will result in wide exposure, this procedure, especially in the rheumatoid patient, has been associated with complication rates as high as 50% (Wolf et al. 1989). If some cartilage is left in the joint, a careful synovectomy should be performed (Førre 1986, personal communication).

The sub-articular granulomas seen in rheumatoid arthritis are a special problem because they can cause collapse of the joint surface above the granuloma. Small granulomas may be grafted with cancellous bone from resected pieces of the joint at the arthroplasty. The treatment of larger bone defects has been discussed previously.

The cortical bone of the proximal tibia is very soft anteriorly and the only good support for a prosthesis is the posterior cortex. This should be remembered when positioning the tibial component.

The Patella

Although there is some controversy whether or not to resurface the patella for all patients with osteoarthrosis undergoing knee replacement, most surgeons agree that for the rheumatoid, patellar replacement is advantageous. Unfortunately there are situations in which what remains of the patella is a thin shell of osteoporotic bone. In those cases it probably is wise not to attempt a patellar resurfacing but rather to merely trim away the edges and smooth the remaining surface as best as possible. If possible we prefer to resurface the patella with a polyethylene implant. Properly performed, we have found better functional results with tricompartmental replacement in rheumatoids as compared to knees in which just the femur and tibia were resurfaced. From a theoretical point of view, it is advantageous to remove the patellar cartilage lest it act as an antigenic stimulus and favor recurrence of synovitis (Førre 1987, personal communication).

Wound Closure and Wound Dressing

Strong number 0 sutures are used to close the fascia and muscle. Two intra-articular vacuum drains are placed and allowed to exit laterally so as not to interfere with the function of the vastus medialis muscle. Great effort is made to make sure that the musculofascial stitches are firm during flexion-extension of the knee. This is done by repeated bending and stretching of the knee joint before the closure of the skin. Again care must be taken handling the skin during the closure.

We use a special dressing of wet gauze to cover the wound. This dressing acts as a sponge to absorb any blood which might be extruded from the incision. The dressing is covered with a thick wad of acrylic extending from the ankle joint to the upper thigh. Finally the entire leg is covered by an elastic compression bandage. The compressing effect of the entire dressing helps to control wound edema. The dressing should be changed after 36 hours, however, since any dried blood can cause it to become rigid and will result in uneven pressure to the leg and damage the skin.

Postoperative Training and Exercises

Active extension as well as small flexion movements are started on the first postoperative day. From the second day, after the drains have been removed, we start the patient on a continuous passive motion machine (Kinetec) for several hours each day. We use the hold-relax method of exercising the knee to increase flexion. Standing and walking are both begun on the third postoperative day for short periods of time with emphasis both on obtaining a normal gait and on flexing and extending the knee while walking.

Swelling of the knee may be the result of soft tissue edema, or intra-articular hematoma. Should the swelling be severe we return the patient to bed rest, elevate the leg, and defer walking for several days. We have used this regimen for over ten years and for over 800 knee arthroplasties and during that time we have had no wound ruptures and only one intra-articular hematoma that required evacuation.

If there is a flexion contracture of the ipsilateral hip the knee with the arthroplasty must be positioned and held so that we can avoid secondary extension lag of the newly performed artificial joint. When there is a hip ankylosis the knee must be positioned over the edge of the bed for flexion exercises.

Walking Aids

We use two crutches until swelling and increased warmth over the joint have abated. Usually by two months after surgery we can discontinue all external support. We like to limit the amount of weight that the patient places on the operative knee. At times, however, if the patient's hands are very weak this may result in full weight bearing on the leg.

Infections

It would appear that from the statistics of the International Swedish Knee Project (Knutson 1985) late infections of the arthroplasty are more common in rheumatoid arthritis than in arthroplasties performed for osteoarthrosis. The patients should be informed about this and told to return to an othopaedic service if there is any suspicion of an infection. The use of prophylactic antibiotics during other types of surgery, especially urologic and dental, is recommended. Many feel that antibiotic cement should always be used for fixation of the prosthesis even if the effect of this in the long run has been questioned (Josefsson 1980; Blomgren 1981; Hedström and Lidgren 1988).

Summary

Knee arthroplasty in severe cases of rheumatoid arthritis demands that the medical, surgical and social resources be optimal. The patient is generally ill, the skin is friable, and deformity and bone loss are often present. A successful knee arthroplasty for such a patient, however, can have an enormous beneficial impact on the patient as a whole with reduction of pain, increase in function, and improvement in the quality of life.

References

Barck A (1988) Uni- and bicompartmental knee replacement. Thesis, Karolinska Institute, Stockholm

Blomgren G (1981) Hematogenous infection of total joint replacement. An experimental study in the rabbit. Acta Orthop Scand 52 [Suppl 187]

Brashear R Jr, Raney B Sr (1978) Chronic arthritis. Shands' handbook of orthopaedic surgery. CV Mosby, St Louis, pp 135–178

Brattström H (1977) Fractures in rheumatoid patients. The Swedish Orthop Association, Stockholm, p 472

Brattström M, Bråfelt I, Hemmingsson I-B, Paulsson K (1977) The reason for the rheumatoid patient to get into the wheelchair. Psykotekniska Institutionen, Stockholm University, no. 92

Calltorp J (1989) Prioritering och beslutsprocess i sjukvårdsfrågor. Thesis, University of Uppsala

Coomes EN (1962) Lateral instability of the knee following polyarthritis. Ann Rheum Dis 21: 378–387

Gschwend N (1977) Die operative Behandlung der kronischen Polyarthritis. Georg Thieme Verlag, Stuttgart, pp 226–227

Hedström S-Å, Lidgren L (1988) Orthopedic infections. Studentlitteratur, Lund, pp 76–83

Helfet A (1974) Disorders of the knee. JB Lippincott Co., Philadelpia, pp 176–184, 255–260

Josefsson G (1980) Gentamicin-impregnated bone cement in total hip replacement. Prevention and treatment of deep infection. Thesis, University of Lund

Karlström G, Wigren A (1978) Hemotogenous infection of arthroplasties. Svenska Läkartidningen 13: 1292–1293

Kaufer H, Karlström G, Wigren A (1980) Hematogenous infection in total joint implants. Clin Orthop 152: 288–291

Knutson K (1985) Survival of knee arthroplasties for rheumatoid arthritis. Acta Orthop Scand 56: 422–425

Kolstad K, Sahlstedt B, Wigren A (1980) Extension deficit and lateral instability in degenerative disease of the knee. Acta Orthop Scand 51: 667–672
Larsen A (1979) Rheumatoid arthritis. Nycomed AS Pharma, PB4284 Torshou, N-0401, Oslo 4
Larsen A, Dale K, Eek M (1977) Radiographic evaluation of rheumatoid arthritis and related conditions by standard reference films. Acta Radiol Diagn 18: 481–491
Laskin R (1988) Total condylar knee replacement in rheumatoid arthritis. A review of patients after ten years. Presented at the Annual Meeting of the American Academy of Orthopaedic Surgeons, Las Vegas, Nev
Lidgren L, Blomgren G, Knutson K, Wigren A, Bengtsson S (1987) Hematogenous infection after knee arthroplasty. Acta Orthop Scand 58: 529–534
Marmor L (1973) The modular knee. Clin Orthop 94: 242–248
Rosendahl Y, Wigren A (1987) Transplantation of cancellous bone – a safe technique in arthroplasty of the knee with rheumatic granulomas. Proceedings of the Scandinavian Orthopaedic Association. In: Acta Orthop Scand 59: 218–222
Sahlberg C (1987) Resection of metatarsal heads in rheumatic arthritis – healing problems. Proceedings of the Scandinavian Podologic Association. In: Acta Orthop Scand 59: 101
Scott R, Siliski (1985) The use of a modified V–Y quadricepsplasty during total knee replacement to gain exposure and improve flexion in the ankylosed knee. Orthopedics 8: 45–48
Smillie IS (1974) Diseases of the knee joint. Churchill Livingstone, Edinburgh, p 330
Wigren A (1987a) Special unit for hip and knee arthroplasty resulted in less waiting time for surgery. In: Leadership in health care. University of Uppsala, Uppsala
Wigren A (1987b) An arthroplasty unit – a profitable investment. Acta Orthop Scand 58: 302–303
Wigren A (1988) Total knee replacement with a modular system. In: The Valbella orthopaedic conference on current concepts in knee surgery
Wigren A, Hakelius L (1986) Soft tissue treatment in orthopaedic surgery. In: New reconstructive possibilities to cover soft tissue defects. Swedish Orthopaedic Association, Stockholm
Wigren A, Kolstad K, Sahlstedt B (1980) Two unusual and serious complications in knee arthroplasties. Proceedings Acta Orthop Scand 51: 379
Wolf A, Hungerford DS, Krackow KA, Jacobs MA (1989) Osteotomy of the tibial tubercle during total knee replacement. J Bone Joint Surg (Am) 71: 848–852

Subject Index

MIX
Papier aus verantwortungsvollen Quellen
Paper from responsible sources
FSC® C105338

If you have any concerns about our products,
you can contact us on
ProductSafety@springernature.com

In case Publisher is established outside the EU,
the EU authorized representative is:
Springer Nature Customer Service Center GmbH
Europaplatz 3, 69115 Heidelberg, Germany

Printed by Libri Plureos GmbH
in Hamburg, Germany